Cancer and the Skeleton

Cancer and the Skeleton

Robert D Rubens MD BSc FRCP

Professor of Clinical Oncology
Department of Clinical Oncology
Guy's Hospital
London
UK

Gregory R Mundy MD

Heyser Professor of Bone and Mineral Metabolism and
Head, Division of Endocrinology and Metabolism
University of Texas Health Science Center
San Antonio
Texas
USA

MARTIN DUNITZ

© Martin Dunitz Ltd 2000

First published in the United Kingdom in 2000 by
Martin Dunitz Ltd
The Livery House
7-9 Pratt Street
London NW1 0AE

All rights reserved. No part of this publication may be reproduced, stored in a retrieval system, or transmitted, in any form or by any means, electronic, mechanical, photocopying, recording or otherwise, without the prior permission of the publisher or in accordance with the provisions of the Copyright Act 1988, or under the terms of any licence permitting limited copying issued by the Copyright Licensing Agency, 33-34 Alfred Place, London WC1E 7DP.

A CIP catalogue record for this book is available from the British Library

ISBN 1-85317-756-3

Distributed in the United States by:
Blackwell Science Inc.
Commerce Place, 350 Main Street
Malden, MA 02148, USA
Tel: 1-800-215-1000

Distributed in Canada by:
Login Brothers Book Company
324 Salteaux Crescent Winnipeg, Manitoba, R3J 3T2
Canada
Tel: 204-224-4068

Distributed in Brazil by:
Ernesto Reichmann, Distribuidora de Livros, Ltda
Rua Coronel Marques 335, Tatuape 03440-000
Sao Paulo
Brazil

Composition by Scribe Design, Gillingham, Kent
Printed and Bound in Spain by Grafos S.A. Arte Sobre papel

Contents

Contributors

Preface

1	Structure and physiology of the normal skeleton *Gregory R Mundy*	1
2	Pathophysiology of myeloma bone disease *Gregory R Mundy and Babatunde O Oyajobi*	21
3	Bone metastases - incidence and complications *Robert D Rubens*	33
4	Pathophysiology of bone metastasis *Gregory R Mundy and Theresa A Guise*	43
5	Bone metastases - morphology *Toru Hiraga, Gregory R Mundy and Toshiyuki Yoneda*	65
6	Hypercalcemia *Vivian Grill and T John Martin*	75
7	Diagnostic nuclear medicine *Gary J R Cook and Ignac Fogelman*	91
8	Radiology and magnetic resonance imaging *David MacVicar*	113
9	Biochemical markers of malignant bone disease *Robert E Coleman*	137
10	Bone metastases - general approaches to systemic treatment *Robert D Rubens*	151
11	Bone metastases - radiotherapy *Philip J Hoskin*	159

12	Clinical use of radioisotopes for bone metastases *Stephen J Houston*	171
13	Pain - mechanisms, assessment, and management *Jana Portnow and Stuart A Grossman*	183
14	Mechanisms of action of bisphosphonates in tumor bone disease *Herbert Fleisch*	201
15	Management of myeloma bone disease *James R Berenson*	215
16	Bisphosphonates in breast cancer and other solid tumors *Jean-Jaques Body*	231
17	Spinal stabilization *Kevin D Harrington*	245
18	Osteoporosis in cancer patients *Aurélie Fontana and Pierre D Delmas*	263
	Index	271

Contributors

James R Berenson MD
Chief of Cancer Research
Associate Director of Research
West Los Angeles VA Medical Center
Professor of Medicine
UCLA School of Medicine
Los Angeles
USA

Jean-Jaques Body
Supportive Care Clinic and
Endocrinology/Bone Diseases Clinic
Institut Jules Bordet
Free University of Brussels
Brussels
Belgium

Robert E Coleman MD FRCP
Professor of Medical Oncology
Division of Oncology and Cellular Pathology
Weston Park Hospital NHS Trust
Sheffield
UK

Gary J R Cook MBBS MRCP FRCR
Clinical Lecturer and Honorary Consultant
Physician
Division of Radiological Sciences
Guy's Hospital
London
UK

Pierre D Delmas MD PhD
Professor of Medicine
INSERM Unite 403, Pavillon F
Hôpital Edouard Herriot
Lyon
France

Herbert Fleisch MD
Professor Emeritus
University of Berne
Avenue Désertes
Pully
Switzerland

Ignac Fogelman MD FRCP
Professor of Nuclear Medicine
Department of Nuclear Medicine
Guy's Hospital
London
UK

Aurélie Fontana MD
INSERM Unite 403, Pavillon F
Hôpital Edouard Herriot
Lyon
France

Vivian Grill MBBS FRACP
Senior Lecturer in Medicine
St Vincent's Institute of Medical Research
Fitzroy
Victoria
Australia

Stuart A Grossman MD
Director, Neuro-Oncology
The Johns Hopkins Oncology Center
Baltimore, MD
USA

Theresa A Guise MD
Associate Professor
Division of Endocrinology
Department of Medicine
University of Texas Health Science Center
San Antonio
Texas
USA

Kevin D Harrington MD
3838 California Street
Suite 516
San Francisco
California
USA

Toru Hiraga DDS PhD
Postdoctoral Fellow
Division of Endocrinology
Department of Medicine
University of Texas Health Science Center
San Antonio
Texas
USA

Philip J Hoskin MD FRCP FRCR
Reader in Oncology
Marie Curie Research Wing for Oncology
Mount Vernon Hospital
Northwood
Middlesex
UK

Stephen J Houston PhD
Lecturer and Honorary Senior Registrar
Department of Medical Oncology
St Luke's Cancer Centre
Royal Surrey County Hospital
Guildford
Surrey
UK

David MacVicar PhD
Consultant Oncological Radiologist
Academic Department of Diagnostic Radiology
The Royal Marsden NHS Trust
Sutton
Surrey
UK

T John Martin MD
Director
St Vincent's Institute of Medical Research
Fitzroy
Victoria
Australia

Gregory R Mundy MD
Heyser Professor of Bone and Mineral Metabolism and
Head, Division of Endocrinology and Metabolism
University of Texas Health Science Center
San Antonio
Texas
USA

Babatunde O Oyajobi MB BCh PhD
Assistant Professor of Medicine
Department of Medicine
University of Texas Health Science Center
San Antonio
Texas
USA

Jana Portnow PhD
The Johns Hopkins Oncology Center
Baltimore, MD
USA

Robert D Rubens MD BSc FRCP
Professor of Clinical Oncology
Department of Clinical Oncology
Guy's Hospital
London
UK

Toshiyuki Yoneda DDS PhD
Professor of Medicine
Division of Endocrinology
Department of Medicine
University of Texas Health Science Center
San Antonio
Texas
USA

Preface

Malignant disease affects the skeleton in a variety of ways. Several types of primary tumours arise in bones, but they are rare compared with the common occurrence of bone metastases from cancers elsewhere. Dissemination of carcinomas of the breast and prostate to the skeleton is particularly prevalent and it is also a notable feature of malignancy originating in the lungs, thyroid and kidneys. Multiple myeloma is a unique neoplastic disorder associated with extensive bone involvement. Other important skeletal problems which arise from cancer are humoral hypercalcaemia and osteoporosis.

Metastatic bone disease is the most common cause of cancer pain and also leads to serious complications such as pathological fracture, hypercalcaemia, spinal cord/cauda equina compression and bone marrow suppression. Management of these problems may necessitate radiation therapy, orthopaedic surgery and specific systemic antitumour agents (endocrine treatment and cytotoxic chemotherapy), the precise approach depending both upon the nature of the primary tumour and individual clinical circumstances. The importance of symptomatic and supportive measures, particularly pain control, cannot be over-emphasised.

The most remarkable recent therapeutic innovation has followed a leap forward in our understanding of how metastatic disease mediates damage to the skeleton. The recognition that skeletal destruction from metastases is a consequence of osteoclastic bone resorption stimulated by tumour-derived cytokines has led to the establishment of bisphosphonates, inhibitors of osteoclastic activity, as an effective approach to the treatment of metastatic bone disease.

Progress in treatment leads to increasing demands upon diagnostic techniques and methods for evaluating response. The mainstay for assessing skeletal disease has been radiological, with isotopic scanning as the principal method to screen for metastases, while important new imaging techniques include computerised tomography and magnetic resource imaging. Of increasing interest in both diagnosis and monitoring of metastatic bone disease are the recently identified specific biochemical markers of bone resorption and formation.

Cancer and the Skeleton brings together these major developments about how cancer affects the skeleton and how the problems this causes are managed. We hope that the diversity of workers in this field of medicine will find it of value.

1

Structure and physiology of the normal skeleton

Gregory R Mundy

Introduction • Natural history of the skeleton • Remodeling of cortical and cancellous bone • The cellular events involved in the remodeling of bone • Origin and cell lineage • Osteoclast apoptosis • Molecular mechanisms of bone resorption • Regulation of osteoclast activity • Cellular events involved in the formation phase of the remodeling sequence • Osteoblastotropic factors which may be involved in the coupling process

INTRODUCTION

All bone diseases are superimposed on the normal process of bone remodeling – the process by which bone renews itself locally in discrete packets which are present on trabecular (cancellous) bone surfaces or in the Haversian systems of cortical (compact) bone. In the case of some diseases (for example Paget's disease, primary hyperparathyroidism, thyrotoxicosis), the processes of bone resorption and bone formation are approximately balanced and there is no major net gain or loss of bone. However, when cancer affects the skeleton, it usually causes disruption of the remodeling process and an imbalance between resorption and formation. In most patients, this imbalance favors resorption and there is loss of bone (osteolytic metastases) around tumor deposits. In a few patients, particularly those with advanced prostate cancer, there is a net gain (osteosclerotic or osteoblastic metastases) around the tumor cells. The mechanisms by which tumors cause these effects will be reviewed in detail in later chapters. In this chapter, the normal physiological process of bone remodeling which occurs in the adult human skeleton, and which underlies the pathologic effects of tumors on bone, will be reviewed.

NATURAL HISTORY OF THE SKELETON

Figure 1.1 represents how total body bone mass changes with age. Bone mass reaches a maximum about 10 years after linear growth stops, probably begins to decrease somewhere in the fourth decade, and declines to half its maximum value by the age of 80. Peak bone mineral density (bone mass), which is reached in the thirties, is less in women than it is in men, and less in Caucasians than in African-Americans. All non-Caucasian women show an additional accelerated phase of bone loss that occurs for about 10 years after the menopause.

The bones of the adult skeleton consist either of cortical (or compact) bone or cancellous (or trabecular) bone. It has been estimated that a woman can expect to lose 35% of her cortical bone and 50% of her cancellous bone as she ages,

2 CANCER AND THE SKELETON

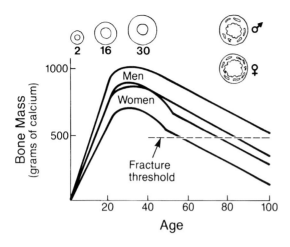

Fig. 1.1 Changes in bone mass which occur with age. Bone mass reaches a peak in young adult life, but then steadily declines. However, the different sexes decline at different rates. In women there is a rapid phase of bone loss caused by estrogen withdrawal at the menopause which lasts for about 10 years.

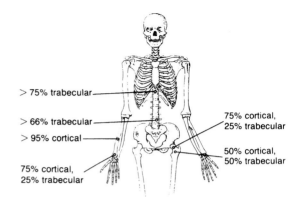

Fig. 1.2 Proportions of cortical and cancellous (also called trabecular) bone in different parts of the skeleton. Note that the axial skeleton, which is where malignant cells are most likely to accumulate, contains relatively more cancellous bone.

and a man can expect to lose about two thirds of these amounts.[1-3] About one half of the loss in cancellous bone is due to estrogen withdrawal at the menopause, and about one half to aging. It remains controversial as to precisely when bone mineral density starts to decline, and whether there is a similar accelerated phase of bone loss in both cancellous and cortical bone after the menopause. Different techniques for measuring parameters of bone mass have given slightly different answers.

Current evidence indicates that cortical bone and cancellous bone do not change with age in exactly the same way, and so they probably should be considered as two separate functional entities. The proportions of cortical and cancellous bone differ at the different sites in the skeleton where osteoporotic fractures frequently occur (Fig. 1.2). Cancellous bone is relatively prominent in the vertebral column, the most common site of fracture associated with osteoporosis, and the abnormality in the remodeling process that predisposes to this type of fracture is important to understand. In the lumbar spine, cancellous bone comprises more than 66% of the total bone. In the intertrochanteric area of the femur, bone consists of 50% cortical and 50% cancellous. In the neck of the femur, the bone is 75% cortical and 25% cancellous. In contrast, in the mid-radius more than 95% of the bone is cortical bone. The differences are most likely to reside in the different environments of the bone cells in cortical or cancellous bone. Bone remodeling cells on cancellous bone surfaces are in intimate contact with the cells of the marrow cavity, which produce a variety of potent osteotropic cytokines. It is likely that the cells in cortical bone, which are more distant from the influences of these cytokines, are influenced more by the systemic osteotropic hormones such as parathyroid hormone and 1,25 dihydroxyvitamin D_3. Osteoclasts and osteoblasts in cancellous bone may be controlled primarily by factors produced by adjacent bone marrow cells. Similar cells in Haversian systems of cortical bone are further removed from the myriad of osteotropic cytokines which are produced by marrow mononuclear cells.

REMODELING OF CORTICAL AND CANCELLOUS BONE

Cortical bone

Cortical bone is the dense or compact bone which comprises 85% of the total bone in the body. It is relatively most abundant in the long bone shafts of the appendicular skeleton. The volume of cortical bone is regulated by periosteal bone formation, by remodeling within Haversian systems, and by endosteal bone resorption. Cortical bone is removed primarily by endosteal resorption and resorption within the Haversian canals. The latter leads to increased porosity of cortical bone. However, periosteal bone formation continues to increase the diameter of cortical bone throughout life. Cortical bone loss probably begins after the age of 40 (according to most studies) and there is an acceleration of cortical bone loss that occurs for 5–10 years after the menopause. This accelerated phase of cortical bone loss continues for 15 years and then gradually slows. There is irrefutable evidence that estrogen replacement therapy after the menopause preserves cortical bone. In later life, women with osteoporosis lose cortical bone at similar rates to those of premenopausal women. Loss of cortical bone is the major predisposing factor for fractures that occur at the hip and around the wrist. Resorption of cortical bone occurs particularly in patients with states of parathyroid hormone (PTH) excess.

Cancellous bone

Although cancellous bone forms only 15% of the skeleton, the changes that occur in this type of bone after the age of 30 determine whether the clinical features of osteoporosis will occur. According to some workers, decline in cancellous bone mass begins in early adult life, occurring earlier than the decline in cortical bone mass.[4] Others have disagreed with these findings, and suggested that the decline in cancellous bone mass begins later, after ovarian function ceases.[5] Riggs and Melton[6] have suggested that the rate of cortical bone loss is relatively greater than cancellous bone loss at the time of the menopause.

Cancellous bone is the type of bone lost predominantly in patients with osteolytic bone disease due to malignancy. In this situation, the malignant cells lodge in the marrow cavity and produce local factors that stimulate adjacent osteoclasts on trabecular plates and on endosteal surfaces of cortical bone.[7,8] The loss of cancellous bone that occurs with aging is not due simply to a generalized thinning of the bone plates, but is rather due to complete perforation and fragmentation of trabeculae.[9,10]

THE CELLULAR EVENTS INVOLVED IN THE REMODELING OF BONE

The process of bone remodeling is the key phenomenon in bone cell biology and understanding the mechanisms which control the remodeling process and its regulation will clarify not only local control of osteoclast and osteoblast function, but also the pathophysiology of age-related bone loss and osteoporosis (Fig. 1.3). The adult skeleton is in a dynamic state, being continually broken down and reformed by the co-ordinated actions of osteoclasts and osteoblasts on trabecular surfaces and

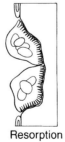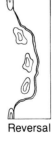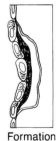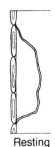

Resorption Reversal Formation Resting

Fig. 1.3 Bone remodeling. Sequence of events involved in normal bone remodeling. Bone remodeling is initiated by an increase in osteoclast activity, which is followed by proliferation of osteoblast precursors, and the differentiation of these cells into mature osteoblasts which lay down new bone and repair the resorption defects caused by osteoclasts. The effects of cancer are superimposed on this remodeling sequence.

in Haversian systems. This turnover or remodeling of bone occurs in focal and discrete packets throughout the skeleton. The remodeling of each packet takes a finite period of time (estimated to be about 3–4 months). The remodeling which occurs in each packet (called a bone remodeling unit by Frost, who first described this sequence almost 30 years ago[11]) is geographically and chronologically separated from other packets of remodeling. This suggests that activation of the sequence of cellular events responsible for remodeling is locally controlled, possibly by an autoregulatory mechanism, perhaps by autocrine or paracrine factors generated in the bone microenvironment. The sequence is always the same – osteoclastic bone resorption followed by osteoblastic bone formation to repair the defect. The new bone which is formed is called a bone structural unit (BSU).[11]

Osteoclast activation is the initial step in the remodeling sequence. Osteoclasts are activated in specific focal sites by mechanisms which are still not understood, but may be initiated by microdamage at that site. The activation of the osteoclast may occur because of interactions that occur between integral membrane proteins (integrins) on osteoclast cell membranes with proteins in bone matrix which contain RGD (arginine-glycine-asparagine) amino acid sequences (such as osteopontin). Miyauchi *et al.*[12] have demonstrated such a phenomenon *in vitro*. Osteoclast activation may also be due to stimulatory signals produced by local cells in the osteoclast microenvironment such as immune cells, but the potential trigger for activation of immune cells is unknown. The resorptive phase of the remodeling process has been estimated to last 10 days (Figs 1.4 and 1.5). This period is followed by repair of the defect by a team of osteoblasts which are attracted to the site of the resorption defect and then presumably proceed to make new bone. This part of the process takes approximately 3 months. The initial events in the formation phase are possibly unidirectional migration (chemotaxis) of osteoblast precursors to the site of the defect followed by enhanced cell proliferation. The complete sequence of cellular events which occur at the bone surface during the remodeling process has been described in detail by Baron *et al.*[13] from studies on the alveolar bone of the rat, and by Boyce *et al.*[14] from the calvarial bone of the mouse. The cellular events which occur in these models are similar to those in adult human bone.

ORIGIN AND CELL LINEAGE

The multinucleated osteoclast is the primary bone resorbing cell. For years, the origin of the osteoclast has been the subject of dispute, although now most workers agree that it is derived from a multipotent precursor it shares with cells of the monocyte–macrophage lineage in the bone marrow (Figs 1.4 and 1.5). A variety of studies have shown that the osteoclast is blood-borne, in contrast to osteoblasts. Walker[15,16] showed that parabiotic linkage of an osteopetrotic mouse with a normal littermate caused a marrow cavity to form due to the formation of osteoclasts. Studies using quail-chick chimeras,[17] in which quail-borne rudiments are grafted on to chick allantoic membrane, have disclosed that the osteoclasts formed are predominantly of host origin. This system takes advantage of the distinctive nuclear morphology of quail and chick cells and permits identification of host and donor cells. Jotereau and LeDouarin[18] have confirmed that osteoclasts in quail-chick chimeras are not bone derived.

Transplantation of hemopoietic tissue into lethally irradiated osteopetrotic recipients suggests that osteoclast precursors must be present in hemopoietic tissues. Walker[19] showed that transplantation of spleen or marrow cells into osteopetrotic mice resulted in removal of excessive bone present in these animals. Marks[20] showed that in the ia osteopetrotic rat, transplantation of spleen cells could cure the disease. Infusion of the mononuclear cell fraction from the spleen[21] was responsible for formation of osteoclasts with ruffled borders, something not seen in untreated ia rats. These studies revealed that transplantation of cells derived from hemopoietic tissue could cure osteopetrosis, and suggest that

STRUCTURE AND PHYSIOLOGY OF THE NORMAL SKELETON 5

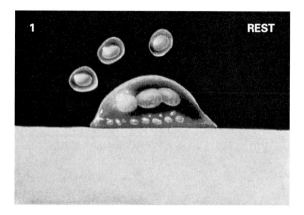
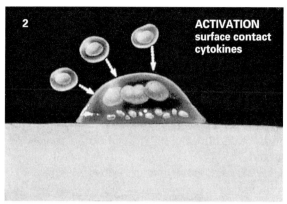
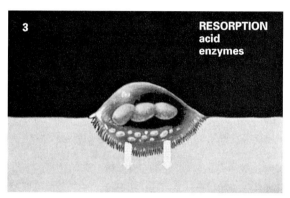
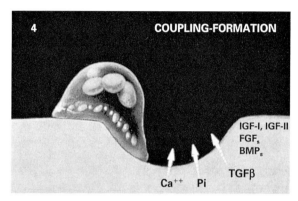

Fig. 1.4 Diagram of early events involved in bone remodeling. (1) Resting osteoclast on a bone surface. (2) Osteoclast activation. The mechanism by which osteoclasts are activated is unknown, but may involve recognition by the osteoclasts of microdamage. Osteoclast activity is modulated by cytokines. (3) As a consequence of activation, the osteoclasts become polarized and produce protons and lysosomal enzymes. (4) Bone resorption leads to the release of local growth regulatory factors for osteoblasts which are capable of stimulating all the subsequent events involved in bone formation. In patiens with cancer, tumor cells may initiate osteoclast activation to lead to osteolysis. There is frequently an impairment in the osteoblast response for reasons which are unclear.

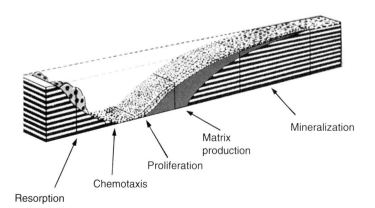

Fig. 1.5 Diagram of the events involved in bone remodeling on a normal cancellous bone surface. Note that these cellular events are depicted chronologically. Bone resorption lasts for less than 2 weeks, but bone formation is prolonged over a period of several months. Note the cellular events involved in the bone formation process. (Redrawn from Eriksen.[119])

the critical cells which are transplanted are osteoclast precursors. However, the results do not exclude the possibility that the transplanted cells act instead by producing a factor which permits normal differentiation of osteopetrotic osteoclasts. Results with transplantation of cells which contained markers showed that osteopetrosis was in fact cured by formation of donor-derived osteoclasts. For example, Coccia and co-workers[22] and Sorell et al.[23] transplanted marrow from HLA-matched male siblings into female patients who had osteopetrosis, and showed by Y-body analysis that the osteoclasts formed in the patients were donor in origin. Studies in osteopetrotic rodents using fetal liver cells[21] and mononuclear cells from thymus,[24] as well as a cell suspension containing hemopoietic stem cells,[25] also indicate that osteopetrosis can be cured by transplantation of hemopoietic cells. These studies all support the concept that the osteoclast precursor is a mononuclear cell derived from hemopoietic tissue.

Osteoclasts form by fusion of mononuclear precursors. This was shown by studies of Kahn and Simmons[17] using quail-chick chimeras, who found that some osteoclasts which formed contained nuclei with both quail and chick characteristics. Young[26] showed in experiments using ^{3}H-thymidine that osteoclasts formed by fusion of mononuclear precursors rather than mitotic division. Using autoradiography, it has been shown that osteoclast-like cells grown in long-term marrow cultures are formed by fusion.[27,28] More recent studies have shown that the cell attachment molecule E-cadherin is involved in the process, since E-cadherin is expressed by osteoclasts as they fuse and either peptide antagonists or neutralizing antibodies to E-cadherin, both of which interfere with the cell attachment function of E-cadherin, block osteoclast formation.[29]

Taken together, these data, derived from diverse experimental systems, all support the notion that the multinucleated osteoclast is formed by fusion of mononuclear cells which are hemopoietic rather than bone derived in origin.

The leading candidate for the mononuclear precursor for the osteoclast appears to be a stem cell of the monocyte–macrophage family. The classic experiments of Fischman and Hay[30] demonstrated in regenerating newt limb that osteoclasts were formed by the fusion of labeled leukocytes which were probably monocytes histologically. Tinkler et al.[31] infused ^{3}H-thymidine-labeled peripheral blood murine monocytes into syngeneic recipients treated with 1,25 dihydroxyvitamin D_3, and observed that the osteoclasts which formed contained labeled nuclei. Similarly, Zambonin Zallone et al.[32] found that some peripheral blood monocytes can fuse with purified osteoclasts in vitro. Burger et al.[33] reported that the osteoclast precursors in mouse marrow cells were immature monocytes by morphologic criteria. Similar nonadherent cells were identified as potential human osteoclast precursors in an entirely different system.[27,34]

We propose the following model of osteoclast development based on the above data (Fig. 1.4). We suggest that the osteoclast arises from a progenitor cell similar to that for other members of the monocyte–macrophage family. In this model, the colony-stimulating factors (CSFs) stimulate the proliferation and differentiation of the granulocyte–macrophage-committed progenitor cells (CFU-GM). These CSFs probably include CSF-1 and GM-CSF, and possibly other cytokines such as interleukin-6 and interleukin-3. This model is consistent with the observations of Burger et al.[33] that incubation of marrow with colony stimulating activity responsible for the proliferation of monocyte–macrophage progenitors, increases the number of osteoclast progenitors, and our finding[28] that recombinant human CSF-1 increased formation of osteoclast-like cells in long-term marrow cultures. CFU-GM stimulated by CSF-1 form promonocytes, which are immature nonadherent progenitors of mononuclear phagocytes and osteoclasts. Also consistent are the studies in op/op osteopetrotic mice, which do not have competent osteoclasts. In this disease, biologically active CSF-1 is not produced and osteoclasts do not form.[35-39] Both Burger et al.[33] and Ibbotson et al.[27] have identified the precursor for these cells as a nonadherent immature monocyte. The promonocyte can presumably proliferate and differentiate along the macrophage pathway and eventually form a tissue macrophage or can differentiate along the osteoclast pathway, depending on the factors to which it is exposed.

The first osteoclast precursors, the early preosteoclasts, can still proliferate and circulate in the peripheral blood. These cells are a specialized subpopulation of peripheral blood monocytes but are morphologically indistinguishable from other monocytes by light microscopy. In this regard, Zambonin Zallone et al.[32] have shown that some peripheral blood monocytes fuse with osteoclasts. The concentration of early preosteoclasts may be increased in states of primary hyperparathyroidism,[40] Paget's disease,[41] or other conditions in which bone resorption or turnover is increased. The early preosteoclast contains nonspecific esterase but not tartrate-resistant acid phosphatase according to the observations of Baron et al.[42] Based on in vitro data with long-term marrow cultures,[40,43,44] PTH, 1,25 dihydroxyvitamin D_3, and other factors such as transforming growth factor alpha (TGFα) and epidermal growth factor (EGF) stimulate the formation of these cells, while calcitonin inhibits their formation. The early preosteoclast gives rise to a late preosteoclast, a step which is regulated by 1,25 dihydroxyvitamin D_3, PTH, or possibly other osteotropic factors. The late preosteoclast has decreased or absent proliferative potential and has lost some of its monocytic surface antigens.

Once the late preosteoclast 'homes' to bone, it expresses osteoclast-specific antigens[45,46] and fuses with other cells to form a multinucleated osteoclast. The late preosteoclast may have ultrastructural features of osteoclasts as reported for mononuclear osteoclasts,[47] and expresses a calcitonin receptor. This cell also has the capacity to bind through integrins to RGD sequences in bone matrix proteins.[12] In this model, mature multinucleated osteoclasts would not express the majority of the monocytic surface antigens, would strongly express osteoclast-specific antigens, and develop all the ultrastructural features of mature osteoclasts. This model is proposed as a continuum rather than as distinct stages of differentiation. Vaananen and colleagues[48] have shown that the cell membrane of the osteoclast is divided into several domains using enveloped viral glycoproteins and lectins as markers. During active resorption, when the osteoclast is polarized, the basolateral domain is distinct from the ruffled border and sealing zone.

OSTEOCLAST APOPTOSIS

Recently, it has been observed that osteoclasts undergo morphologic apoptosis at the conclusion of the resorbing phase of the bone remodeling process.[49] The morphologic characteristics of osteoclast apoptosis are condensation of the nuclear chromatin, darker staining of the osteoclast cytoplasm, loss of ruffled border and detachment from the mineralized bone matrix, and cessation of bone resorption. Osteoclast apoptosis is a common occurrence at reversal sites and may be precipitated by resorption inhibitors such as estrogen and bisphosphonates, and also by TGFβ.[50] Regulation of the process of osteoclast apoptosis may be potentially important during bone resorption, since this represents a step by which bone resorption could be regulated.

MOLECULAR MECHANISMS OF BONE RESORPTION (FIGURE 1.6)

Osteoclasts resorb bone by the production of proteolytic enzymes and hydrogen ions in the localized environment under the ruffled border of the cell. Hydrogen ions are generated in the cell by the enzyme carbonic anhydrase Type II. They are then pumped across the ruffled border by a proton pump, apparently related but not identical to the proton pump in the intercalated cells of the kidney.[51] Lysosomal enzymes are also released by the osteoclast, and the hydrogen ions produced by the proton pump provide an optimal environment for these proteolytic enzymes to degrade the bone matrix.

The production of protons under the ruffled border of the osteoclast is required for normal bone resorption. This probably occurs because

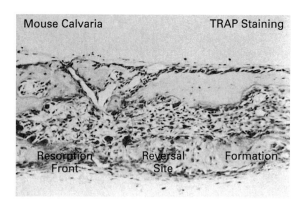

Fig. 1.6 Cells involved in the remodeling sequence demonstrated after local injection of interleukin-1 over the murine calvaria. Osteoclasts at the reversal site are undergoing apoptosis (Boyce et al.[14]).

the osteoclast needs to release mineral from the bone matrix, and provide an optimal environment for the maximal proteolytic activity of lysosomal enzymes as well as activation of growth factors such as transforming growth factor β and the insulin-like growth factors. A molecular mechanism for the translocation of protons from the osteoclast cytosol to the area under the ruffled border has recently been identified by several workers. This molecular mechanism may be a variation of the complex vacuolar ATPase found in the intercalated cells of the kidney,[51] although there has been some controversy on this point.[52] Although this ATPase may not be typical of the renal ATPase, this is a complex enzyme and pharmacologic inhibition may depend on the specific subunit composition of the enzyme.

There are a number of ion exchangers, pumps, and channels in the basolateral membrane of the osteoclast which are required for the extrusion of protons across the ruffled border of the cell (apical surface). These are required to maintain the electrochemical balance of the osteoclast. These ion exchangers, pumps, and channels include an Na^+/H^+ antiporter, an Na^+/K^+ ATPase, a HCO_3^-/Cl^- exchanger, a Ca^{++} ATPase, and a K^+ channel.

There has been considerable controversy over the capacity of osteoclasts to produce collagen-degrading enzymes. For many years it has been thought that the osteoblast was the major source of collagenase activity in the microenvironment of the resorbing osteoclast,[53] and that osteoclasts caused matrix degradation by the production of lysosomal cysteine proteinases, which caused collagen degradation at low pH.[54,55] Using immunolocalization studies, Delaisse et al.[56] have demonstrated the presence of intracellular collagenase (matrix metalloproteinase-1) as well as collagenase in the extracellular subosteoclastic resorbing compartment, using anti-mouse antibodies. These more recent studies on matrix metalloproteinases have suggested that the osteoclast itself may be a rich source of collagen-digesting enzymes, which certainly makes sense for a cell responsible for resorbing the bone matrix, which comprises more than 90% Type I collagen. Other enzymes are likely important in bone resorption. Cathepsin K has been recently identified in osteoclasts.[57] It has significant primary sequence homology to members of the papain cysteine protease superfamily, including cathepsins S, L, and B. Cathepsin K is a potential target for inhibitors of bone destruction.[58]

The osteoclast is a motile cell. It resorbs bone to form a lacuna and then moves across the bone surface to resorb a separate area of bone. The tracks of its path can often be followed.[59] Periods of locomotion are not associated with resorption. When the cell stops moving, it usually starts resorbing bone.

Disruption of any of the critical molecular mechanisms responsible for bone resorption causes osteopetrosis. For example, it has recently been shown that there is an unusual form of inherited osteopetrosis in children in which there is a deficiency of the carbonic anhydrase Type II isoenzyme.[60] The osteoclasts in this disease are incompetent, bone is not resorbed, and the bone marrow cavity is not formed. Children with this disease also have renal tubular acidosis, due to a similar enzyme defect in renal tubular cells leading to impairment of hydrogen ion secretion. In another well-studied model of osteopetrosis which occurs in mice, the op/op variant, it has recently been found that osteopetrosis is due to a defect in osteoclast formation caused by an abnormality in the coding region for CSF-1. As a consequence of this genetic abnormality, defective CSF-1 is produced by stromal cells in the osteoclast microenvironment, and osteoclast formation is impaired. The disease can be cured by treatment with exogenous CSF-1.[37,39]

Osteopetrosis has been a very informative disease for studying molecular mechanisms responsible for osteoclast formation and action. Not only has the study of this disease led to observations that carbonic anhydrase Type II and CSF-1 are required for normal osteoclast function, but recently it has been shown that the expression of the proto-oncogenes src and fos is also necessary for osteoclasts to function.[61-63] This has been demonstrated by targeted disruption of the normal proto-oncogenes for src and fos in embryonic stem cells followed by homologous recombination and observations in mutant mice which fail to express these oncogenes. In both cases, osteopetrosis occurs. In the case of src, the defect is not in osteoclast formation but in osteoclast action:[64] src is a nonreceptor tyrosine kinase bound to the cytoplasmic plasma membrane which may be involved in polarization and activation of the osteoclasts. There are approximately 40 or 50 proteins inside cells which are phosphorylated on tyrosine residues by src, and the essential substrate in the osteoclast or in any other cells remains unknown. Two possibilities have recently been suggested. A cytoskeletal protein associated with actin which is phosphorylated by src is localized to the ruffled border in active osteoclasts and may be important.[64] Boyce has favored the notion that cortactin, a cytoskeletal protein expressed in the ruffled border of the osteoclast, may be an essential src substrate. Tanaka et al.[65] have suggested that another cytoskeletal protein, c-cbl, is an important 120 kilodalton substrate for src in osteoclastic resorption, and showed by immunofluorescence studies and confocal microscopy that c-cbl and c-src may co-localize. It is possible that a number of important cytoskeletal proteins are responsible for the effects of src during the

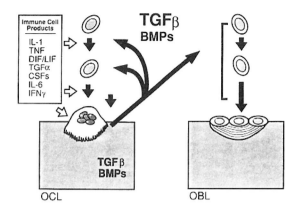

Fig. 1.7 Potential role of TGFβ and related factors in the remodeling process. These growth factors are produced in active form as a consequence of bone resorption. They are then available locally to control subsequent events involved in bone formation. In osteolytic bone disease, this coupling phenomenon is frequently impaired.

bone resorption process. Similarly, it has been shown that PI3 kinase, an enzyme involved in phosphoinositol metabolism which is activated by interactions between osteopontin and the $\alpha_V\beta_3$ integrin receptor on osteoclasts, co-precipitates with src in osteoclast lysates.[66] A model integrating the role of c-src into the mechanisms by which osteoclasts resorb bone is shown in Fig. 1.7.

The early response gene c-fos is essential for normal osteoclast formation. Gene knockout experiments have shown in mice that null mutations for c-fos introduced into the germ line lead to mice with absent osteoclast formation and severe osteopetrosis.[62,67] Since the defect is in the osteoclast lineage, this type of osteopetrosis is different from either op/op osteopetrosis (where the defect in accessory cells is critical) or from c-src deficiency (where osteoclasts form but have impaired functional capacity). Surprisingly, overexpression of c-fos leads to osteogenic sarcomas and related mesenchymal tumors.[68] In this case, the defect seems to be specific for the osteoblast lineage. The relationship between defects caused by overexpression of c-fos and lack of expression of c-fos remains unclear.

Adhesion molecules on osteoclast cytoplasmic membranes are clearly important for normal osteoclast function and particularly for bone resorption. These integral membrane proteins (integrins) have been shown recently to bind to molecules present in the bone matrix such as osteopontin through specific RGD (Arg-Gly-Asp) amino acid sequences, an event which leads to osteoclast activation, accumulation of intracellular calcium, and activation of the phosphoinositol pathway.[12] Several other RGD-containing matrix proteins have been identified, including collagen Type I and bone sialoprotein II, which could act as integrin-binding proteins in bone.[69] A major integrin on the osteoclast surface is the $\alpha_V\beta_3$ dimer, which appears to be closely related to the vitronectin receptor.[70] The importance of this process in bone resorption has recently been demonstrated by Sato et al.[71] who have found that synthetic peptide antagonists to RGD sequences inhibit osteoclastic bone resorption in vitro. Recently, it has been shown that echistatin, which inhibits binding to RGD sequences in vivo, also blocks bone resorption in vivo.[72] Surprisingly, the $\alpha_V\beta_3$ integrin is expressed predominantly at the basolateral membrane, suggesting that other integrins may be important at the apical (ruffled border) membrane.[73]

Several other processes may be involved in the complex mechanism of osteoclastic bone resorption. Some workers have suggested that the surface of the bone is prepared for the osteoclast by the actions of collagenase released by bone lining cells or osteoblasts.[74] The osteoclasts then produce acid and lysosomal enzymes which complete the process. Since osteoblasts have the capacity to produce enzymes which could activate latent collagenase such as plasminogen activator, such a mechanism is possible. However, Boyde has claimed that studies with scanning electron microscopy show that osteoclasts do not necessarily require osteoblast preparation of the bone surface for resorption to occur, and isolated osteoclasts can resorb bone surfaces without the support of any other cells.

It appears that oxygen-derived free radicals are also involved in the resorption of bone by osteoclasts.[75] Many degradative processes by phagocytic cells are associated with free radical production, and bone resorption seems another. The use of radical generating systems in vivo and in vitro shows that enzymes which deplete tissues of radicals such as superoxide dismutase block osteoclastic bone resorption stimulated by parathyroid hormone or interleukin-1. Staining reactions with nitroblue tetrazolium show that radical generation occurs within osteoclasts. Radicals could be involved in the degradation of bone under the ruffled border. However, the demonstration that radical generation is associated with new osteoclast formation in vivo suggests that radicals also have a cellular effect on the formation of osteoclasts.[75] There is some debate over the relative importance of specific reactive oxygen species.[76,77] However, Steinbeck et al.[78] have clearly shown expression of NADPH-oxidase in osteoclasts, as well as the capacity of osteoclasts actively to produce superoxide.

Nitric oxide has recently been shown to be a potential intermediate in the mode of action of some cytokines on bone resorption.[79–83] Nitric oxide synthase inhibitors block bone resorption which is stimulated by IL-1 or TNF, suggesting that nitric oxide is in part responsible for the effects of these cytokines. However, larger concentrations of nitric oxide inhibit bone resorption, and this may be relevant to the inhibitory effects of gamma interferon on osteoclastic bone resorption stimulated by cytokines.

REGULATION OF OSTEOCLAST ACTIVITY

Osteoclasts lie on bone surfaces in a bed of elliptical or fusiform spindle-shaped cells called lining cells, which are probably members of the osteoblast lineage. When exposed to a bone resorbing agent, the first response is that these lining cells retract and the osteoclasts insinuate

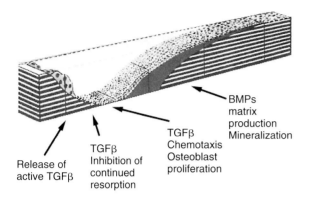

Fig. 1.8 Potential role of the TGFβ superfamily in the remodeling process. TGFβ is the most abundant factor in the bone matrix and is produced in large amounts in an active form during bone resorption. It may then trigger osteoblast chemotaxis and proliferation, leading to a autocrine/paracrine production of other growth regulatory factors for osteoblasts, including BMPs, FGFs, and IGF-I and IGF-II. These factors may work as a cascade to complete the process of osteoblast differentiation and bone formation. (Redrawn from Eriksen.[119])

themselves into the retracted area, a ruffled border forms, and bone is resorbed at the exposed surface.[59] The molecular mechanisms by which these complicated processes are controlled are unknown. Why lining cells retract at specific sites and how the osteoclast is activated are still not clear (Fig. 1.8). Although some have suggested that the osteoclast is activated by a soluble signal released from the lining cell,[84,85] it is possible that the major mechanism for activation of the mature cell may be by interactions between integrins on osteoclast cell membranes with extracellular bone constituents such as osteopontin.[12]

Many hormones and local factors have not been shown to stimulate osteoclast activity directly. Their mechanisms of action differ. Osteoclastic resorption may be stimulated by factors which enhance proliferation of osteoclast progenitors, which cause differentiation of committed precursors into mature cells or activation of the mature multinucleated cell to resorb bone.[86] Similarly, osteoclasts could be inhibited by agents which block proliferation of precursors, which inhibit differentiation or fusion, or which inactivate the mature multinucleated resorbing cell. Current evidence indicates that most factors which stimulate or inhibit osteoclasts act on at least two of these steps. The factors which regulate osteoclastic bone resorption are considered in Chapter 5.

Recently, a member of the TNF receptor superfamily has been identified as inhibiting bone resorption independently of the stimulus by two groups.[87,88] This protein has been named osteoclastogenesis inhibitory factor (OCIF) or osteoprotegerin (OPG), and represents a peptide which is a soluble secreted form of the TNF receptor and acts as an antagonist to osteoclastic bone resorption both *in vitro* and *in vivo*. Even more recently, the ligand for this endogenous antagonist has been identified as the putative osteoclastogenesis differentiation-inducing factor (ODIF) which acts directly on osteoclasts. It appears to be identical or at the very least related to RANK ligand (also called TRANCE).[89] This peptide, which has a membrane-bound form, is also a ligand for OPG/OCID[90] and has been shown to stimulate osteoclastic bone resorption in marrow cultures by acting directly on cells in the osteoclast lineage. This has led to the concept that osteoprotegerin or OCIF inhibits bone resorption by binding directly to TRANCE/ODIF, the final common mediator of osteoclastic bone resorption.

All the diseases of bone are superimposed on this normal cellular remodeling sequence. In diseases such as primary hyperparathyroidism, hyperthyroidism, and Paget's disease, in which osteoclasts are activated, there is a compensatory and (relatively) balanced increase in the formation of new bone. However, there are also a number of well described conditions in which osteoblast activity does not completely repair the defect left by previous resorption by replacing all the bone removed. One example is myeloma, usually characterized by punched-out lytic bone lesions with little new bone formation.[91] In myeloma, there appears to be a specific effect in osteoblast maturation.[92] There are probably increased numbers of osteoblasts around the edges of the lytic lesions, but the osteoblasts fail (in the great majority of patients) to synthesize more than thin osteoid seams. In solid tumors associated with malignancy, there is also a failure of bone formation to repair resorptive defects especially in patients dying from their malignancy.[93] In elderly patients with osteoporosis, there is a decrease in mean wall thickness, presumably reflecting the inability of osteoblasts to repair adequately the resorptive defects made during normal osteoclastic resorption.[94] It should also be stressed that progressive bone loss, beginning at about 35 years of age (depending on the bone), occurs in all humans, and is indicative of a 'physiological' imbalance between resorption and formation.

Although bone formation usually occurs on sites of previous osteoclastic resorption in normal adult humans, there are several special situations in which osteoblasts may lay down new bone on surfaces not previously resorbed. Two examples are osteoblastic metastases associated with tumors such as carcinoma of the prostate and breast, and during prolonged exposure to pharmacological doses of fluoride therapy. However, in most physiological and pathological circumstances, the coupling of bone formation to previous bone resorption occurs faithfully. The cellular and humoral mechanisms which are responsible for mediating the coupling process (or disrupting it, as in the diseases described above) are still not clear. Several theories have been proposed to account for coupling. Almost 20 years ago, Rasmussen and Bordier[95] suggested that the osteoclast, once it finishes the resorptive phase of the remodeling sequence, undergoes fission to form mononuclear cells which are the precursors of osteoblasts. However, it is now widely accepted that osteoclasts and osteoblasts have different origins. Osteoclasts arise from hematopoietic stem cells or at least stem cells in the marrow environment which have the capacity to circulate. Osteoblasts, in contrast, arise from stromal mesenchymal cells. Many workers have favored the notion that coupling is humorally mediated, that an osteoblast-stimulating factor (such as IGF-I, IGF-II, or TGFβ) is released from bone matrix during the process of osteoclastic bone resorption, and the stimulation of osteoblast activity leads to new bone formation.[96] A variation on this humoral concept is that the factor which stimulates resorption also acts directly (but slowly) on osteoblasts to cause their activation and subsequent new bone formation. There is an alternative to the humoral hypothesis to explain coupling. It is possible that since osteoblasts normally line bone surfaces, once the phase of osteoclastic resorption is over and osteoclasts disappear from the resorption site, osteoblasts and their precursors repopulate the resorption site and merely reline the bone surface. They may thus repair the resorptive defect without the necessity for involvement of a humoral mediator which is specifically generated as a consequence of resorption. Manolagas and Jilka[97] have alternatively proposed that coupling does not involve sequential signals released during the process of bone remodeling, but rather that factors that work through the GP-130 signal transduction mechanism are responsible for simultaneous stimulation of osteoclast and osteoblast lineages.

Obviously, understanding this sequence of cellular events may lead to clarification of the mechanism of decreased osteoblast activity which occurs in age-related bone loss, and possibly the pathophysiology of osteoporosis, as well as the specific defects in osteoblast function which occur in malignancies such as myeloma, breast cancer, and prostate cancer. Based on observations that have been made possible in recent years of the effects of stimulatory factors such as TGFβ on bone *in vivo*,[98] and interpretation of the data available, a hypothesis for how coupling may be mediated will be proposed here. Before this model is described, the events which are likely to be important in the formation phase of the remodeling sequence will be reviewed, and the local osteotropic factors which may be responsible for mediating these events.

CELLULAR EVENTS INVOLVED IN THE FORMATION PHASE OF THE REMODELING SEQUENCE

The specific cellular events following the phase of osteoclastic resorption are osteoclast apoptosis, followed by osteoblast chemotaxis, proliferation, and differentiation, which in turn is followed by formation of mineralized bone and cessation of osteoblast activity. The initial event is likely osteoclast apoptosis, which can be enhanced by active TGFβ.[50] This is followed by chemotactic attraction of osteoblasts or their precursors to the sites of the resorption defect. This attraction is also likely mediated by local factors produced during the resorption process. Resorbing bone has been shown to produce chemotactic factors for cells with osteoblast characteristics in vitro.[99,100] One mediator which may be responsible for this effect is TGFβ (Fig. 1.7), since active TGFβ is released by resorbing bone cultures.[101] Structural proteins such as collagen or the bone Gla protein could also be involved, since Type I collagen and bone Gla protein and their fragments cause the same effect.[99,100] TGFβ, which is enriched in the bone matrix and released as a consequence of bone resorption, is also chemotactic for bone cells.[102] However, TGFβ is not the only potential chemoattractant in bone. Platelet-derived growth factor is chemotactic for some mesenchymal cells, monocytes, neutrophils, and smooth muscle cells.[103–106] Perhaps a combination of chemotactic factors is responsible for the attraction of osteoblast precursors to resorption sites.

The next event involved in the formation phase of the coupling phenomenon is proliferation of osteoblast precursors. This is likely to be mediated by local osteoblast growth factors released during the resorption process. There are several leading candidates for these factors, which represent autocrine and paracrine factors. These include members of the TGFβ superfamily (TGFβs I and II). In addition, PDGF causes proliferation of cells with osteoblast characteristics. The insulin-like growth factors I and II and the heparin-binding fibroblast growth factors also cause osteoblast proliferation. All these factors are stored in the bone matrix.

The next sequential event during the formation phase is the differentiation of the osteoblast precursor into the mature cell. Several of the bone-derived growth factors can cause the appearance of markers of the differentiated osteoblast phenotype, including expression of alkaline phosphatase activity, Type I collagen, and osteocalcin synthesis. Most prominent of these are IGF-I and BMP-2. Active TGFβ inhibits osteoblast differentiation *in vitro*, which suggests its role may be to 'trigger' the process, after which it is removed or becomes inactivated, allowing the increased pool of precursors to undergo differentiation.

The final phase of the formation process must be cessation of osteoblast activity. The resorption lacunae are usually repaired either completely or almost completely. It is not known how this is achieved. One possibility is that factors produced during this process decrease osteoblast activity. Under the appropriate circumstances, again, one such factor could be TGFβ. Active TGFβ decreases differentiated function in osteoblasts, and as noted above is expressed by osteoblasts as they differentiate.[107]

OSTEOBLASTOTROPIC FACTORS WHICH MAY BE INVOLVED IN THE COUPLING PROCESS

Osteotropic factors which could be involved in the coupling phenomenon are TGFβ, BMPs, insulin-like growth factors-I and II, platelet-derived growth factor, and heparin-binding fibroblast growth factors. This area has also been reviewed by Canalis *et al*.[108] These factors are likely to be released locally from bone as it resorbs, or by bone cells activated as a consequence of the resorption process. They may then act in a sequential manner to regulate all the cellular events required for the formation of bone.

The TGFβ superfamily may be particularly important in the coupling which links bone formation to prior bone resorption (Fig. 1.8). Prolonged primary cultures of fetal rat calvarial osteoblasts show that the BMPs are expressed as these cells differentiate to form new bone, in parallel with other differentiation markers such as osteocalcin and alkaline phosphatase. Transient exposure of these cells to TGFβ stimulates proliferation of the osteoblasts (continued exposure inhibits the formation of mineralized bone expression of differentiation markers). Addition of BMPs to culture leads to increased numbers of mineralized nodules. We suggest that the following events (Figs 1.5 and 1.7) occur during normal bone remodeling based on our *in vitro* observations. Bone resorption leads to the release of active TGFβ, as has been shown previously.[101] TGFβ causes cessation of further osteoclastic bone resorption by causing osteoclasts to undergo apoptosis.[50] Osteoblast precursors are recruited to the site of resorption. Exposure of osteoblast precursors to active TGFβ causes increased proliferation. However, this exposure to active TGFβ is transient, and as a consequence, the proliferating cells undergo differentiation and express bone morphogenetic proteins. This is also associated with expression of osteoblast differentiation markers such as alkaline phosphatase, Type I collagen, and osteocalcin. Osteoid matrix becomes mineralized resulting in new bone. Thus, the bone resorption process results in a cascade of growth factors which are responsible for the subsequent events. Initially, one of the most abundant growth factors in the bone matrix, namely TGFβ, is released in an active form as a consequence of resorption. TGFβ then attracts osteoblast precursors to the site of the resorption defect and stimulates proliferation of osteoblast precursors.[102,109] The proliferating osteoblasts then begin to differentiate to form more mature osteoblasts and express differentiation markers such as alkaline phosphatase and osteocalcin, but also the bone morphogenetic proteins. These bone morphogenetic proteins then are responsible for an autostimulatory effect on the osteoblasts and the formation of mineralized bone. Of course, it is unlikely that the TGFβ superfamily members are acting alone. Other growth factors such as the insulin-like growth factors and the heparin-binding fibroblast growth factors (FGFs) and the platelet-derived growth factors are also likely to be having effects on osteoblast proliferation and differentiation. These factors are all bone growth stimulants. Recently, it has been shown that FGFs have comparable osteoblast stimulating effects on bone to those of TGFβ.[110]

The most convincing evidence that IGF-I may play a role as a coupling factor has been provided by the work of Canalis *et al.*[111] in cultures of embryonic rat calvariae. This group showed that PTH stimulated expression of IGF-I by calvarial cultures. Thus, this mechanism has been suggested for the anabolic effect of PTH. In other words, PTH may stimulate bone cells to produce IGF-I upon transient exposure, and this production of IGF-I is responsible for subsequent bone formation. However, this is unlikely to be the only mechanism involved, and it remains unclear whether this is the mechanism responsible for the anabolic effect of IGF-I *in vivo*.

Hence, like hematopoiesis and differentiation of multipotent hematopoietic stem cells, bone formation may represent a complex multihierarchical organization of the cells in the osteoblast lineage. It is possible that the actions of these factors could be co-ordinated in a similar way to that which has been suggested for the hematopoietic growth factors. These factors may work as a cascade, as suggested above for TGFβ and the BMPs, or they may act in concert together. It is likely that there exists a hierarchical modulation of receptors, and potential for alteration by one growth factor of the target osteoblast's responses to other growth factors is modulated by some growth factors altering expression of receptors for other factors, and therefore osteoblast responsivity. There is much evidence to suggest that there are synergistic as well as inhibitory interactions between the growth factors which act on osteoblasts. For example, TGFβ, PDGF, IGF-I and -II, FGF-I and -II, and BMPs may all influence osteoblasts directly, but also may modulate osteoblast responsivity to each other growth factor.[112–118] Although the potential interactions between these factors are extraordinarily complex, possibly even as complex as the interactions between the CSFs on hematopoiesis, it will be essential to unravel them to understand the local control of bone formation. It is likely that the complicated interactions between these factors released locally in active form as a consequence of the resorption process are responsible for the carefully co-ordinated formation of new bone which occurs at these sites.

In summary, then, cancer affects bone by altering the activities of the normal bone cells involved in remodeling of bone. In most cases this leads to unbalanced resorption and subsequent osteolysis, but in some to enhanced formation (sclerosis). Cancer seems to uncouple the resorption and formation by mechanisms which are not understood. It is possible that better understanding of these mechanisms may help in our understanding of the normal physiological process of remodeling.

REFERENCES

1. Mazess RB. On aging bone loss. *Clin Orthop* (1982) **165**: 239–52.
2. Riggs BL, Wahner HW, Dunn WL *et al*. Differential changes in bone mineral density of the appendicular and axial skeleton with aging: relationship to spinal osteoporosis. *J Clin Invest* (1981) **67**: 328–35.
3. Smith DM, Khairi MRA, Johnston CC Jr. The loss of bone mineral with aging and its relationship to risk of fracture. *J Clin Invest* (1975) **56**: 311–18.
4. Riggs BL, Wahner HW, Melton LJ III *et al*. Rates of bone loss in the axial and appendicular skeletons of women: evidence of substantial vertebral bone loss prior to menopause. *J Clin Invest* (1986) **77**: 1487–91.
5. Genant HK, Cann CE, Ettinger B *et al*. Quantitative computed tomography of vertebral spongiosa: a sensitive method for detecting early bone loss after oophorectomy. *Ann Intern Med* (1982) **97**: 699–705.
6. Riggs BL, Melton LJ III. Involutional osteoporosis. *N Engl J Med* (1986) **314**: 1676–86.
7. Mundy GR, Luben RA, Raisz LG *et al*. Bone-resorbing activity in supernatants from lymphoid cell lines. *N Engl J Med* (1974) **290**: 867–71.
8. Mundy GR, Raisz LG, Cooper RA *et al*. Evidence for the secretion of an osteoclast stimulating factor in myeloma. *N Engl J Med* (1974) **291**: 1941–6.
9. Parfitt AM, Mathews CHE, Villanueva AR *et al*. Relationships between surface, volume, and thickness of iliac trabecular bone in aging and in osteoporosis. *J Clin Invest* (1983) **72**: 1396–409.
10. Kleerekoper M, Villanueva AR, Stanciu J *et al*. The role of three dimensional trabecular microstructure in the pathogenesis of vertebral compression fractures. *Calcif Tissue Int* (1985) **37**: 594–7.
11. Frost HM. Dynamics of bone remodeling. In *Bone Biodynamics* (Boston, MA: Little, Brown, 1964): 315.
12. Miyauchi A, Alvarez J, Greenfield EM *et al*. Recognition of osteopontin and related peptides by an $\alpha v \beta 3$ integrin stimulates immediate cell signals in osteoclasts. *J Biol Chem* (1991) **266**: 20 369–74.
13. Baron R, Vignery A, Horowitz M. Lymphocytes, macrophages and the regulation of bone remodeling. In Peck WA (ed) *Bone and Mineral Research* (Amsterdam: Elsevier, 1984): 175–243.
14. Boyce BF, Aufdemorte TB, Garrett IR *et al*. Effects of interleukin-1 on bone turnover in normal mice. *Endocrinology* (1989) **125**: 1142–50.
15. Walker DG. Congenital osteopetrosis in mice cured by parabiotic union with normal siblings. *Endocrinology* (1972) **91**: 916–20.
16. Walker DG. Osteopetrosis cured by temporary parabiosis. *Science* (1973) **180**: 875.
17. Kahn AJ, Simmons DJ. Investigation of the cell lineage in bone using a chimera of chick and quail embryonic tissue. *Nature* (1975) **258**: 325–7.
18. Jotereau FV, LeDouarin NM. The developmental relationship between osteocyte and osteoclasts: a study using quail-chick nuclear marker in endochondral ossification. *Dev Biol* (1978) **63**: 255–65.
19. Walker DG. Control of bone resorption by hematopoietic tissue. The induction and reversal of congenital osteopetrosis in mice through the use of bone marrow and splenic transplants. *J Exp Med* (1975) **142**: 651–63.
20. Marks SC Jr. Osteopetrosis in the ia rat cured by spleen cells from a normal littermate. *Am J Anat* (1976) **146**: 331–8.
21. Marks SC Jr. Studies of the cellular cure for osteopetrosis by transplanted cells. Specificity of

22. Coccia PF, Krivit W, Cervenka J et al. Successful bone marrow transplantation for infantile malignant osteopetrosis. *N Engl J Med* (1980) **302**: 701–8.
23. Sorell M, Kapoor N, Kirkpatrick D et al. Marrow transplantation for juvenile osteopetrosis. *Am J Med* (1981) **70**: 1280–7.
24. Marks SC Jr, Schneider GB. Evidence for a relationship between lymphoid cells and osteoclasts: bone resorption restored in ia (osteopetrotic) rats by lymphocytes, monocytes and macrophages from a normal littermate. *Am J Anat* (1978) **152**: 331–41.
25. Loutit JF, Nisbit NW. The origin of osteoclasts. *Immunobiology* (1982) **161**: 193–203.
26. Young RW. Cell proliferation and specialization during endochondral osteogenesis in young rats. *J Cell Biol* (1962) **41**: 357–70.
27. Ibbotson KJ, Roodman GD, McManus LM et al. Identification and characterization of osteoclast-like cells and their progenitors in cultures of feline marrow mononuclear cells. *J Cell Biol* (1984) **94**: 471–80.
28. MacDonald BR, Mundy GR, Clark S et al. Effects of human recombinant CSF-GM and highly purified CSF-1 on the formation of multinucleated cells with osteoclast characteristics in long-term bone marrow cultures. *J Bone Miner Res* (1986) **1**: 227–33.
29. Mbalaviele G, Chen H, Boyce BF et al. The role of cadherin in the generation of multinucleated osteoclasts from mononuclear precursors in murine marrow. *J Clin Invest* (1995) **95**: 2757–65.
30. Fischman DA, Hay ED. Origin of osteoclasts from mononuclear leukocytes in regenerating newt limbs. *Anat Res* (1962) **143**: 329–38.
31. Tinkler SMB, Williams DM, Johnson NW. Osteoclast formation in response to intraperitoneal injection of 1, alpha hydroxycholecalciferol in mice. *J Anat* (1981) **133**: 91–7.
32. Zambonin Zallone A, Teti A, Primavera MV. Monocytes from circulating blood fuse in vitro with purified osteoclasts in primary culture. *J Cell Sci* (1984) **66**: 335–42.
33. Burger EH, Vander Meer JWM, Gevel JS et al. In vitro formation of osteoclasts from long-term cultures, bone marrow and splenic transplants. *J Exp Med* (1982) **192**: 651–63.
34. Kurihara N, Chenu C, Civin CI et al. Identification of committed mononuclear precursors for osteoclast-like cells formed in long-term marrow cultures. *Endocrinology* (1990) **126**: 2733–41.
35. Wiktor-Jedrzejczak W, Bartocci A, Ferrante AWJ et al. Total absence of colony-stimulating factor 1 in the macrophage-deficient osteopetrotic (op/op) mouse. *Proc Natl Acad Sci* (1990) **87**: 4828–32.
36. Yoshida H, Hayashi S, Kunisada T et al. The murine mutation osteopetrosis is in the coding region of the macrophage colony stimulating factor gene. *Nature* (1990) **345**: 442–4.
37. Felix R, Cecchini MG, Fleisch H. Macrophage colony stimulating factor restores in vivo bone resorption in the op/op osteopetrotic mouse. *Endocrinology* (1990) **127**: 2592–4.
38. Felix R, Cecchini MG, Hofstetter W et al. Impairment of macrophage colony-stimulating factor production and lack of resident bone marrow macrophages in the osteopetrotic op/op mouse. *J Bone Miner Res* (1990) **5**: 781–9.
39. Kodama H, Yamasaki A, Nose M et al. Congenital osteoclast deficiency in osteopetrotic (op/op) mice is cured by injections of macrophage colony-stimulating factor. *J Exp Med* (1991) **173**: 269–72.
40. MacDonald BR, Takahashi N, McManus LM et al. Formation of multinucleated cells with osteoclastic characteristics in long-term human bone marrow cultures. *Endocrinology* (1987) **120**: 2326–33.
41. Demulder A, Singer F, Roodman GD. Granulocyte macrophage progenitors (CFU-GM) are abnormal in Paget's disease. *J Bone Miner Res* (1991) **6**: 433 (abst).
42. Baron R, Neff L, Tran Van PT et al. Kinetic and cytochemical identification of osteoclast precursors and their differentiation into multinucleated osteoclasts. *Am J Pathol* (1986) **121**: 363–78.
43. Roodman GD, Ibbotson KJ, MacDonald BR et al. 1,25(OH)2 vitamin D3 causes formation of multinucleated cells with osteoclast characteristics in cultures of primate marrow. *Proc Natl Acad Sci* (1985) **82**: 8213–17.
44. Takahashi N, MacDonald BR, Hon J et al. Recombinant human transforming growth factor alpha stimulates the formation of osteoclast-like cells in long term human marrow cultures. *J Clin Invest* (1986) **78**: 894–8.
45. Oursler MJ, Bell LV, Clevinger B et al. Identification of osteoclast specific monoclonal antibodies. *J Cell Biol* (1985) **100**: 1592–1600.

46. Horton MA, Lewis D, McNulty K et al. Human fetal osteoclasts fail to express macrophage antigens. *Br J Exp Pathol* (1985) **66**: 103–8.
47. Ries WL, Gong JK. A comparative study of osteoclasts: in situ versus smear specimens. *Anat Rec* (1982) **203**: 221–32.
48. Salo J, Metsikko K, Palokangas H et al. Bone-resorbing osteoclasts reveal a dynamic division of basal plasma membrane into two different domains. *J Cell Sci* (1996) **109**: 301–7.
49. Hughes DE, Wright KR, Uy HL et al. Bisphosphonates promote apoptosis in murine osteoclasts in vitro and in vivo. *J Bone Miner Res* (1995) **10**: 1478–87.
50. Hughes DE, Tiffee JC, Li HH et al. Estrogen promotes apoptosis of murine osteoclasts – mediated by TGFβ. *Nat Med* (1996) **7**: 1132–6.
51. Blair HC, Teitelbaum SL, Ghiselli R et al. Osteoclastic bone resorption by a polarized vacuolar proton pump. *Science* (1989) **245**: 855–7.
52. Chatterjee D, Chakraborty M, Leit M et al. Sensitivity to vanadate and isoforms of subunits A and B distinguish the osteoclast proton pump from other vacuolar H+ ATPases. *Proc Natl Acad Sci U S A* (1992) **89**: 6257–61.
53. Sakamoto S, Sakamoto M. Isolation and characterization of collagenase synthesized by mouse bone cells in culture. *Biomed Res* (1984) **5**: 39–45.
54. Vaes E. The action of parathyroid hormone on the excretion and synthesis of lysosomal enzymes and on the extracellular release of acid by bone cells. *J Cell Biol* (1968) **39**: 676–97.
55. Eilon G, Raisz LG. Comparison of the effects of stimulators and inhibitors of resorption on the release of lysosomal enzymes and radioactive calcium from fetal bone in organ culture. *Endocrinology* (1978) **103**: 1969–75.
56. Delaisse JM, Eeckhout Y, Neff L et al. (Pro)collagenase (matrix metalloproteinase-1) is present in rodent osteoclasts and in the underlying bone-resorbing compartment. *J Cell Sci* (1993) **106**: 1071–82.
57. Drake FH, Dodds RA, James IE et al. Cathepsin K, but not cathepsins B, L, or S, is abundantly expressed in human osteoclasts. *J Biol Chem* (1996) **271**: 12 511–16.
58. Bossard MJ, Tomaszek TA, Thompson SK et al. Proteolytic activity of human osteoclast cathepsin K – expression, purification, activation, and substrate identification. *J Biol Chem* (1996) **271**: 12 517–24.
59. Jones SJ, Boyde A, Ali NN et al. A review of bone cell substratum interactions. *Scanning* (1985) **7**: 5–24.
60. Sly WS, Whyte MP, Sundaram V et al. Carbonic anhydrase II deficiency in 12 families with the autosomal recessive syndrome of osteopetrosis with renal tubular acidosis and cerebral calcification. *N Engl J Med* (1985) **313**: 139–45.
61. Soriano P, Montgomery C, Geske R et al. Targeted disruption of the c-src proto-oncogene leads to osteopetrosis in mice. *Cell* (1991) **64**: 693–702.
62. Johnson RS, Spiegelman BM, Papaloannou V. Pleiotropic effects of a null mutation in the c-fos proto-oncogene. *Cell* (1992) **71**: 577–86.
63. Wang ZQ, Ovitt C, Grigoriadis AE et al. Bone and haematopoietic defects in mice lacking c-fos. *Nature* (1992) **360**: 741–5.
64. Boyce BF, Yoneda T, Lowe C et al. Requirement of pp60^{c-src} expression of osteoclasts to form ruffled borders and resorb bone. *J Clin Invest* (1992) **90**: 1622–7.
65. Tanaka S, Amling M, Neff L et al. c-Cbl is downstream of c-Src in a signalling pathway necessary for bone resorption. *Nature* (1996) **383**: 528–31.
66. Hruska KA, Rolnick F, Huskey M. Occupancy of the osteoclast $\alpha_v\beta_3$ integrin by osteopontin stimulates a novel src associated phosphatidylinositol 3 kinase (P13 kinase) resulting in phosphatidylinositol trisphosphate (PIP$_3$) formation. *J Bone Miner Res* (1992) **7 (Suppl 1)**: 55 (abst).
67. Grigoriadis AE, Wang ZQ, Cecchini MG et al. c-Fos: a key regulator of osteoclast-macrophage lineage determination and bone remodeling. *Science* (1994) **266**: 443–8.
68. Ruther U, Garber C, Komitowski D et al. Deregulated c-fos expression interferes with normal bone development in transgenic mice. *Nature* (1987) **325**: 412–16.
69. Teti A, Rizzoli R, Zallone AZ. Parathyroid hormone binding to cultured avian osteoclasts. *Biochem Biophys Res Commun* (1991) **174**: 1217–22.
70. Davies J, Warwick J, Totty N et al. The osteoclast functional antigen, implicated in the regulation of bone resorption, is biochemically related to the vitronectin receptor. *J Cell Biol* (1989) **109**: 1817–26.
71. Sato Y, Tsuboi R, Lyons R et al. Characterization of the activation of latent TGFβ by co-cultures of endothelial cells and pericytes or smooth muscle cells – a self regulating system. *J Cell Biol* (1990) **111**: 757–63.
72. Fisher JE, Caulfield MP, Sato M et al. Inhibition of osteoclastic bone resorption in vivo by echistatin,

an arginyl-glycyl-aspartyl (RGD)-containing protein. *Endocrinology* (1993) **132**: 1411–13.
73. Baron R, Chakraborty M, Chatterjee D. The biology of the osteoclast. In Mundy GR, Martin TJ (eds) *Physiology and Pharmacology of Bone. Handbook of Experimental Pharmacology* (Berlin: Springer-Verlag, 1993): 111–47.
74. Chambers TJ. The pathobiology of the osteoclast. *J Clin Pathol* (1985) **38**: 241–52.
75. Garrett IR, Boyce BF, Oreffo ROC et al. Oxygen-derived free radicals stimulate osteoclastic bone resorption in rodent bone in vitro and in vivo. *J Clin Invest* (1990) **85**: 632–9.
76. Suda N, Morita I, Kuroda T. Participation of oxidative stress in the process of osteoclast differentiation. *Biochim Biophys Acta* (1993) **1157**: 318–23.
77. Fraser JHE, Helfrich MH, Wallace HM. Hydrogen peroxide, but not superoxide, stimulates bone resorption in mouse calvariae. *Bone* (1996) **19**: 223–6.
78. Steinbeck MJ, Appel WH, Verhoeven AJ et al. NADPH-oxidase expression and in situ production of superoxide by osteoclasts actively resorbing bone. *J Cell Biol* (1994) **126**: 765–72.
79. Ralston SH, Ho LP, Helfrich MH et al. Nitric oxide: a cytokine-induced regulator of bone resorption. *J Bone Miner Res* (1995) **10**: 1040–9.
80. MacIntyre I, Zaidi M, Alam ASMT et al. Osteoclastic inhibition – an action of nitric oxide not mediated by cyclic GMP. *Proc Natl Acad Sci U S A* (1991) **88**: 2936–40.
81. Lowik CWGM, Nibbering PH, Vanderuit M. Inducible production of nitric oxide in osteoblast-like cells and in fetal mouse bone explants is associated with suppression of osteoclastic bone resorption. *J Clin Invest* (1994) **93**: 1465–72.
82. Brandi ML, Hukkanen M, Umeda T et al. Bidirectional regulation of osteoclast function by nitric oxide synthase isoforms. *Proc Natl Acad Sci U S A* (1995) **92**: 2954–8.
83. Evans DE, Ralston SH. Nitric oxide and bone. *J Bone Miner Res* (1996) **11**: 300–5.
84. Rodan GA, Martin TJ. Role of osteoblasts in hormonal control of bone resorption – a hypothesis. *Calcif Tissue Int* (1981) **33**: 349–51.
85. McSheehy PMJ, Chambers TJ. Osteoblastic cells mediate osteoclastic responsiveness to parathyroid hormone. *Endocrinology* (1986) **118**: 824–8.
86. Mundy GR, Roodman GD. Osteoclast ontogeny and function. In Peck W (ed) *Bone and Mineral Research. Volume V* (Amsterdam: Elsevier, 1987): 209–80.
87. Simonet WS, Lacey DL, Dunstan CR et al. Osteoprotegerin: a novel secreted protein involved in the regulation of bone density. *Cell* (1997) **89**: 309–19.
88. Tsuda E, Goto M, Mochizuki S et al. Isolation of a novel cytokine from human fibroblasts that specifically inhibits osteoclastogenesis. *Biochem Biophys Res Commun* (1997) **234**: 137–42.
89. Wong BR, Josien R, Lee SY et al. TRANCE (tumor necrosis factor (TNF)-related activation-induced cytokine), a new TNF family member predominantly expressed in T cells, is a dendritic cell-specific survival factor. *J Exp Med* (1997) **186**: 2075–80.
90. Yasuda H, Shima N, Nakagawa N et al. Osteoclast differentiation factor is a ligand for osteoprotegerin/osteoclastogenesis-inhibitory factor and is identical to TRANCE/RANKL. *Proc Natl Acad Sci* (1998) **95**: 3597–602.
91. Snapper I, Kahn A. *Myelomatosis* (Basel: Karger, 1971).
92. Valentin-Opran A, Charhon SA, Meunier PJ et al. Quantitative histology of myeloma induced bone changes. *Br J Haematol* (1982) **52**: 601–10.
93. Stewart AF, Vignery A, Silvergate A et al. Quantitative bone histomorphometry in humoral hypercalcemia of malignancy – uncoupling of bone cell activity. *J Clin Endocrinol Metab* (1982) **55**: 219–27.
94. Darby AJ, Meunier PJ. Mean wall thickness and formation periods of trabecular bone packets in idiopathic osteoporosis. *Calcif Tissue Int* (1981) **33**: 199–204.
95. Rasmussen H, Bordier P. *The Physiological and Cellular Basis of Metabolic Bone Disease* (Baltimore, MD: Williams & Wilkins, 1974).
96. Howard GA, Bottemiller BL, Turner RT et al. Parathyroid hormone stimulates bone formation and resorption in organ culture: evidence for a coupling mechanism. *Proc Natl Acad Sci* (1981) **78**: 3204–8.
97. Manolagas SC, Jilka RL. Mechanisms of disease: bone marrow, cytokines, and bone remodeling – emerging insights into the pathophysiology of osteoporosis. *N Engl J Med* (1995) **332**: 305–11.
98. Marcelli C, Yates, AJP, Mundy GR. In vivo effects of human recombinant transforming growth factor beta on bone turnover in normal mice. *J Bone Miner Res* (1990) **5**: 1087–96.
99. Mundy GR, Rodan SB, Majeska RJ et al. Unidirectional migration of osteosarcoma cells with osteoblast characteristics in response to

99. products of bone resorption. *Calcif Tissue Int* (1982) **34**: 542–6.
100. Mundy GR, Poser JW. Chemotactic activity of the gamma-carboxyglutamic acid containing protein in bone. *Calcif Tissue Int* (1983) **35**: 164–8.
101. Pfeilschifter J, Mundy GR. TGFβ stimulates osteoblast activity and is released during the bone resorption process. In Cohn DV, Martin TJ, Meunier PJ (eds) *Calcium Regulation and Bone Metabolism: Basic and Clinical Aspects* (Amsterdam: Elsevier, 1987): 450–4.
102. Pfeilschifter J, Wolf O, Naumann A et al. Chemotactic response of osteoblast-like cells to transforming growth factor β. *J Bone Miner Res* (1990) **5**: 825–30.
103. Deuel TF, Senior RM, Huang JS et al. Chemotaxis of monocytes and neutrophils to platelet-derived growth factor. *J Clin Invest* (1982) **69**: 1046–9.
104. Grotendorst GR, Seppa HEJ, Kleinman HK et al. Attachment of smooth muscle cells to collagen and their migration toward platelet-derived growth factor. *Proc Natl Acad Sci* (1981) **78**: 3669–72.
105. Seppa H, Grotendorst G, Seppa S et al. Platelet-derived growth factor is chemotactic for fibroblasts. *J Cell Biol* (1982) **92**: 584–8.
106. Senior RM, Griffin GL, Huang JS et al. Chemotactic activity of platelet alpha granule proteins for fibroblasts. *J Cell Biol* (1983) **96**: 382–5.
107. Dallas SL, Park-Snyder S, Miyazono K et al. Characterization and autoregulation of latent TGFβ complexes in osteoblast-like cell lines: production of a latent complex lacking the latent TGFβ-binding protein (LTBP). *J Biol Chem* (1994) **269**: 6815–21.
108. Canalis E, McCarthy T, Centrella M. Growth factors and the regulation of bone remodeling. *J Clin Invest* (1989) **81**: 277–81.
109. Gehron-Robey PG, Young MF, Flanders KC et al. Osteoblasts synthesize and respond to transforming growth factor type beta (TGFβ) in vitro. *J Cell Biol* (1987) **105**: 457–63.
110. Dunstan C, Boyce B, Izbicka E et al. Acidic and basic fibroblast growth factors promote bone growth in vivo comparable to that of TGFβ. *J Bone Miner Res* (1993) **8 (Suppl 1)**: 250 (abst).
111. Canalis E, Centrella M, Burch W et al. Insulin-like growth factor I mediates selective anabolic effects of parathyroid hormone in bone cultures. *J Clin Invest* (1989) **83**: 60–5.
112. Assoian RK, Grotendorst GR, Miller DM et al. Cellular transformation by coordinated action of three peptide growth factors from human platelets. *Nature* (1984) **309**: 804–6.
113. Bowen-Pope DF, Dicorletto PE, Ross R. Interactions between the receptors for platelet-derived growth factor and epidermal growth factor. *J Cell Biol* (1983) **96**: 679–83.
114. Seyedin SM, Thomas TC, Thompson AY et al. Purification and characterization of two cartilage-inducing factors from bovine demineralized bone. *Proc Natl Acad Sci* (1985) **82**: 2267–71.
115. Massague J. Transforming growth factor β modulates the high affinity receptors of epidermal growth factor and transforming growth factor α. *J Cell Biol* (1985) **100**: 1508–14.
116. Massague J, Kelly B, Mottola C. Stimulation by insulin-like growth factors is required for cellular transformation by type β transforming growth factor. *J Biol Chem* (1985) **260**: 4551–4.
117. Roberts AB, Anzano MA, Wakefield LM et al. Type β transforming growth factor: a bifunctional regulator of cellular growth. *Proc Natl Acad Sci* (1985) **82**: 119–23.
118. Tucker RF, Shipley GD, Moses HL et al. Growth inhibitor from BSC-1 cells closely related to platelet type B transforming growth factor. *Science* (1984) **226**: 705–7.
119. Eriksen EF. Normal and pathological remodeling of human trabecular bone: three dimensional reconstruction of the remodeling sequence in normals and in metabolic bone disease. *Endocr Rev* (1986) **7**: 379–408.

2

Pathophysiology of myeloma bone disease

Gregory R Mundy and Babatunde O Oyajobi

History of myeloma bone disease • Epidemiology of myeloma bone disease • Nature of the bone disease • Pathophysiology of the bone lesions • Potential factors involved in the bone destruction of myeloma • Animal models of human myeloma bone disease • Hypercalcemia in myeloma bone disease • Bone markers in myeloma bone disease • Management of myeloma

Myeloma is characterized by a unique form of bone disease which occurs in the majority of patients. Bone destruction in myeloma is responsible for the most prominent and distressing clinical features of this disease, namely intractable bone pain, fractures occurring either spontaneously or following trivial injury, and hypercalcemia with its attendant symptoms and signs. Although myeloma is a disease with Protean features resulting from the effects of the disease on multiple organ systems including the kidney, the hematopoietic bone marrow, humoral immunity, and other organ systems, perhaps its most important clinical manifestation, and certainly the one which most often heralds the onset of the disease, is its effects on the skeleton. In this chapter, the pathophysiology of the bone lesions will be discussed, and in Chapter 15 the role of the bisphosphonates in the prevention and treatment of myeloma bone disease is reviewed.

HISTORY OF MYELOMA BONE DISEASE

Myeloma bone disease was first described in 1848 in a London tradesman called Thomas Alexander McBean.[1] The patient was a 42-year-old man who suffered a severe and debilitating form of bone disease which was called by his physicians *mollities and fragilitas ossium* (disease with soft bones). He was also found to have a novel substance in his urine which had special chemical properties, and which subsequently came to be known as Bence Jones protein.[2] It is now recognized to be monoclonal free light chains of immunoglobulin molecules produced by myeloma cells. This interesting and unique form of bone disease was first called multiple myeloma by Rusitzky[3] and later in Europe became, and still is widely referred to as, 'Kahler's disease'.[4]

EPIDEMIOLOGY OF MYELOMA BONE DISEASE

Although myeloma is not a common malignancy, there are probably about 40 000 patients in the USA and over 50 000 in western Europe with this condition at any one point in time, and almost all of them have myeloma bone disease. Myeloma occurs mostly in the middle-aged or elderly. Patients under the age of 40 are relatively uncommon, certainly less than 10% of the total. It is more prominent in blacks than in whites (ratio 2:1) and slightly more common in males than in females. There is a probable real increase in incidence of the disease in recent years. There are no etiologic factors that are as yet well defined, although certain chemical toxins and a Kaposi's sarcoma-related herpes virus have recently been implicated.[5] Myeloma is probably grossly under-registered, which makes assessment for risk factors difficult. However, there is no apparent clustering and no clear-cut familial incidence. Since the average life-span for patients with myeloma is about 3 years and approximately 90% of patients have overt bone disease, the approximate prevalence of myeloma bone disease in the USA at any point in time is about 40 000 cases. Although the median survival is 3 years, there is great variability in life-span following diagnosis. About 15–20% of patients survive 5 years, 7% 10 years, and 1–2% of patients are alive at 15 years. No convincing cures have as yet been reported.

The extent of the bone lesions is an important factor in the prognosis of a patient with myeloma. Eighty per cent of patients present with bone pain as a predominant symptom.[6] The bone lesions occur in several patterns. Occasionally, patients develop single osteolytic lesions that are associated with solitary plasmacytomas. Some patients have diffuse osteopenia, which mimics the appearance of osteoporosis, and is due to the myeloma cells being spread diffusely throughout the axial skeleton. In most patients there are multiple discrete lytic lesions occurring at the site of deposits or nests of myeloma cells. Hypercalcemia occurs as a consequence of bone destruction in about one third of patients with advanced disease. Rarely, patients with myeloma do not have lytic lesions or bone loss, but rather have an increase in the formation of new bone around myeloma cells. This rare situation is known as osteosclerotic myeloma.

NATURE OF THE BONE DISEASE

Bone remodeling is profoundly disturbed in almost all patients with myeloma. Although occasional patients with other malignancies have skeletal manifestations, they are rarely as severe and certainly not as common as in myeloma. Bone destruction in myeloma is responsible for the most prominent and distressing clinical features of this disease. As noted above, 80% of patients present with bone pain as a predominant symptom.[6] Patients with myeloma bone disease are susceptible to fractures occurring either spontaneously or following trivial injury. The bone pain is often intractable, but occasionally fluctuates in intensity for reasons which are unknown. Pathological fractures may involve the vertebrae, ribs, and long bones (most commonly), but occasionally occur in other sites such as the sternum and pelvis. Hypercalcemia occurs in about 30% of patients, and is accompanied by its characteristic attendant symptoms and signs, and usually by concomitant renal failure. The bone lesions occur in several patterns. Occasionally, patients develop single osteolytic lesions that are associated with solitary plasmacytomas and others generalized osteopenia when the myeloma cells occur throughout the bone marrow.

PATHOPHYSIOLOGY OF THE BONE LESIONS

The most common bone manifestation in patients with myeloma is osteolysis, which may occur as sharply discrete lesions or as diffuse osteopenia. Osteolytic bone lesions are by far the most common bone lesions in patients with myeloma. Although the precise molecular mechanisms remain unclear, observations over the past 30 years have revealed the following:

1) The cellular mechanism of osteolysis in myeloma is due to an increase in osteoclast activity (Fig. 2.1). This is the only cellular mechanism for bone destruction which is clearly evident in myeloma.
2) Osteoclast activity in myeloma occurs adjacent to collections of myeloma cells (Fig. 2.1). In some patients, the bone disease occurs in adjacent nests of myeloma cells and the result is a discrete osteolytic lesion. In other patients, the myeloma cells are spread more diffusely throughout the marrow, and the result is osteopenia. Thus, it appears that the mechanism by which

PATHOPHYSIOLOGY OF MYELOMA BONE DISEASE 23

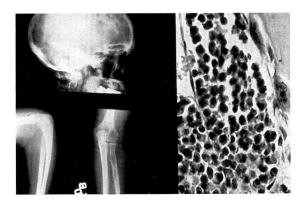

Fig. 2.1 Histologic section of bone from a patient with osteolytic bone lesions caused by myeloma. Myeloma cells are present in the bone marrow cavity immediately adjacent to active bone resorbing osteoclasts. Osteoclasts are not increased at sites distant from the myeloma cells. (Reproduced from Mundy et al.[54])

osteoclasts are stimulated in myeloma is a local one, whereby myeloma cells (or host cells) produce local factors (cytokines) responsible for increasing osteoclast formation and activation.

3) It has been known now for many years that cultures of human myeloma cells *in vitro* express and secrete several osteoclast activating factors into the cell culture media. Several of these local mediators have been identified, and include lymphotoxin (tumor necrosis factor β), interleukin-1β, and interleukin-6. The mediator appears to depend on the culture conditions. This has remained a controversial area. More recent information suggests that enhanced bone resorbing activity is produced when myeloma cells are in contact with marrow stromal cells and the bone marrow microenvironment of patients with myeloma.[7]

4) Hypercalcemia occurs in many patients with myeloma sometime during the course of the disease. The frequency before the use of powerful bisphosphonates became common was probably 30%, but is now likely lower. Hypercalcemia is almost always associated with markedly increased bone resorption and frequently with impaired renal function which is fixed and due to the effects of the disease on renal function. Glomerular filtration may be further compromised by volume depletion and hypercalcemia.

5) Bone formation rates are often reduced in myeloma, and the increase in osteoclastic bone resorption in myeloma is usually associated with impaired osteoblast function. Alkaline phosphatase activity in the serum is decreased or in the normal range, unlike patients with other types of osteolytic bone disease, and radionuclide scans do not show evidence of increased uptake, indicating the lack of an osteoblast response to the increase in bone resorption, in contrast with what is found in other types of osteolytic bone disease such as breast cancer.

6) Occasional patients with myeloma show predominantly an increase in new bone formation with subsequent osteosclerosis. This is often associated with POEM's syndrome (polyneuropathy, organomegaly, endocrinopathy, M protein, and skin changes) (see below).

Bartl et al.[8] and Bartl and Frisch[9] have classified the morphologic picture of myeloma in the bone marrow and correlated the patterns they observed with the presence of osteolysis and survival. The patterns they identified are: 1) interstitial infiltration of the marrow; 2) interstitial infiltration, but also with sheets of cells; 3) interstitial infiltration of the marrow with myeloma cells but with additional discrete nodules; 4) a nodular pattern alone; and 5) diffusely packed bone marrow. Interstitial and interstitial with sheet patterns are associated with the lowest frequency of osteolysis and nodular-packed with the highest. The latter are also associated with the poorest prognosis. Not all morphologists agree that these patterns really represent different types of myeloma behavior, and the usefulness of this sort of classification is not clear at the present time. However, these notions do emphasize again that there may be important interactions which occur between myeloma cells and neighboring cells in the marrow microenvironment, both for the growth of the myeloma and possibly other effects, such as destruction of bone.

POTENTIAL FACTORS INVOLVED IN THE BONE DESTRUCTION OF MYELOMA

Bone lesions in myeloma are caused by increased production of local osteoclastotropic cytokines which are overproduced in the bone marrow microenvironment of patients with myeloma. It has proven very difficult to identify these cytokines, although this mechanism has been recognized for over 20 years. It is now becoming apparent that the reason may be that in patients with myeloma there are complex interactions between myeloma cells and the marrow microenvironment and bone cells or stromal cells that exist in their immediate vicinity which, together, form a complex neoplastic unit which produces active bone resorbing factors. This may explain why it has been so difficult to determine the mechanism of bone destruction in myeloma. A number of cytokines have been implicated in myeloma bone disease. These include lymphotoxin, interleukin-1, interleukin-6, and parathyroid hormone-related protein (PTH-rP). Lymphotoxin is a normal activated lymphocyte product which is also produced by lymphoid cell lines in culture, and in particular by B-lymphoblastoid cell lines. It has now been found that in a number of cell culture lines isolated from patients with myeloma, the tumor cells express lymphotoxin messenger RNA and contain biologic activity in the conditioned media which can be ascribed to lymphotoxin.[10] The conditioned media also contain bone resorbing activity which can be partially neutralized by lymphotoxin-neutralizing antibodies.

Lymphotoxin increases bone resorption[11] and stimulates the formation of osteoclasts from precursors in marrow cell cultures.[12] Moreover, lymphotoxin activates mature isolated osteoclasts to form resorption pits on bone slices.[13] Lymphotoxin has identical effects to those of tumor necrosis factor α and interleukin-1α and β on bone resorption. Repeated injections of recombinant human lymphotoxin cause hypercalcemia in normal mice.[10]

Interleukin-1α and β are powerful stimulators of osteoclastic bone resorption,[14-16] and in addition cause hypercalcemia *in vivo* through this mechanism.[17,18] They have also been implicated in myeloma bone disease. Freshly isolated marrow cells from patients with myeloma, which contain both myeloma cells and stromal cells, have been shown to produce interleukin-1β in the conditioned media.[19,20] Bone resorbing activity produced by these cultures can be neutralized by antibodies to interleukin-1β. In contrast, established cell lines from patients with myeloma do not express interleukin-1β.[10,21] The reason for these discrepancies probably relates to the nature of the cells which are studied. Artifacts could occur in both models. Established cell lines could have changed in culture to produce factors that the parent cells *in situ* did not. Alternatively, the freshly isolated cells (which contain dead and dying elements) likely release factors that are not released *in situ* (as has been shown previously for prostaglandins).

Interleukin-6 is a multifunctional cytokine which may play an important role in the pathophysiology of myeloma. There is considerable evidence that suggests it may be an important growth factor in myeloma, and neutralizing antibodies to interleukin-6 may have important effects on the course of the disease.[22-24] We have found that interleukin-6 has effects on bone resorption and calcium homeostasis which are different from those of interleukin-1 and tumor necrosis factor *in vitro* and *in vivo*.[25] Interleukin-6 does not stimulate osteoclastic bone resorption in organ cultures of fetal rat long bones or neonatal mouse calvariae. However, in other types of organ culture it has been shown to stimulate osteoclastic bone resorption.[26,27] Interleukin-6 causes mild hypercalcemia *in vivo*, much less prominent than that caused by interleukin-1 or lymphotoxin. When interleukin-6 is stably transfected into Chinese hamster ovarian cells, these cells from tumors in nude mice express interleukin-6. Mice carrying tumors with CHO cells expressing interleukin-6 develop increasing levels of interleukin-6 in the serum as the tumor grows. These mice become progressively hypercalcemic, and in addition develop leukocytosis, thrombocytosis, and cachexia.[25]

Interleukin-6 may also have effects in the bone microenvironment which are different from those of the other cytokines. Although bone cells isolated from trabecular bone surfaces (bone lining cells) express cytokines such as interleukin-1, tumor necrosis factor, colony-stimulating factors, and interleukin-6, it is only in the case of interleukin-6 that these bone cells produce more of a cytokine when exposed to osteotropic factors such as parathyroid hormone, interleukin-1, and tumor necrosis factor.[28] In the case of the other cytokines, production by bone cells may be enhanced by nonphysiologic stimuli such as bacterial lipopolysaccharide. In addition, bone cell expression of interleukin-6 can be decreased by incubation of the bone cells with estrogen.[29,30]

Parathyroid hormone-related protein (PTHrP) has also been implicated in the destructive bone lesions associated with myeloma.[31-33] PTHrP has been identified by immunohistochemistry and by *in situ* hybridization in the bone marrow biopsies from patients with myeloma, and has also been measured in increased amounts in the peripheral blood of some patients.[33] Its specific role relative to other cytokines which are likely important in myeloma has yet to be clarified. However, PTHrP does have synergistic effects with interleukin-6 on bone resorption and hypercalcemia.[34]

One recent advance in myeloma pathogenesis may be relevant to the bone disease. Rettig *et al.*[5] had suggested that marrow dendritic cells in patients with myeloma harbor a virus related to the Kaposi sarcoma virus. This virus expresses a biologically active form of interleukin-6 which could be related to the increased osteoclast formation which occurs in patients with myeloma. However, this work is controversial and although another group has similar findings,[35] some have had difficulty confirming it.[36-40]

The most important of these cytokines in the pathophysiology of the bone lesions associated with myeloma remains unknown. It is possible that a combination of these cytokines works in concert to enhance bone resorption in myeloma, and it is also possible that other factors may be involved. These factors have been difficult to identify by traditional factor identification methods from cell cultures, possibly in part because important cell–cell interactions in the bone microenvironment are involved (see below).

Many efforts have been directed to identify the responsible cytokine produced by myeloma cells which stimulates osteoclasts to resorb bone. However, interactions between myeloma cells and bone cells are likely more complicated than simple excess production of a factor by myeloma cells which stimulates osteoclasts. Recent data have suggested that the avidity with which myeloma cells grow in bone compared with other hematologic malignancies may be influenced by products produced as a consequence of osteoclastic bone resorption, and in particular the cytokine interleukin-6, which is a major growth regulatory factor for myeloma cells. Thus, bone may not be simply a passive bystander in this disease, but rather may act to amplify the growth of myeloma cells in bone. If this concept is correct, then a vicious cycle could exist between myeloma cells and osteoclastic bone resorption whereby myeloma cells stimulate osteoclasts to resorb bone by the production of osteotropic cytokines such as tumor necrosis factor β, interleukin-1β, and interleukin-6 (IL-6), but that as a consequence of this increase in osteoclast activity the cytokine IL-6 is generated in large amounts by cells involved in the resorption process and this further enhances the growth of myeloma cells in bone. This vicious cycle could mean that the greater the bone destruction, the more aggressive the behavior of myeloma cells, which then may cause even greater bone destruction.

This concept is based on the recent information that osteoclasts produce considerably more

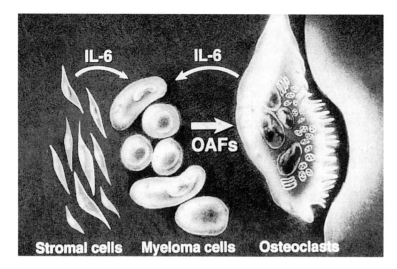

Fig. 2.2 Postulated relationship between myeloma cells, stromal cells, and osteoclasts. Myeloma cells and stromal cells adhere through VCAM-1/α4β1 integrin connections, resulting in increased expression of cytokines such as interleukin-6, and possibly other cytokines such as RANK ligand. This results in activation of osteoclasts, which in turn produce cytokines such as interleukin-6 which enhance myeloma cell growth. These important cell–cell contacts between myeloma cells and stromal cells can be inhibited by neutralizing antibodies to α4 integrin.

IL-6 than any other cell, and certainly more than other types of bone cells. The only cells which produce comparable amounts of IL-6 are endometrial cells. However, osteoclasts are much fewer in number than are other cells. It is possible that production of IL-6 in the bone microenvironment may be related to direct cellular interactions between myeloma cells and other cells such as stromal cells, osteoblasts or even osteoclasts.[41]

Recently, Michigami et al.[7] have shown preliminary data that suggest that complex interactions between myeloma cells and marrow stromal cells mediated by VCAM-1 and α4β1 integrin receptors on myeloma cells may be responsible for the bone lesions. VCAM-1 is expressed on the stromal cells. Soluble VCAM ligands stimulate myeloma cells to produce bone resorbing activity, and this bone resorbing activity produced by myeloma cells can be blocked by neutralizing antibodies either to VCAM-1 or to α4β1 (Fig. 2.2). This likely explains why it has been so difficult to determine which cytokines are most important in causing stimulation in patients with myeloma. Such important cell–cell interactions in myeloma have also been described by others.[42]

ANIMAL MODELS OF HUMAN MYELOMA BONE DISEASE

One major drawback to studying the mechanisms responsible for myeloma bone disease has been the lack of suitable animal models of the human disease. In contrast to solid tumors associated with the hypercalcemia of malignancy, human myeloma cells do not grow well in nude mice and it has not been easy to mimic the human disease in animal models. This has meant that it has been difficult to establish an acceptable animal model of the human disease to study pathogenetic mechanisms and determine the efficacy of various forms of therapy. However, the recent development of two animal models of human myeloma bone disease may circumvent these problems. One is a murine model of myeloma characterized by Radl et al.,[43] who have described a myeloma bone disease which occurs spontaneously in aging mice of the C57BL/KaLwRij strain (Fig. 2.3). Myeloma occurs at the rate of approximately 1 in every 200 of these mice as they age, and causes a monoclonal gammopathy with features reminiscent of the human disease, including bone marrow myeloma cells and, most important for this discussion, characteristic myelomatous

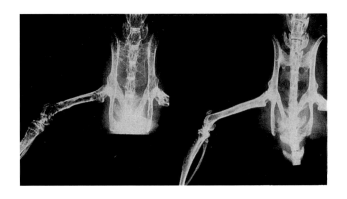

Fig. 2.3 The 5T model of human myeloma bone disease described by Radl et al.[43] The osteolytic bone disease and osteopenia which occurs in mice bearing this murine myeloma are identical to the bone lesions seen in patients with myeloma. Rarely, an osteosclerotic variant of the 5T model has been found.

skeletal lesions. Osteolytic lesions are found in most mice, and in occasional mice osteosclerotic lesions are found. We,[24] as well as Manning et al.,[44] have developed cell lines from these myeloma cells which can be studied both *in vitro* and *in vivo*. Either freshly dispersed myeloma cells from the bone marrow or involved organs of myeloma-bearing mice can be transplanted into fresh mice by tail vein injection into the recipients of the same strain, or by bone marrow inoculation. The disease is faithfully transmitted from mouse to mouse. In order to develop a more convenient animal model of the human myeloma bone disease, the cell line that we have established from tumor-bearing mice was subcloned and fully characterized after inoculation and passage in mice.[24] The cell line causes characteristic osteolytic bone lesions in mice when injected via the tail vein. The cell line also produces the monoclonal protein and IL-6, but its growth is independent of exogenously added IL-6. Some mice carrying these myeloma cells become mildly hypercalcemic, again reminiscent of the human myeloma bone disease. The osteolytic bone lesions are characterized by an increase in osteoclast numbers and activity. Identical results are found when these tumor cells are inoculated into immunodeficient (NU/BG/XID) mice. We have also been involved recently in the development of a second animal model of human myeloma bone disease.[21] In this model, human myeloma cells are inoculated into immunocompromised mice, which have severe combined immunodeficiency (SCID) but in addition are irradiated. Under these circumstances, ARH-77 human myeloma cells cause typical osteolytic bone lesions characteristic of myeloma in addition to mild hypercalcemia. Mice carrying ARH-77 cells also develop hind limb paralysis 28–35 days after tumor cell inoculation.

HYPERCALCEMIA IN MYELOMA BONE DISEASE

Hypercalcemia in myeloma is due primarily to increased osteoclastic bone resorption caused by local cytokines released by the myeloma cells, which in turn leads to osteolysis and entry of calcium into the extracellular fluid. This entry of the calcium into the extracellular fluid overwhelms the patient's capacity to maintain normal calcium homeostasis, and the result is hypercalcemia. However, the pathogenesis of hypercalcemia is even more complex than this. First, not all patients with myeloma bone disease develop hypercalcemia.[6] Approximately 20–40% of patients develop hypercalcemia, usually late in the course of the disease, but not always. This frequency may be decreasing slightly in recent years with the advent of bisphosphonate therapy. By and large, hypercalcemia occurs in those patients who have the largest tumor volume, although not all patients with large tumor burdens develop hypercalcemia. The reasons for this are unclear, but may be related to the amount of bone resorbing activity produced by the myeloma cells, as well as the status of glomerular filtration. We have found that measurements of total body myeloma cell number together with production of bone resorbing activity by cultured bone marrow myeloma cells *in vitro* do not correlate closely with hypercalcemia, although they do correlate with the extent of osteolytic bone lesions.[45] Thus, there are clearly other factors which are involved in the pathogenesis of hypercalcemia in addition to osteoclast activation. Probably the most important of these is the impairment of renal function which occurs frequently in patients with myeloma. Impaired renal function in myeloma occurs for multiple reasons, including uric acid nephropathy, amyloid nephropathy, myeloma kidney due to Bence Jones protein excretion, chronic pyelonephritis, and hypercalcemia itself. In addition to impaired glomerular filtration, increased renal tubular calcium reabsorption may also be a contributing factor to the pathophysiology of hypercalcemia.[46] It is unclear why patients with myeloma have this increase in renal tubular calcium reabsorption. The differences between hypercalcemia which occurs in myeloma and hypercalcemia in patients with solid tumors are sometimes of assistance in the differential diagnosis. For example, in patients with hypercalcemia due to myeloma, there is almost always impaired renal function and an increase in the serum phosphorus which is associated with decreases in glomerular filtration rate. Markers of bone formation such as serum alkaline phosphatase are usually not increased in patients with myeloma, since bone formation is not increased and in fact may be impaired for reasons which are not clear. Patients with hypercalcemia due to myeloma usually respond very rapidly to treatment with corticosteroids and calcitonin, unlike patients with hypercalcemia due to solid tumors.[47]

BONE MARKERS IN MYELOMA BONE DISEASE

Bone markers may eventually be important for monitoring the progress of osteolytic bone disease. The current most useful marker for bone resorption is the measurement of deoxypyridinoline crosslinks of collagen.[48] These can be readily measured in the urine either by chemical assay or by ELISA, and likely will soon be readily measurable in the serum. This measurement provides a very accurate and precise parameter of osteoclastic bone resorption which is much improved over previous markers such as urinary hydroxyproline or fasting urine calcium.

Parameters of bone formation such as serum alkaline phosphatase are often decreased in patients with myeloma, unless the patient has an active fracture undergoing repair. Measurements of osteocalcin (bone Gla protein) show a large scatter. Serum osteocalcin is usually decreased in patients with advanced disease and more extensive bone lesions. Earlier in the disease in patients who have less aggressive or obvious bone disease, serum osteocalcin levels may be normal or even increased.[49]

MANAGEMENT OF MYELOMA

For a number of years, clinicians have attempted to devise therapeutic approaches in myeloma that would relieve disabling symptoms due to skeletal destruction. An earlier approach was the use of fluoride and later calcium and fluoride, although this combination was ineffective and, in fact, probably detrimental because of the associated side-effects. More recently, several groups have shown that the newer generation bisphosphonates relieve bone pain, and produce a rapid, sustained, and significant decrease in the urinary excretion of calcium and hydroxyproline indicating decreased bone turnover.[50,51] This was shown first with pamidronate[50] and then with clodronate.[51] Pamidronate has recently been approved by the FDA for this use in myeloma patients with bone disease and without hypercalcemia. This was based primarily on a large study by Berenson *et al.*[52] which showed that in several hundred patients with myeloma, there was a satisfactory response in bone pain, reduced need for radiation therapy, and prevention of fractures. This study confirmed other large studies in Europe, and the results of the sixth MRC myeloma trial, in which clodronate was the bisphosphonate used.[53] The majority of patients with myeloma are now being treated with regular infusions of pamidronate. Outstanding residual questions include which is the best bisphosphonate for this purpose, what is the ideal dose, for how long should it be administered, should it be given to patients early in the course of the disease, and most importantly do these drugs have a beneficial effect on survival. Active research in this area is likely soon to lead to the introduction of other suitable and nontoxic agents of this class that will be useful as oral forms of therapy to relieve the symptoms caused by bone destruction and its complications in patients with myeloma. This topic will be considered in more detail in Chapter 15.

There are other important issues in the management of myeloma bone disease. This crippling form of bone disease is associated with the most severe and intractable bone pain, as well as frequent fractures following trivial injury. When the bone pain is localized to specific areas such as in the vertebral spine or the ribs, a course of local radiation therapy may be very effective. Analgesics should be used liberally for the severe pain. Patients require frequent counseling because of the bone pain, deformity, and loss of height associated with progressive myeloma bone disease, and will in general manage their symptoms best when they understand the nature of the bone disease and those activities which put them at risk for further complications. Similar principles that guide the lifestyles of patients with osteoporosis also apply to myeloma bone disease. For example, patients should avoid those situations that are risky for the development of fractures such as climbing ladders, slipping on ice, or slipping on loose bathroom rugs. They should also be made aware of local support groups which are located in some of the world's major cities, as well as the International Myeloma Foundation, which was founded in 1990 and is dedicated to improving the quality of life for multiple myeloma patients. This foundation has a hot-line and runs seminars for patients and family members as well as physicians and health professionals, and serves as a resource center for information for patients with this unfortunate condition.

REFERENCES

1. MacIntyre W. Case of mollities and fragilitas ossium accompanied with urine strongly charged with animal matter. *Med Chir Soc Tr* (1850) **33**: 211.
2. Bence Jones H. Papers on chemical pathology: prefaced by the Gulstonian lectures, read at the Royal College of Physicians. Proc Royal Society London. *Lancet* (1847) **ii**: 88.
3. Rusitzky J. Multiple myeloma (in German). *Z F Chir* (1873) **3**: 102.
4. Kahler O. On the symptomatology of multiple myeloma. Observations of albumosuria (in German). *Prager Med Wschr* (1989) **14**: 33–45.
5. Rettig MB, Ma HJ, Vescio RA *et al*. Kaposi's sarcoma-associated herpesvirus infection of bone marrow dendritic cells from multiple myeloma patients. *Science* (1997) **276**: 1851–4.
6. Snapper I, Kahn A. *Myelomatosis* (Basel: Karger, 1971).
7. Michigami T, Dallas SL, Mundy GR *et al*. Interactions of myeloma cells with bone marrow stromal cells via α4β1 integrin-VCAM-1 is required for the development of osteolysis. *J Bone Miner Res* (1997) **12 (Suppl 1)**: S128 (abst).
8. Bartl R, Frisch B, Burkhardt R *et al*. Bone marrow histology in myeloma: its importance in diagnosis, prognosis, classification and staging. *Br J Haematol* (1982) **51**: 361–75.
9. Bartl R, Frisch B. Bone marrow histology in multiple myeloma: prognostic relevance of histologic characteristics. *Hematol Rev* (1989) **3**: 87.
10. Garrett IR, Durie BGM, Nedwin GE *et al*. Production of the bone resorbing cytokine lymphotoxin by cultured human myeloma cells. *N Engl J Med* (1987) **317**: 526–32.
11. Bertolini DR, Nedwin GE, Bringman TS *et al*. Stimulation of bone resorption and inhibition of

12. Pfeilschifter J, Chenu C, Bird A et al. Interleukin-1 and tumor necrosis factor stimulate the formation of human osteoclast-like cells in vitro. *J Bone Miner Res* (1989) **4**: 113–18.
13. Thomson BM, Mundy GR, Chambers TJ. Tumor necrosis factors alpha and beta induce osteoblastic cells to stimulate osteoclastic bone resorption. *J Immunol* (1987) **138**: 775–9.
14. Gowen M, Wood DD, Ihrie EJ et al. An interleukin-1 like factor stimulates bone resorption in vitro. *Nature* (1983) **306**: 378–80.
15. Gowen M, Meikle MC, Reynolds JJ. Stimulation of bone resorption in vitro by a non-prostanoid factor released by human monocytes in culture. *Biochem Biophys Acta* (1983) **762**: 471–4.
16. Gowen M, Nedwin G, Mundy GR. Preferential inhibition of cytokine stimulated bone resorption by recombinant interferon gamma. *J Bone Miner Res* (1986) **1**: 469–74.
17. Sabatini M, Boyce B, Aufdemorte T et al. Infusions of recombinant human interleukin-1 α and β cause hypercalcemia in normal mice. *Proc Natl Acad Sci* (1988) **85**: 5235–9.
18. Boyce BF, Aufdemorte TB, Garrett IR et al. Effects of interleukin-1 on bone turnover in normal mice. *Endocrinology* (1989) **125**: 1142–50.
19. Cozzolino F, Torcia M, Aldinucci D et al. Production of interleukin-1 by bone marrow myeloma cells. *Blood* (1989) **74**: 380–7.
20. Kawano M, Tanaka H, Ishikawa H et al. Interleukin-1 accelerates autocrine growth of myeloma cells through interleukin-6 in human myeloma. *Blood* (1989) **73**: 2145–8.
21. Alsina M, Boyce B, Devlin RD et al. Development of an in vivo model of human multiple myeloma bone disease. *Blood* (1996) **87**: 1495–501.
22. Klein B, Zhang XG, Jourdan M et al. Cytokines involved in human multiple myeloma. *Monoclonal Gammopathies* (1989) **12**: 55–9.
23. Bataille R, Jourdan M, Zhang XG et al. Serum levels of interleukin-6, a potent myeloma cell growth factor, as a reflection of dyscrasias. *J Clin Invest* (1989) **84**: 2008–11.
24. Garrett IR, Dallas S, Radl J et al. A murine model of human myeloma bone disease. *Bone* (1997) **20**: 515–20.
25. Black K, Garrett IR, Mundy GR. Chinese hamster ovarian cells transfected with the murine interleukin-6 gene cause hypercalcemia as well as cachexia, leukocytosis and thrombocytosis in tumor-bearing nude mice. *Endocrinology* (1991) **128**: 2657–9.
26. Lowik CWGM, Vanderpluijm G, Bloys H et al. Parathyroid hormone (PTH) and PTH-like protein (Plp) stimulate interleukin-6 production by osteogenic cells. A possible role of interleukin-6 in osteoclastogenesis. *Biochem Biophys Res Commun* (1989) **162**: 1546–52.
27. Ishimi Y, Miyaura C, Jin CH et al. IL-6 is produced by osteoblasts and induces bone resorption. *J Immunol* (1990) **145**: 3297–303.
28. Feyen JHM, Elford P, DiPadova FE et al. Interleukin-6 is produced by bone and modulated by parathyroid hormone. *J Bone Miner Res* (1989) **4**: 633–8.
29. Girasole G, Jilka RL, Passeri G et al. 17β-estradiol inhibits interleukin-6 production by bone marrow-derived stromal cells and osteoblasts in vitro. A potential mechanism for the antiosteoporotic effect of estrogens. *J Clin Invest* (1992) **89**: 883–91.
30. Jilka RL, Hangoc G, Girasole G et al. Increased osteoclast development after estrogen loss. Medication by interleukin-6. *Science* (1992) **257**: 88–91.
31. Budayr AA, Nissenson RA, Klein RF et al. Increased serum levels of a parathyroid hormone-like protein in malignancy-associated hypercalcemia. *Ann Intern Med* (1989) **11**: 807–12.
32. Suzuki A, Takahashi T, Okuno Y et al. Production of parathyroid hormone-related protein by cultured human myeloma cells. *Am J Hematol* (1994) **45**: 88–90.
33. Firkin F, Seymour JF, Watson AM et al. Parathyroid hormone-related protein in hypercalcemia associated with haematological malignancy. *Br J Haematol* (1996) **94**: 486–92.
34. De La Mata J, Uy H, Guise TA et al. IL-6 enhances hypercalcemia and bone resorption mediated by PTH-rP in vivo. *J Clin Invest* (1995) **95**: 2846–52.
35. Agbalika F, Mariette X, Marolleau JP et al. Detection of human herpesvirus-8 DNA in bone marrow biopsies from patients with multiple myeloma and Waldenstrom's macroglobulinemia. *Blood* (1998) **91**: 4393–4.
36. Parravicini C, Lauri E, Baldini L et al. Kaposi's sarcoma-associated herpesvirus infection and multiple myeloma. *Science* (1997) **278**: 1969–73.
37. Cathomas G, Stalder A, Kurrer MO et al. Multiple myeloma and HHV-8 infection. *Blood* (1998) **91**: 4391–3.
38. Cull GM, Timms JM, Haynes AP et al. Dendritic cells cultured from mononuclear cells and CD34

cells in myeloma do not harbour human herpesvirus 8. *Br J Haematol* (1998) **100**: 793–6.
39. Tarte K, Olsen SJ, Lu ZY et al. Clinical-grade functional dendritic cells from patients with multiple myeloma are not infected with Kaposi's sarcoma-associated herpesvirus. *Blood* (1998) **91**: 1852–7.
40. Yi Q, Ekman M, Anton D et al. Blood dendritic cells from myeloma patients are not infected with Kaposi's sarcoma-associated herpesvirus (KSHV/HHV-8). *Blood* (1998) **92**: 402–4.
41. Lokhorst HM, Lamme T, de Smet M et al. Primary tumor cells of myeloma patients induce interleukin-6 secretion in long-term bone marrow cultures. *Blood* (1994) **84**: 2269–77.
42. Teoh G, Anderson KC. Interaction of tumor and host cells with adhesion and extracellular matrix molecules in the development of multiple myeloma. *Hematol Oncol Clin North Am* (1997) **11**: 27–42.
43. Radl J, Croese JW, Zurcher C et al. Animal model of human disease. Multiple myeloma. *Am J Pathol* (1988) **132**: 593–7.
44. Manning LS, Berger JD, O'Donoghue HL et al. A model of multiple myeloma: culture of 5T33 murine myeloma cells and evaluation of tumorigenicity in the C57BL/KalwRij mouse. *Br J Cancer* (1992) **66**: 1088–93.
45. Durie BGM, Salmon SE, Mundy GR. Relation of osteoclast activating factor production to the extent of bone disease in multiple myeloma. *Br J Haematol* (1981) **47**: 21–30.
46. Tuttle KR, Kunau RT, Loveridge N et al. Altered renal calcium handling in hypercalcemia of malignancy. *J Am Soc Nephrol* (1991) **2**: 191–9.
47. Binstock ML, Mundy GR. Effects of calcitonin and glucocorticoids in combination in hypercalcemia of malignancy. *Ann Intern Med* (1980) **193**: 269–72.
48. Delmas PD. Clinical use of biochemical markers of bone remodeling in osteoporosis. *Bone* (1992) **13**: S17.
49. Bataille R, Delmas PD, Chappard D et al. Abnormal serum bone gla protein levels in multiple myeloma. Crucial role of bone formation and prognostic implications. *Cancer* (1990) **66**: 67–72.
50. Van Breukelen FJM, Bijvoet OLM, Van Oosterom AT. Inhibition of osteolytic bone lesions by (3-amino-1-hydroxypropylidene)-1,1-bisphosphonate (APD). *Lancet* (1979) **i**: 803–5.
51. Siris ES, Sherman WH, Baquiran DC et al. Effects of dichloromethylene diphosphonate on skeletal mobilization of calcium in multiple myeloma. *N Engl J Med* (1980) **302**: 310–15.
52. Berenson JR, Lichtenstein A, Porter L et al. Efficacy of pamidronate in reducing skeletal events in patients with advanced multiple myeloma. *N Engl J Med* (1996) **334**: 488–93.
53. McCloskey EV, MacLennan IC, Drayson MT et al. A randomized trial of the effect of clodronate on skeletal morbidity in multiple myeloma. MRC Working Party on Leukaemia in Adults. *Br J Haematol* (1998) **100**: 317–25.
54. Mundy GR, Raisz LG, Cooper RA et al. Evidence for the secretion of an osteoclast stimulating factor is myeloma. *N Engl J Med* (1974) **291**: 1041–6.

3

Bone metastases – incidence and complications

Robert D Rubens

Incidence • Clinical features • Complications • Conclusion

INCIDENCE

Metastatic bone disease is a much more frequent cause of malignancy in the skeleton than primary bone cancer. Tumours arising in the breast and prostate gland are particularly likely to disseminate to bone; some 70% of patients dying from these cancers having evidence of skeletal deposits at post-mortem examination (Table 3.1). Carcinomas of the thyroid, kidney, and bronchus also commonly give rise to bone metastases with an incidence at autopsy of 30–40%. Tumours of the gastrointestinal tract, on the other hand, rarely produce bone metastases, and are seen in only about 5% of patients dying from these malignancies.[1]

Although this variability in metastatic patterns from different primary cancers probably reflects aspects of the underlying molecular and cellular behaviour of both the tumour cells and the tissues to which they spread, it is also likely to be dependent, at least in part, on other mechanisms. The predominant distribution of bone metastases in the axial skeleton which contains most of the red bone marrow suggests that the slow blood flow here could facilitate the attachment of metastatic cells. By contrast, metastatic disease in the kidneys, in which the circulation is rapid, is extremely rare.

Table 3.1 Incidence of bone metastases at post-mortem examination in different cancers

Primary tumour	Incidence of bone metastases (%)
Breast	73
Prostate	68
Thyroid	42
Kidney	35
Lung	36
Alimentary tract	5

Source: Galasko.[1]

Nevertheless, slow blood flow alone does not adequately account for metastatic disease in the bone marrow. The high incidence of bone metastases from cancers arising in the breast and prostate without associated lesions in the lung has raised questions about the precise route taken by cancer cells from the primary tumour to the skeleton. In the absence of lung deposits, it

Table 3.2 Epidemiology in the UK of common primary cancers frequently associated with bone metastases

Carcinoma	Annual incidence	Prevalence	Deaths per annum	5-year survival (all stages) (%)
Breast	26 000	105 000	16 000	64
Prostate	14 000	28 000	10 000	46
Lung	42 000	30 000	37 000	< 10

is unlikely that malignant cells could have passed from the venous system through the pulmonary circulation to bone. Even if the lung parenchyma is not receptive to the establishment of metastatic disease, the relatively large size of tumour cells makes it unlikely that they could have passed through the narrow pulmonary capillaries, particularly if aggregated in the form of tumour emboli. A useful explanation for the predilection of metastatic disease from breast and prostate cancer to the skeleton came from the experiments of Batson conducted in animals and human cadavers which led to the demonstration of the vertebral-venous plexus.[2]

The experiments revealed how venous blood from the pelvis and the breasts flowed, not only towards the venae cavae, but also into the vertebral venous plexus. The flow into the vertebral veins was shown to predominate when intra-thoracic or intra-abdominal pressure was increased. These experiments provided a satisfactory explanation for the particular tendency of prostatic and breast cancers, as well as those arising in the kidney, thyroid, and lung, to produce metastases in the axial skeleton and limb girdles.

Given the high prevalence of carcinomas of the breast, prostate, and lung, these cancers probably account for at least 80% of the incidence of metastatic bone disease (Table 3.2). In geographical regions of highest incidence of breast cancer, this tumour alone accounts for 10% of malignant tumours and is the one most often associated with metastatic bone disease. Because this cancer often follows a prolonged clinical course, even after its dissemination, morbidity from skeletal metastases makes particularly heavy demands on the resources available for the provision of health care.

CLINICAL FEATURES

Radiologically, bone metastases from breast cancer are usually seen to be a mixture of osteolytic and osteosclerotic lesions. Osteolysis usually predominates predisposing these metastases to the serious complications of pathological fracture and hypercalcaemia. By contrast, osteosclerotic disease predominates in prostatic cancer although computerized tomography often demonstrates lytic areas within it. With osteosclerotic lesions, the complications of hypercalcaemia and pathological fracture are less common, which re-emphasizes the supreme importance of breast cancer as a cause of morbidity from metastatic bone disease. A comparison of the radiological appearances of bone metastases from breast, prostate, and lung cancer, and survival from their diagnosis, is given in Table 3.3.

In a detailed report of 587 patients dying from breast cancer, 69% had radiological evidence of skeletal metastases before death;[3] comparative figures for lung and liver metastases were each

Table 3.3 Comparison of the radiological appearances of bone metastases and survival from their diagnosis in breast, prostate, and lung cancer

Carcinoma	Common radiological appearance	Median survival from diagnosis of bone metastases
Breast	Mixed lytic/blastic	24 months
Prostate	Osteoblastic	20 months
Lung	Osteolytic	3 months

Table 3.4 Frequency of sites involved by recurrent and/or metastatic disease at first relapse of breast cancer in 681 patients of the Guy's Hospital Breast Unit (%)[3]

Local recurrence	36
Distant metastases	
bone	24
distant soft tissue	11
lung	7
pleura	4
liver	3
brain	1
other	4

27%. The report also described 2240 patients who had presented with breast cancer over a 10-year period, 681 (30%) of whom had relapsed after a median follow-up of 5 years, 395 (58%) with distant metastases (Table 3.4). The first relapse was in bone in 184, which accounted for 47% of all those with first distant relapse, 27% of the total with any relapse (local and/or distant), and 8% of the total study population. There were no strong predictors of which patients were at particular risk of developing skeletal disease, but the incidence of bone metastases was found to be significantly raised in association with oestrogen receptor positive and well differentiated tumours.

In breast cancer, survival of patients with metastases confined to the skeleton differs markedly from that in patients with visceral disease. After first relapse in bone, median survival in the above study was 20 months, compared with only 3 months after first relapse in liver[3] (Fig. 3.1). If metastatic disease had remained confined to the skeleton, the median duration of survival rose to 24 months, 20% of patients still being alive after the development of metastases. These results emphasize the prolonged clinical course that metastatic breast cancer can follow, which is also a feature of prostatic cancer after the development of bone metastases.[4] The prognosis after first relapse of breast cancer in bone is, however, influenced by other factors as demonstrated in a further series of 367 patients.[5] Some 139 of these women whose disease remained confined to the skeleton were significantly older, more likely to have

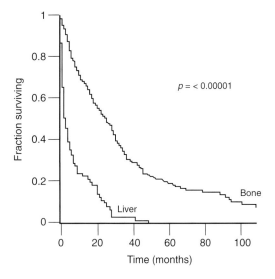

Fig. 3.1 Survival of patients with breast cancer after first relapse in bone compared to survival after first relapse in the liver[3]

Table 3.5 Characteristics of patients with breast cancer with first relapse of disease in bone in relation to the concomitant or subsequent development of extraosseous metastases[5]

	Metastases		
	Bone only (n = 139)	Bone + other sites (n = 228)	p
Mean age	59%	54%	< 0.001
Premenopausal	24%	37%	
Postmenopausal	63%	43%	< 0.009
Axillary node involvement			
negative	29%	18%	
1–3 positive	24%	19%	
≥ 4 positive	16%	30%	< 0.02
Histological type/grade			
ductal grade I	2%	1%	
II	39%	38%	
III	19%	32%	< 0.0001
lobular	21%	12%	< 0.04

lobular cancers, and to have presented with little or no axillary lymph node involvement (Table 3.5). The 228 women who subsequently developed extraosseous metastases were more likely to have had poorly differentiated tumours and heavy nodal involvement at primary diagnosis. Favourable factors for a longer survival after first relapse in bone were low histological grade, positive oestrogen receptor status, long postoperative disease-free interval, and lack of development of extraosseous disease (Fig. 3.2).

The clinical problem of metastatic bone disease in lung cancer is significantly different. At autopsy, the incidence of bone metastasis is similar in the four main histological types (squamous cell, small cell, large cell anaplastic, and adenocarcinoma) at about 30%.[6] Less than 10% of patients with lung cancer remain alive 5 years after diagnosis. When metastatic disease becomes apparent, most patients die within a few weeks or months. Although bone metastases from lung cancer are usually osteolytic, because of poor survival prospects, morbidity from skeletal complications is much less of a

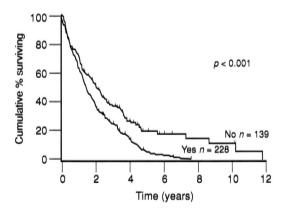

Fig. 3.2 Survival after the diagnosis of bone metastases according to the concomitant or subsequent development of nonosseous metastases[5]

long-term health-care problem than is the case for either breast or prostatic cancer.

The diagnosis of bone metastases is usually straightforward, but sometimes difficulties arise. Confusion with benign bone pathology is a particular problem in elderly patients, especially women, in whom degenerative disease and osteoporosis are common. For example, in elderly women with painful vertebral collapse and a past history of breast cancer, it may be difficult to distinguish between osteoporotic collapse and metastatic destruction. In elderly men with prostatic cancer, pelvic pain and associated radiological sclerotic changes could be attributable to either metastases or Paget's disease of bone. Notwithstanding these difficulties, careful attention to the results of imaging tests and biochemical profiles normally enables the correct diagnosis to be ascertained.[7]

COMPLICATIONS (TABLE 3.6)

Pain

Bone metastases are the most common cause of pain from cancer.[8] It arises from either mechanical or chemical stimulation of pain receptors in the periosteum and endosteum. Pressure effects from an expanding tumour mass, cytokine release, and the formation of microfractures probably all contribute as do mechanical instability and pathological fracture. Spread of tumour from bone to surrounding neurological structures such as the spinal cord, nerve roots, and brachial and lumbosacral plexuses are all significant causes of pain and neurological disability.

Different sites of bone metastases are associated with distinct clinical pain syndromes and neurological sequelae. Common sites of metastatic involvement associated with pain are the base of the skull (in association with cranial nerve palsies, neuralgias, and headache), vertebral metastases (producing neck and back pain with or without neurological complications secondary to epidural extension), and pelvic and femoral lesions producing pain in the low back and lower limbs (often associated with mechanical instability and incident pain).

The spine is the most common site of metastatic spread from breast and prostatic cancer. Pain at the site of bone involvement is common and may be associated with radicular pain if the tumour involves adjacent nerve roots. Extension of the tumour into the epidural space may lead to spinal cord compression with associated motor, sensory, and autonomic signs. Certain distinct referred pain patterns have been described. Damage to the lower cervical and upper thoracic spine may be referred to the interscapular region, while involvement of the lower thoracic and upper lumbar spine may cause unilateral or bilateral pain in the region of the iliac crest or sacroiliac joints. Upper cervical lesions should be suspected in any patient with neck pain and neurological symptoms or signs in the arms or legs. At other sites of vertebral body metastases, local or radicular pain may be indicative of incipient spinal cord compression. Meticulous neurological examination is therefore essential in such patients, with appropriate imaging, because prompt intervention with high-dose steroids, radiotherapy, or surgical decompression may prevent the establishment of severe and permanent disability.

Bone pain may be poorly localized. It often has a deep boring quality which aches and is accompanied by episodes of stabbing discomfort. Pain worsened by movement, weight-bearing, or changes in body position or posture often occurs when metastases involve the pelvis, femora, or vertebrae. This so-called incident

Table 3.6 Complications of bone metastases

Pain
Pathological fracture
Spinal cord and cauda equina compression
Cranial nerve palsies
Hypercalcaemia
Bone marrow suppression

pain is difficult to manage and sometimes requires orthopaedic stabilization.

Evaluation of pain is difficult because of its subjective nature, but is important in order to monitor the effectiveness of treatment. Various methods have been developed including linear analogue scales and categorical systems. The latter take into account the described intensity of pain, analgesia consumption, and mobility. Scoring can be applied to these recordings to enable a semi-quantitative assessment of pain to be developed and are particularly useful in the interpretation of clinical trials.[9] An example of one such method is given in the table in Chapter 10.

Pain and its management are discussed in detail in Chapter 13.

Pathological fracture

Pathological fracture is a major, sometimes catastrophic, complication of metastatic bone disease which causes severe pain and often prolonged disability. Fractures of long bones have the most serious consequences and occur in approximately 10% of patients with bone metastases from breast cancer.[3] Adding fractures at other sites, particularly the ribs and vertebrae, brings the incidence of pathological fracture to about 50% in patients with metastatic bone disease. Although survival after pathological fracture may be prolonged after orthopaedic surgery followed by radiotherapy and appropriate systemic treatment, the median survival after a long bone fracture in patients with breast cancer is about 12 months. In a large series of 1800 patients with metastatic bone disease, 150 (8%) had fracture of either the femur or humerus.[10] In this series, carcinoma of the breast was responsible for 53% of the fractures, kidney for 11%, lung for 8%, thyroid and lymphoma each for 4%, and prostatic cancer for 3%; a variety of other cancers accounted for the remainder.

Distinguishing benign from pathological fractures radiologically is usually easy to do as the latter normally occur in the presence of previously diagnosed bone metastases.

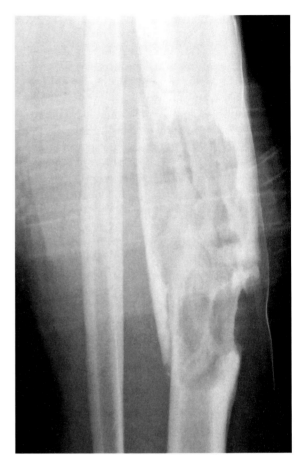

Fig. 3.3 Pathological fracture through an osteolytic metastasis in the tibia. (Reproduced from Rubens and Fogelman (eds), p.69,[9] with permission.)

However, occasionally, a pathological fracture in a solitary metastasis may be the first presentation of metastatic bone disease irrespective of whether or not a primary diagnosis of cancer elsewhere has been made. In such circumstances, the pathological nature of the fracture is normally apparent on plain radiographs as they occur through rarefied bone with trabecular destruction and endosteal scalloping (Fig. 3.3). Histological material obtained at the time of surgical fixation of the fracture will usually confirm the diagnosis.

After the occurrence of long bone fracture, pain is severe, admission to hospital is urgent, and surgery is needed at a time when the patient's general medical condition is poor and not ideal for general anaesthesia. Furthermore, because of the greater difficulty in stabilizing an established, rather than an impending, fracture, perioperative morbidity is high. An important objective in the management of metastatic bone disease is, therefore, prophylactic surgical fixation of a bone deemed to be at high risk of fracture before it occurs.

Prediction of impending pathological fracture is controversial.[11] Factors taken into account have included pain, the anatomical site of the lesion, its radiological characteristics, and size. Although intensity of pain, which is difficult to quantify, is not clearly associated with fracture risk, pain aggravated by function does appear to be an important predictor of impending fracture. Presumably functional pain indicates reduction in the mechanical strength of a bone and in one series was found invariably to be followed by fracture.[11] There is a general understanding that radiologically lytic lesions are at a considerably higher risk of fracture than those that are either mixed or sclerotic. Hence, a particularly high fracture rate occurs with metastases from lung cancer but, given the poor prognosis of this tumour, such fractures rarely result in prolonged disability. By contrast, in breast cancer, which follows a more prolonged course, pathological fracture is an important cause of chronic disability. In prostatic cancer, with its predominantly sclerotic nature, pathological fracture is relatively uncommon.

Radiological assessment also gives information on the size of the lesion and the extent to which the bone is destroyed. When less than two thirds of the diameter of a long bone is affected, pathological fracture is relatively unusual, but above this size the fracture rate increases markedly with an incidence of about 80% for such lesions. A practical scoring system which incorporates the above factors has been described and gives useful guidance in selecting patients for prophylactic fixation.[11]

Rib fractures are a common cause of chest pain, often pleuritic in character. They are frequently localized as an area of severe tenderness on palpation. Rib fractures, although distressing, do not usually have serious sequelae and can effectively be treated by analgesics and a single fraction of radiotherapy. Rarely, multiple rib fractures interfere with the integrity of the chest wall and result in impairment of respiratory function. A now rare cause of rib fracture in patients with breast cancer is radionecrosis of bone following radiotherapy to the chest wall.

Vertebral body fractures are common in patients with bony metastases leading to loss of height of, often several, vertebrae. Acute vertebral collapse is associated with severe pain which usually remits following radiotherapy. The pain is frequently a combination of localized bony pain associated with a radicular component as a consequence of compression of spinal nerve roots. A serious consequence of vertebral fractures is extension of tumour into the theca leading to spinal cord or cauda equina compression. Vertebral fracture from metastatic disease may be difficult to distinguish from osteoporotic collapse. This is particularly so in middle-aged and elderly women with breast cancer who are physiologically at increased risk of osteoporosis. Additionally, treatments which are prescribed for breast cancer such as ovarian ablation, chemotherapy-induced ovarian failure, and corticosteroids, predispose to osteoporosis.

Orthopaedic surgical approaches to spinal stabilization are discussed in Chapter 17.

Spinal cord and cauda equina compression

Compression of the spinal cord or cauda equina in patients with metastatic disease of the spine is a medical emergency needing prompt recognition and treatment. Its causes include pressure from an enlarging extradural mass, spinal angulation following vertebral collapse, vertebral dislocation following pathological fracture, or, rarely, intradural metastases (Table 3.7). For

Table 3.7 Causes of spinal cord and cauda equina compression
Extradural mass
Vertebral collapse/spinal angulation
Vertebral dislocation postfracture
Intradural metastasis

Table 3.8 Clinical features of spinal cord compression
Pain
local spinal
radicular
Motor weakness
Sensory loss
Autonomic dysfunction

its diagnosis, contrast myelography has been widely replaced by magnetic resonance imaging (MRI). Compression may occur at multiple vertebral levels (Fig. 3.4).

Back pain is experienced by most patients with spinal cord compression and is often the symptom heralding this complication (Table 3.8). Two types of pain are recognized: local spinal and radicular. The site of radicular pain depends on the location of the tumour, and is particularly common in the cervical and lumbosacral regions, but less so with thoracic lesions. Both local spinal and radicular pain occur in close proximity to the site of the lesion identified at MRI. Motor weakness, sensory loss, and autonomic dysfunction are common features of spinal cord or cauda equina compression. The primary tumours which most often cause this complication are, in order of decreasing frequency, carcinoma of the breast, lung cancer, prostatic cancer, lymphoma, and renal carcinoma.[12]

Spinal cord compression complicating breast cancer has been studied in detail in a series of 70 patients, an incidence of 4% in the 1684 patients with metastatic disease who were observed.[13] The median time to the development of spinal cord compression from diagnosis of breast cancer was 42 months. All patients had radiological evidence of bone metastases and only five were not known to have had bone metastases previously. The most frequent symptom was motor weakness (96%), followed by pain (94%), sensory disturbance (79%), and sphincter disturbance (61%). Ninety-one per cent of patients had had at least one of these symptoms for more than a week. Radiotherapy was the primary treatment for 43 patients whilst 21 had decompressive

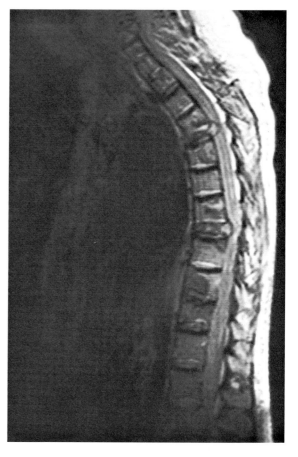

Fig. 3.4 Magnetic resonance image of the thoracic spine showing spinal cord compression at two levels in association with vertebral metastases. (Reproduced from Rubens and Fogelman (eds), p.88,[9] with permission.)

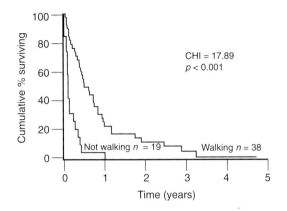

Fig. 3.5 Survival from diagnosis of spinal cord compression in patients with breast cancer according to ambulatory status after treatment[13]

surgery, seven of whom subsequently had postoperative radiotherapy; six patients were too unwell for either treatment. Following treatment, 96% of those who were ambulant before treatment maintained the ability to walk. In those unable to walk, 45% regained ambulation, radiotherapy and surgery being equally effective in achieving this result. Median survival following cord compression was 4 months with no significant difference being seen between those treated by either radiotherapy or surgery. The most important predictor of survival was the ability to walk after treatment (Fig. 3.5). The conclusion from the study was that the majority of patients had had previous warning symptoms of cord compression and nearly all had prior evidence of spinal bone metastases before the complication occurred. These findings stress the importance of prompt presentation, diagnosis, and treatment and they suggest that earlier diagnosis and interventions could improve outcome.

Cranial nerve palsies

Cranial nerve palsies are a common consequence of metastases in the base of the skull. They are frequently associated with head, neck, or facial pain and may be aggravated by neck movements. Frontal, periorbital, or retro-orbital pain may be caused by orbital or parasellar lesions and may be accompanied by proptosis and/or diplopia. Involvement of the sphenoid or ethmoid sinuses may cause bifrontal, bitemporal, or retro-orbital pain sometimes associated with feelings of fullness in the head, nasal stuffiness, or diplopia. Neurological symptoms and signs may enable the precise anatomical site of a metastasis to be determined. For example, tumours near the jugular foramen often produce occipital pain radiating to the vertex or ipsilateral side of the neck or shoulder and are accompanied by dysfunction of the ninth, tenth, and eleventh cranial nerves producing hoarseness, dysarthria, and dysphagia. Middle fossa and foramen ovale involvement can produce trigeminal neuropathy and facial nerve involvement, leading to sensory loss in the chin and face and facial weakness. Clival and hypoglossal nerve involvement results in dysphagia, dysarthria, and weakness of the tongue.

Hypercalcaemia

Hypercalcaemia, covered in detail in Chapter 6, is common in patients with malignant disease of bone. It is seen particularly frequently in multiple myeloma, about a third of patients developing this metabolic complication. It is also common in breast cancer, in which it affects approximately 20% of patients with bone metastases. Hypercalcaemia can also develop in the absence of metastatic involvement of the skeleton, as a result of the production of parathyroid hormone-related protein (PTHrP) by the tumour.

Irrespective of the cause of hypercalcaemia, either from metastatic deposits or humorally induced, osteoclastic bone resorption is the underlying mechanism. In association with bone metastases, urinary calcium excretion is markedly elevated, but in humoral hypercalcaemia it is low as a consequence of excessive renal tubular reabsorption of calcium under the influence of PTHrP.

Hypercalcaemia may initially be asymptomatic, but as the blood calcium level rises a variety of symptoms appear. Although usually a gradual process, its development may be rapid and life-threatening. Common symptoms include lassitude, anorexia, nausea, and constipation. Thirst and polyuria frequently develop with, as the condition advances, vomiting, dehydration, drowsiness, psychosis, coma, renal failure, and cardiac arrest.

Bone marrow suppression

Infiltration of the bone marrow by metastatic cells leads to impaired haemopoiesis and the development of a leucoerythroblastic anaemia characterized by the appearance of immature red blood cells and granulocytes in the peripheral blood. Associated leukopenia and thrombocytopenia predispose to infection and haemorrhage respectively. In its severest form, diffuse involvement of the bone marrow by metastatic cells can result in either marrow fibrosis or necrosis which may be associated with splenomegaly and immature cells of all lineages being seen in the peripheral blood.[14] Radiotherapy, often needed in the treatment of metastatic bone disease, can exacerbate this problem. The presence of bone metastases, particularly when irradiation has been administered, may compromise significantly the ability to give effective chemotherapy; animal experiments have shown that cytotoxic drugs may interfere with osteoblast function and new bone formation.[15]

CONCLUSION

Metastatic bone disease is a major cause of morbidity in patients with cancer. The principal problems that arise are pain, pathological fractures, spinal cord compression, cranial nerve palsies, hypercalcaemia, and bone marrow suppression. Together these problems are responsible for a particularly high proportion of days spent in hospital as a result of cancer. To some extent, it is possible to predict which patients with bone metastases are at high risk of developing the most severe complications and this can assist in the selection of patients for optimal treatment and contributes to the prevention of serious morbidity.

REFERENCES

1. Galasko CSB. The anatomy and pathways of skeletal metastases. In Weiss L, Gilbert AH (eds) *Bone Metastases* (Boston, MA: GK Hall, 1981): 49–63.
2. Batson OV. The role of the vertebral veins in metastatic processors. *Ann Intern Med* (1942) **16**: 38–45.
3. Coleman RE, Rubens RD. The clinical course of bone metastases from breast cancer. *Br J Cancer* (1987) **55**: 61–6.
4. Clain A. Secondary malignant bone disease. *Br J Cancer* (1965) **19**: 15–29.
5. Coleman RE, Smith P, Rubens RD. Clinical course and prognostic factors following bone recurrence from breast cancer. *Br J Cancer* (1998) **77**: 336–40.
6. Muggia FM, Chervu LR. Lung cancer: diagnosis in metastatic sites. *Semin Oncol* (1974) **1**: 217–28.
7. Rubens RD, Coleman RE. Bone metastases. In Abeloff MD, Armitage JO, Lichter AS, Niederhuber JE (eds) *Clinical Oncology* (New York: Churchill Livingstone, 1995): 643–65.
8. Houston SJ, Rubens RD. Metastatic bone pain. *Pain Rev* (1994) **1**: 138–52.
9. Coleman RE. Assessment of response to treatment. In Rubens RD, Fogelman I (eds) *Bone Metastases: Diagnosis and Treatment* (London: Springer-Verlag, 1991): 99–120.
10. Higinbotham NL, Marcove RC. The management of pathological fractures. *J Trauma* (1965) **5**: 792–8.
11. Mirels H. Metastatic disease in long bones. *Clin Orthop Related Res* (1989) **249**: 256–64.
12. Gilbert RW, Kim J-H, Posner JB. Epidural spinal cord compression from metastatic tumour: diagnosis and treatment. *Ann Neurol* (1978) **3**: 40–51.
13. Hill ME, Richards MA, Gregory WM, Smith P, Rubens RD. Spinal cord compression in breast cancer: a review of 70 cases. *Br J Cancer* (1993) **68**: 969–73.
14. Kiraly JF, Wheby MS. Bone marrow necrosis. *Am J Med* (1976) **60**: 361–8.
15. Friedlander GE, Tross RB, Doganis AC, Kirkwood JM, Baron R. Effects of chemotherapeutic agents on bone. I. Short term methotrexate and doxorubicin (adriamycin) treatment in a rat model. *J Bone Joint Surg* (1984) **66**: 602–7.

4

Pathophysiology of bone metastasis

Gregory R Mundy and Theresa A Guise

Classification of bone metastases • Frequency of bone metastases • Favored sites of skeletal involvement by malignant disease • Clinical consequences of skeletal involvement by cancer • Pathophysiology of the metastatic process • Tumor cell mediation of bone destruction at the metastatic site • Mechanisms of osteoclast stimulation at the metastatic site • Bone-derived tumor growth factors at the metastatic site • Potential treatment of metastatic osteolytic bone disease • Osteoblastic metastases

The skeleton is one of the most favored sites for metastasis of solid tumors. Bone metastasis is a catastrophic complication for most patients, although in the early stages it may be occult and inapparent. It usually means that the malignant process is incurable, and it causes not only intractable pain but also other local complications such as fracture after trivial injury and nerve compression. Extensive bone destruction can lead to hypercalcemia, the most rapidly fatal complication. In this chapter, the pathophysiologic mechanisms responsible for bone metastasis will be reviewed.

CLASSIFICATION OF BONE METASTASES

Tumors cause two distinct (but overlapping) types of skeletal lesions when they spread to bone (Fig. 4.1). The most common form of bone metastasis is the destructive or osteolytic lesion. In this type of metastatic bone lesion, tumor products distort the normal remodeling sequence so that there is an increase primarily in osteoclast activity and subsequent bone destruction. The secondary osteoblast response seen in normal bone remodeling is almost always impaired, so that the lesion is predominantly lytic. Less common is the predominantly osteoblastic response which occurs without prior resorption at the same site. The mechanisms which are responsible for tumors causing distinctive and discrete effects on osteoblasts and osteoclasts involved in normal bone remodeling remain obscure, although recent information is providing some clarification.

FREQUENCY OF BONE METASTASES

The commonest malignant tumors which affect humankind involve the skeleton. Approximately 700 000 people die of cancer in the USA each year,[1] and at least two thirds of these have bone metastases. Over 220 000 people die with lung and breast cancer, and the frequency of bone metastases in these patients is even greater. Although bone metastasis occurs frequently with nearly all tumors, there are some cancers which have a special predilection for the skeleton. The best examples are breast cancer and prostate cancer, which almost always metastasize to the skeleton. Other common solid tumors such as lung cancer frequently cause bone metastases, whereas other common cancers such

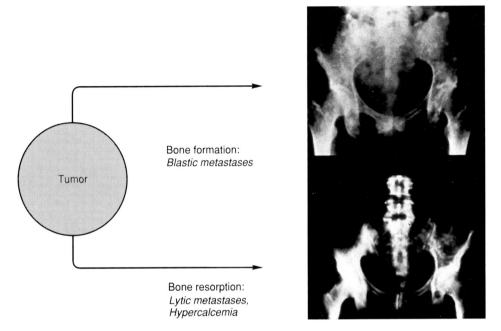

Fig. 4.1 Tumors have two effects on the skeleton: either to cause osteolytic lesions and, in some patients, hypercalcemia or osteoblastic lesions. Osteolytic lesions are far more common than osteoblastic lesions.

as thyroid, renal, and colon cancers rarely do. This special pattern of types of solid tumors which are associated with metastatic bone lesions is exemplified in Table 4.1 and Fig. 4.2.

However, these estimates of the frequency of metastasis depend on the sensitivity of the diagnostic technique utilized to detect them. The techniques which have been mostly used are

Table 4.1 Distribution of bone metastases detected by scintigraphy

Primary tumour	Distribution of skeletal metastases (%)				
	Skull	Spine	Rib cage	Pelvis	Appendicular skeleton
Breast	28	60	59	38	32
Lung	16	43	65	25	27
Prostate	14	60	50	57	38
Cervix	26	26	22	43	43
Bladder	13	47	53	47	7
Rectum	21	36	29	43	43

Source: Tofe *et al.*[124]

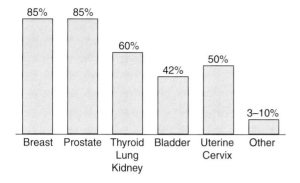

Fig. 4.2 Frequency of bone metastases associated with common malignancies. These represent patients with advanced disease.

bone scans, X-rays, and histologic examination of autopsy specimens. Both radiologic and histologic assessments are limited by the extent of the sample evaluated. Bone scans survey the whole body, but because isotope accumulation depends on osteoblast activity, those lesions with very little osteoblastic component cannot be detected. Possibly even more importantly, they depend on the length of time the patient lives. For example, patients with disseminated breast cancer may live some years and are more likely to develop bone metastases than patients with lung cancer, who have a much shorter life expectancy.

Skeletal involvement is also common in some hematologic malignancies, most notably myeloma. Myeloma almost always causes osteolytic lesions, which are present in at least 95% of cases.[2] In some patients with myeloma there may be a mixture of discrete osteolytic and diffuse osteopenic lesions. For example, it is common to find patients who have multiple discrete osteolytic lesions in the skull and diffuse osteopenia resembling radiological osteoporosis in the vertebral column. Hypercalcemia occurs late in the disease in approximately 30% of patients with myeloma,[3] although this frequency is probably decreasing with the widespread use of pamidronate. Both osteolytic and osteoblastic lesions can occur in patients with lymphomas, particularly Hodgkin's disease, but these are not as common as they are in patients with myeloma. In a small percentage of patients with myeloma, osteosclerosis occurs due to a generalized stimulation of osteoblast activity.

FAVORED SITES OF SKELETAL INVOLVEMENT BY MALIGNANT DISEASE

Tumor cells most frequently affect those parts of the skeleton which are the most heavily vascularized, and in particular the red bone marrow of the axial skeleton and the proximal ends of the long bones, the ribs, and the vertebral column. This is true in both hematologic malignancies and for all solid tumors. Although metastases to the appendicular skeleton occur less frequently, they may be seen particularly in patients with melanoma and renal cancer. Breast cancer cells sometimes metastasize to the posterior clinoid processes. The precise reasons for these unusual distributions of bone lesions are not clear. Galasko[4,5] has reviewed in detail the distribution of skeletal metastases from various solid tumors. One of the major, but certainly not the sole, determinants of the site of metastasis is blood flow from the primary site. Since some common cancers frequently metastasize to the vertebral column, it was suggested 50 years ago that access through the vertebral venous plexus (Batson's plexus) for prostate and breast cancers may be important. Batson's plexus is a low-pressure, high-volume system of vertebral veins which can communicate with the intercostal veins and runs up the spine. Batson's vertebral plexus has been suggested as being responsible for the distribution of prostate tumor cell metastasis to the spine. This plexus has extensive intercommunications which apparently function independently of other major venous systems such as the pulmonary, caval and portal systems.[6] It has been studied by the injection of dye into the dorsal vein of the penis in cadavers and experimental animals.[6] A number of workers have suggested that this system may be important for the spread of tumor cells to the axial skeleton.[7,8] However, Dodds et al.[9] have questioned whether prostate cancer cells do in fact spread preferentially through this paravertebral plexus to the spine.

CLINICAL CONSEQUENCES OF SKELETAL INVOLVEMENT BY CANCER

Bone pain

Frequent bone pain is common in patients with either osteolytic or osteoblastic lesions. The mechanisms responsible for bone pain are unclear, and bone may undergo remissions and exacerbations without apparent change in nature or behavior of the underlying metastasis. Bone pain is a major symptomatic problem in patients with bone metastases. Nelson *et al.*[10] have suggested that tumor production of the vasoactive peptide endothelin-1 in bone may mediate not only the osteoblastic response observed in prostate cancer but also pain.

Pathologic fractures

Pathologic fractures following trivial injury occur commonly in patients with metastatic bone disease, and particularly in those with osteolytic lesions, and are a major cause of morbidity. These fractures occur most frequently in the vertebral bodies, the ribs, and the proximal ends of long bones, at the common sites of osteolytic metastases.

Nerve compression syndromes

Nerve compression syndromes may occur because of tumors which impinge directly on the spinal cord, but occur more frequently because severe destructive osteolytic lesions lead to nerve fracture and fragility of the vertebral body and compression of the cord as a result of the subsequent deformity. Nerve compression syndromes also occur occasionally in patients with osteoblastic lesions because of bony overgrowth which impinges directly on nerves or causes narrowing of foramina or canals. Similar syndromes can occur because of direct tumor invasion from the extradural space. Prostate cancer which metastasizes to the vertebral spine is an important cause of spinal cord compression, cauda equina syndromes, and paraparesis, and metastases to the base of the skull can impinge on cranial nerve foramena.

Hypercalcemia

Hypercalcemia occurs commonly in patients with metastatic bone disease, and particularly in patients with osteolytic lesions. It is very common in patients with prostate cancer. Approximately 30% of patients with breast cancer will develop hypercalcemia at some time during the course of the disease, and usually late in the disease,[11] although this figure is decreasing now that the bisphosphonates are becoming so widely used. Hypercalcemia is almost always due primarily to an increase in bone resorption, which is caused in turn by the production of bone-active agents by the tumor cells which stimulate osteoclastic bone resorption. However, in almost all these patients, there is an impairment of the kidney's capacity to compensate for this increased calcium load.

Although hypercalcemia usually occurs in association with osteolytic bone lesions, it also occurs without evidence of localized osteolysis. In most patients with cancer, hypercalcemia is caused by one (or more) systemic factors produced by the tumor cells which stimulate osteoclastic bone resorption and increase renal tubular calcium reabsorption. This type of hypercalcemia has frequently been referred to as the humoral hypercalcemia of malignancy. It is not particularly helpful to distinguish hypercalcemia due to localized bone destruction from hypercalcemia associated with metastasis. In some patients with osteolytic lesions, it is clear that systemic mediators are produced by the tumor cells and they are likely to play a major role in the pathophysiology of hypercalcemia. These factors may be particularly important if they are produced in large enough amounts locally at the primary or metastatic sites that they circulate in in relatively high concentrations. In the past, a distinction between humoral hypercalcemia and osteolytic hypercalcemia has been made by some groups. These distinctions have been determined by measurements of nephrogenous cyclic AMP,[12] a parameter of PTH-rP production. However, PTH-rP is not the only factor associated with the hypercalcemia of malignancy, and some patients with humoral hypercalcemia do not have increased nephrogenous cyclic AMP. More importantly, PTH-rP is often secreted by metastatic tumor cells in bone which are associated with osteolytic lesions, and is probably the cause. Thus, PTH-rP may be a local mediator of bone destruction in osteolytic lesions even in the absence of hypercalcemia in increased plasma PTH-rP concentration.

Studies by Tuttle et al.[13] have shown that renal tubular calcium reabsorption is increased not only in patients with humoral hypercalcemia but also almost universally in patients with the hypercalcemia of malignancy, and even in patients with hypercalcemia due to myeloma. It had previously been recognized that renal tubular calcium reabsorption was frequently increased in patients with solid tumors associated with hypercalcemia,[14] but widely thought that hypercalcemia associated with osteolytic lesions or with myeloma and breast cancer was not usually associated with increased renal tubular calcium reabsorption. The studies of Tuttle et al.[13] and the earlier studies of Percival et al.[15] have refuted that conclusion. Gallacher et al.[16] also showed that in patients with breast cancer there was frequently an increase in reabsorption of calcium in the renal tubules which could not be accounted for by PTH-rP. In the studies of Tuttle et al.,[13] the glomerular filtration rate and hydration status were carefully measured, and renal tubular calcium reabsorption was compared with control patients who were matched for impairment of renal function. The mechanisms responsible for the increase in renal tubular calcium reabsorption in hypercalcemic patients with cancer are not entirely clear, although increased production of PTH-rP is likely responsible in some patients. In those patients who do not produce PTH-rP, the mechanism is likely related to other factors which have not yet been identified or characterized. Harinck et al.[17] suggested that calcium reabsorption may be due to changes in volume status caused by chronic hypercalcemia, so that subsequent volume depletion increased sodium reabsorption in the proximal tubules and this is associated with increased calcium reabsorption. However, Tuttle et al.[13] showed that increased renal tubular calcium reabsorption was essentially universal in patients with the hypercalcemia of malignancy independent of PTH-rP status and the increase in renal tubular calcium reabsorption also occurred independent of hydration status.

PATHOPHYSIOLOGY OF THE METASTATIC PROCESS

The metastasis of tumor cells to specific sites in the skeleton is clearly not a simple random event determined solely by blood flow, but rather a directed and multistep process which is dependent on specific properties of the tumor cells as well as factors in the bone microenvironment which favor metastasis. Liotta and colleagues have suggested that, although the distribution of metastases in distant organs can be predicted by the anatomic distribution of blood flow from the primary site in 30% of cases, in the majority there are specific properties of the tumor cell and features at the metastatic site which determine whether the metastasis can become established.[18] Over 100 years ago, this nonrandom concept for tumor metastasis was recognized by Paget,[19] who used the term 'seed and soil' to explain the phenomenon of tumor spread to specific sites in the body.

Since tumor metastasis is a multistep process involving separate discrete steps, interruption of one or more of these steps can inhibit the metastatic process. Each of these discrete steps represents cellular interactions caused by specific determinants of both the tumor and the tissue.[18,20] The steps involved in the shedding of tumor cells from the primary site involve detachment of tumor cells from adjacent cells, followed by invasion of adjacent tissue in the primary organs. The cells then enter tumor capillaries (stimulated by specific angiogenesis factors produced by the tumor) and via these

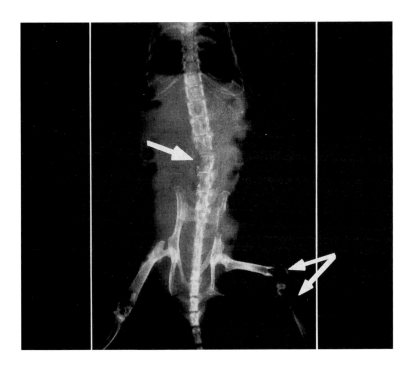

Fig. 4.3 Osteolytic lesions formed by human melanoma cells after injection into the left ventricle of the heart of nude mice after 3 weeks. (Reproduced from Nakai et al.[32])

capillaries reach the general circulation.[21] The steps involved in entering the tumor blood vessels at the primary site are similar to those which are involved in exit from the vasculature in the bone marrow cavity. These steps include the attachment of the tumor cells to basement membrane, the secretion of proteolytic enzymes which enable tumor cells to disrupt the basement membrane, and then migration of the tumor cells through the basement membrane.[22–24]

Attachment of tumor cells to other cells and to extracellular structures is critical for the metastatic process. Cell adhesion molecules (CAMs) such as laminin and E-cadherin are particularly likely to be important in those events involved in cancer cell invasion and metastasis. CAMs mediate cell-to-cell and cell-to-substratum communications. Cancer cell adhesion to normal host cells and to extracellular matrix through CAMs has been shown to regulate tumor cell invasiveness and proliferation.[25]

At the primary site, loss of CAMs causes disruption of the interconnections between cancer cells and promotes the detachment of cancer cells from the primary tumor which results in initiation of local invasion and eventually in the development of metastasis. In contrast, at the metastatic site, elevated expression of CAMs might be responsible for the arrest of cancer cells by attachment to the extracellular matrix. Subsequently, expression of CAMs might be diminished, which may free cancer cells from direct contact-mediated regulation by host immune cells. Recent studies have demonstrated that metastatic breast and ovarian cancers show heterogeneous expression of E-cadherin[26] and E-cadherin expression in these cancer cells may be reversibly modulated according to culture conditions *in vitro*[27] and environmental factors *in vivo*.[28] Therefore, cancer cells may express either decreased or increased levels of CAMs depending on the stage of metastasis development and sites of metastasis. We think it likely that the CAMs E-cadherin and laminin are involved in bone metastasis (see below).

Integrins are the most abundant CAMs and are responsible for a variety of cell–cell and

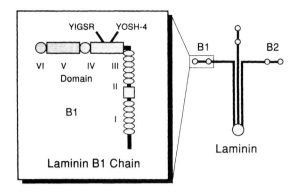

Fig. 4.4 The laminin molecule, indicating specific sites in the glycoprotein to which antagonists and the control peptides used by Nakai et al.[32] were derived. The domain designated YIGSR is critical for bone metastasis.

cell–matrix interactions,[29] and have been implicated in hematogenous dissemination.[30] In cancer metastasis, integrins have been shown to mediate cancer cell attachment to vascular endothelial cells and to matrix proteins such as laminin and fibronectin which underlie endothelium, an initial step in tumor colonization.[25] For example, it has recently been demonstrated that A375 human melanoma cells express high levels of the $\alpha_v\beta_3$ integrin (vitronectin receptor) on the cell surface when they bind to and invade the basement membrane matrix matrigel.[31]

Because of their complex structural and functional diversity, it seems unlikely at the present time that multiple integrins could potentially be involved in bone metastasis.

Laminin

We have found that synthetic antagonists to laminin inhibit osteolytic bone metastasis formation by A375 cells in nude mice.[32] These studies were performed with a model for bone metastasis based on the *in vivo* technique first described by Arguello et al.[33] to study metastasis to bone of murine tumor cells. We inoculated human melanoma cells into the left ventricle of nude mice and examined the formation of osteolytic metastases by radiographs and histology. This process was prevented by a synthetic antagonist to laminin (Figs 4.3–4.5).

We are aware that our bone metastasis model does not allow us to study the roles of CAMs in the steps *before* cancer cell entry into the circulation since we inject cells into the left ventricle of the heart. However, we will be able to examine CAMs for their importance in the events involved specifically after intravasation of cancer cells. In these steps, increased expression of integrins may be required for cancer cells to arrest and form microfoci at metastatic sites.

E-cadherin

E-cadherin (uvomorulin) is a 120 kd cell surface glycoprotein involved in calcium-dependent

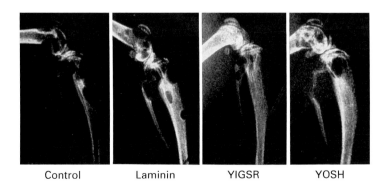

Fig. 4.5 Effects of laminin antagonists on bone resorption. Note that control mice, mice treated with laminin, and mice treated with control peptide (YOSH) all have multiple osteolytic lesions, most pronounced with laminin. However, in the mice treated with the synthetic laminin antagonist (YIGSR), there was reduction in the number of metastases. (Reproduced from Nakai et al.[32])

epithelial cell-specific cell adhesion. E-cadherin has homophilic properties in cell–cell adhesion and thus causes homotypic cell aggregation, which may be important in controlling embryogenesis and morphogenesis.[34] Recent evidence has shown that E-cadherin also plays a role in cancer invasion and metastasis. Treatment of epithelial noninvasive Madin–Darby canine kidney (MDCK) cells with monoclonal antibodies to E-cadherin rendered these cells more invasive.[35] Overexpression of the E-cadherin gene in highly invasive cancer cells dramatically suppressed their invasiveness and, conversely, introduction of E-cadherin-specific antisense RNA rendered noninvasive epithelial cells invasive.[36] E-cadherin expression was increased in populations of MCF-7 breast cancer cells with reduced invasiveness, whereas relatively low levels of E-cadherin were detected in the highly invasive human breast cancer cells, MDA-231.[37]

We have examined the capacity of the human breast cancer cell lines MCF-7 (high E-cadherin expression) and MDA-231 cells (low E-cadherin expression) to form bone metastases.[38] We have found that MDA-231 cells are much more effective at forming osteolytic bone lesions *in vivo*. This experiment has been performed multiple times on a total of 50 mice for MDA-231 cells and 40 mice for MCF-7 cells. Whereas MDA-231 cells form obvious osteolytic lesions by 4 weeks after inoculation into the left ventricle, MCF-7 cells take more than 8 weeks to form similar lesions. At 4 weeks, no lesions are apparent in mice inoculated with MCF-7 cells. However, when MDA-231 cells were transfected with E-cadherin cDNA, their capacity to form osteolytic bone lesions was markedly reduced.[38]

Secretion of proteolytic enzymes by the tumor cells or by host cells may be responsible for disruption of the basement membranes of blood vessels and the tissue stroma, processes which are required for tumor cell egress from the circulation. These enzymes may include Type IV collagenase as well as other proteolytic enzymes. Tumor cells may cross the basement membrane by a process of directed migrational chemotaxis, but increased random movement (or chemokinesis) may also be responsible. Tumor cells produce motility factors which can increase their locomotive capacity and result in increased migration through defects in the basement membrane.[23] Tumor cells have varying capacity for metastasis. Primary tumors comprise heterogeneous populations of cells which have been shown in many studies to have differing invasive properties and different metastatic potential.[39-43] Tumor cells are unstable phenotypically for reasons which are not completely understood, although this has been the subject of many studies.[44,45] As tumors grow, they undergo rapid clonal diversification.[46] Some of the possibilities for this variability in individual tumor behavior include a host selection process, which may be due to some cells having the capability of surviving naturally occurring immune defense mechanisms, or the effects of treatment with anti-cancer drugs or radiation therapy which may lead to acquired genetic variability. It is now well recognized that the genetic component of tumor cells can greatly influence their metastatic potential as well as their invasive capabilities and tumorigenicity.[18,47] In breast cancers, expression of the Her-2/Neu oncogene occurs in parallel with aggressive behavior of the cells.[48] In some tumors, particularly melanoma, expression of the NM23 oncogene appears to inhibit the capability of the tumor to metastasize.[24,49] As already noted, the expression of laminin receptors on tumor cells may cause enhanced metastatic capabilities. Deletions of chromosomal material on chromosome 11p have been noted in aggressive breast cancers[50] and deletions of chromosomes 17 and 18 may be found in colon carcinomas which arise from colonic polyps.[51,52]

There are multiple mechanisms which protect against tumor metastasis. Current evidence suggests that less than 1% of tumor cells survive in the circulation.[18] Tumors probably survive best in the circulation as aggregates, which may prevent the loss of individual cells in the circulation from mechanical shear forces or from anoxia.

The blood coagulation mechanism appears to be important in promoting tumor cell metastasis.[53-55] Anticoagulants of the coumadin class have been tested over many years for their capacity to inhibit metastasis and promote survival, although the data remain inconclusive and controversial. Once within the bone marrow cavity, tumor cells pass through wide-channeled marrow sinusoids. The cellular and molecular events involved in their passage from the marrow sinusoid to the bone surface are similar to the events involved in their escape from the primary site. Again, the tumors must attach to basement membranes of blood vessels, disrupt these basement membranes by the production of proteolytic enzymes, and then migrate through the basement membrane to invade the tissue stroma. A fourth step is involved in the pathophysiology of the bone metastasis, and this involves the destruction of bone. There is some controversy over the mechanisms by which this may occur (see below). Recently, we have studied several human tumors (A375 melanoma cells and cultured breast cancer cells) to determine their capability of growing metastases in bone using a modification of the technique described by Arguello et al.[33] We have used inhibitors of specific cell adhesion molecules to determine their effects on the metastatic process. Tumor cells bind to basement membranes on endothelial cells at the metastatic site[56] through specific cell adhesion molecules such as fibronectin and laminin. We have used synthetic antagonists of laminin which interfere with the binding of laminin to laminin receptors on the tumor cells to determine the effects on the formation of the bone metastasis. We have found that a synthetic antagonist YIGSR totally inhibits this process in bone. A similar result was found when this antagonist was used in a lung metastasis model.[57] There may be a 50-fold increase in laminin receptors on the surface of high invasive and metastatic tumor cells compared with other tumor cells which do not have the capability of metastasis or invasion.[58]

Secretion of proteolytic enzymes

Tumor cells produce proteolytic enzymes to degrade basement membranes and traverse the vessels to enter the tissue stroma. This process can involve direct production of proteolytic enzymes by tumor cells such as Type IV collagenase, or even production of proteolytic enzymes by host cells. Garbisa et al.[47] have pointed out the potential role of the production of Type IV collagenase by tumor cells and its potential for degradation of the capillary basement membrane. Basset et al.[59] have shown that host cells associated with some invasive breast carcinomas expressed a gene which encodes a metalloproteinase. This gene was expressed by fibroblasts and stromal cells which were present adjacent to the breast cancer cells. Expression of this metalloproteinase was stimulated by growth factors produced by the breast cancer cells such as PDGF, TGFα, and bFGF.

Cell motility

Tumor cells may be attracted from the vasculature toward bone surfaces by a number of chemotactic factors. Bone itself contains multiple factors with chemotactic potential for tumor cells. These include fragments of Type I collagen which have been shown to cause unidirectional migration of tumor cells[60] and fragments of the bone protein osteocalcin which may cause chemotaxis of tumor cells and monocytes.[61] The conditioned media harvested from resorbing or remodeling bones contain chemotactic activity which stimulates the unidirectional migration of rat and human tumor cells.[62,63] The nature of the factor responsible has not been identified, but may be TGFβ which is present in abundant amounts in bone.[64] Further evidence supporting a role for cell motility in the development of bone metastases can be gleaned from experiments using the previously described mouse bone metastasis model. Human breast cancer cell line MDA-MB-231, which overexpresses the small heat shock protein 27 (hsp 27), has decreased cell motility *in vitro* and caused fewer bone metastases *in vivo*.[65]

TUMOR CELL MEDIATION OF BONE DESTRUCTION AT THE METASTATIC SITE

The cellular mechanism responsible for local destruction of bone by tumor cells has been a

52 CANCER AND THE SKELETON

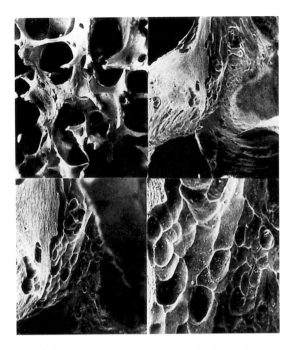

Fig. 4.6 Demonstration that osteoclasts are the major mechanism by which solid tumors cause bone destruction. Multiple Howship's lacunae are seen in this scanning electron micrograph of the cancellous bone surface of a vertebral body in this patient with metastatic pancreatic cancer (from Boyde et al.[66]). This figure shows successively higher powers of the same site on the cancellous bone surface.

controversial issue for some years. Although definitive proof is still not available, it is likely that the predominant mechanism for bone destruction is an increase in osteoclast activity. In other words, tumors produce local factors which stimulate osteoclasts which then in turn are responsible for the resorption of bone. The alternative possibility is that tumor cells may destroy bone directly without the addition of osteoclasts. The evidence in favor of osteoclastic bone resorption being the predominant mechanism is twofold. First, when looked for carefully using techniques such as scanning electron microscopy, osteoclasts are invariably found to be present adjacent to tumor deposits[66] (Fig. 4.6). Moreover, distinctive osteoclast resorption lacunae are universally present. Such studies show no evidence of smaller resorption lacunae corresponding to the size of the tumor cells. Secondly, drugs which effectively inhibit osteoclast activity such as the bisphosphonates, plicamycin, and gallium nitrate work very effectively in the hypercalcemia of malignancy which is due predominantly to increased bone resorption caused by tumors and in decreasing morbidity from breast cancer metastases to bone. These data suggest that since these drugs work through the inhibition of osteoclast function, osteoclasts are major (possibly sole) mediators of the bone destruction. Nevertheless, there is *in vitro* evidence which suggests that breast cancer cells have the capacity to cause bone resorption *in vitro*. When breast cancer cells have been added to devitalized bone, they cause both mineral release and matrix degradation.[67]

MECHANISMS OF OSTEOCLAST STIMULATION AT THE METASTATIC SITE

As indicated above, the major cellular mechanism for bone destruction in osteolytic bone disease is osteoclastic. Consequently, there is interest in determining the mediator that is responsible for this increase in osteoclast activity. Recent studies suggest that the factor which is responsible in at least some patients is PTH-rP, the tumor peptide which has been associated with humoral hypercalcemia of malignancy. This is so even though many of these patients do not have increased plasma PTH-rP or increased nephrogenous cyclic AMP, indicating the absence of these latter parameters does not mean that PTH-rP is unimportant. It has been shown by immunohistochemistry that there is increased expression of PTH-rP in bone sites compared with either soft tissue metastases or primary tumors in patients with carcinoma of the breast.[68,69] We have studied the human breast cancer cell line MDA-MB-231, which has been inoculated into the left cardiac ventricle of nude mice and of osteolytic lesions developed following 4–6 weeks. We found that there is an increase in PTH-rP expression in the tumor cells which metastasize to bone, similar to what has been

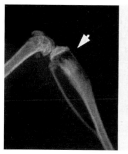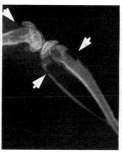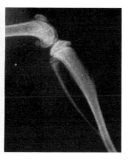

Fig. 4.7 Effects of neutralizing antibodies to PTH-rP on capacity of human MDA-MB-231 breast cancer cells to cause osteolytic bone lesions following intracardiac injection in nude mice. The neutralizing antibodies to PTH-rP prevent the development of osteolytic lesions (Guise et al.[70]).

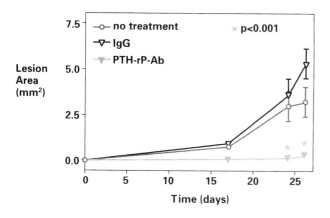

Fig. 4.8 Quantitation of lesion area from experiment described in Fig. 4.7 (Guise et al.[70]). Impairment of the development of osteolytic lesions is caused by neutralizing antibodies to PTH-rP.

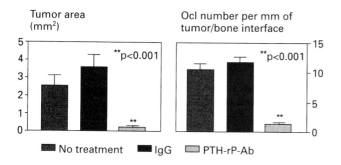

Fig. 4.9 Histomorphometric analysis of data shown in Figs 4.7 and 4.8. Neutralizing antibodies to PTH-rP not only reduces the number of osteoclasts adjacent to metastatic human breast cancer cells but also markedly reduces tumor burden in bone.

described in patients.[68] This is also associated with the development of typical osteolytic bone lesions which are seen in patients with the disease. When tumor-bearing nude mice are treated with neutralizing antibodies to PTH-rP, not only is there a decrease in the development of the osteolytic bone lesions but there is also a decrease in the tumor burden in bone[70] (Figs 4.7–4.9). The most likely explanation for the increase in PTH-rP production in the bone microenvironment is that bone provides a fertile environment for the growth of tumor cells and also enhances the production of PTH-rP. More recent studies have shown that a likely mechanism responsible for this effect is production of transforming growth factor β (TGFβ) which is

TYPE	CONCENTRATION (ng/g)
Insulin-like Growth Factor II	1500
Transforming Growth Factor β	450
Insulin-like Growth Factor I	100
Platelet-Derived Growth Factor	60
Basic Fibroblast Growth Factor	50
Acidic Fibroblast Growth Factor	10
Bone Morphogenic Protein	1–2

Fig. 4.10 Growth factors which are stored in the bone matrix are released during the process of resorption in active form,[71] and are thus available to modulate tumor growth and activity at the sites of metastatic deposits in bone.[64]

released from bone in active form when bone resorbs.[71] Studies by Yin et al.[72] have shown that when MDA-MB-231 cells are transfected with a dominant-negative type II TGFβ receptor which makes the cells unresponsive to TGFβ, PTH-rP production is not enhanced in the bone microenvironment and the development and progression of osteolytic bone lesions are significantly less compared with this metastasis caused by parental MDA-MB-231. TGFβ is probably not the only bone-derived growth factor whose production in the marrow site and effects on metastatic tumor cells are important (see below). It is also likely that there are other mechanisms for bone destruction associated with tumor cells which metastasize to bone. These may involve production by the tumor cells or by host immune cells in the bone microenvironment of mediators such as transforming growth factor α, interleukin 1α, tumor necrosis factor, and interleukin-6, each of which acting alone or in combination with PTH-rP represents a strong stimulus to increase bone resorption.[73–75]

BONE-DERIVED TUMOR GROWTH FACTORS AT THE METASTATIC SITE

Bone provides a very favorable niche for tumor cells and it is clear that in this microenvironment many tumors grow very well. In part, the reason may be that bone is a large repository or storehouse for growth regulatory factors[64] (Fig. 4.10). In particular, bone is rich in TGFβ but also stores other growth regulatory factors which may act as tumor growth factors, including bone morphogenetic proteins, heparin-binding fibroblast growth factors, platelet-derived growth factors, and insulin-like growth factors I and II. These factors are presumably the reason bone is resorbed so avidly in metastases. They may be made available locally through bone resorption. This has been shown particularly in the case of TGFβ. TGFβ may alter the behavior of many tumor cells, and in particular breast cancer cells, to enhance the production of PTH-rP.[76–78]

Another factor which may be important in tumor cell behavior in the bone microenvironment is calcium. Calcium released by resorbing bone may alter tumor cell proliferation.[79] Unfortunately, there is still little information on this topic.

One of the major difficulties which has limited the study of bone metastasis has been the lack of suitable animal models. Although this has retarded the accumulation of knowledge in the pathophysiology of bone metastasis, it has not been a problem in investigating other types of metastases and in particular lung metastases.[42] Arguello et al.[33] devised a technique where tumor cells are injected directly into the left ventricle of mice. This leads to the colonization of bone in regions containing

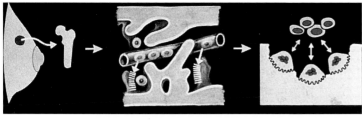

- CAMs
- MMPs

- CAMs
- MMPs

- PTH-rP
- Cytokines
- src

Fig. 4.11 Molecular mechanisms involved in breast cancer cell metastasis to bone. Some of these steps are general steps and some are steps which are specific for bone. These molecular mechanisms have been clarified by recent studies of Yoneda and Guise.[70,88]

hematopoietic bone marrow by appropriate tumor cells with potential to metastasize to bone. This leads to multiple lytic lesions resembling those seen in patients with cancer. In these models, bone metastasis occurs when tumor cells have ready access to the arterial circulation. We have modified this model by the use of human tumor cells in nude mice.[32] By inoculating human breast cancer cells into the left ventricle of nude mice, we have been able to characterize a number of steps involved in osteolytic bone metastasis. We have treated the animals with antagonists or antibodies to specific molecules involved in the process (for example E-cadherin, PTH-rP), transfected the tumor cells with specific genes (for example E-cadherin, TIMP-2, src, and PTH-rP) to show their role in this process, and treated the animals with agents (for example bisphosphonates, growth factors) which regulate normal bone cell function thereby determining the interaction between bone cells and tumor cells in the bone microenvironment. Some of the molecular mechanisms likely involved in the process of breast cancer metastasis to bone which have been identified using this technique are shown diagrammatically in Fig. 4.11. With a special modification of this technique, Yoneda *et al.*[80] have developed a method for specifically examining metastasis to the calvarium to give a better picture of the progressive development of bone metastasis (Fig. 4.12).

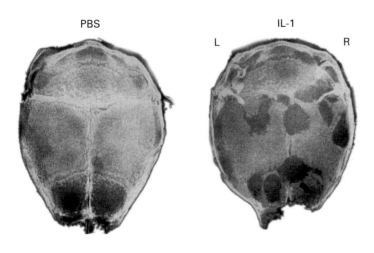

PBS

IL-1

L   R

Fig. 4.12 Effects of increasing local bone turnover on the development of osteolytic bone lesions in nude mice. In this experiment, interleukin-1 was administered for 3 days over the calvaria of a nude mouse to increase bone turnover. Following interleukin-1 injections, the mice were inoculated with MDA-MB-231 cells into the left cardiac ventricle. Note the obvious development of osteolytic lesions in the calvarium in which bone turnover was stimulated by interleukin-1, compared with a calvarium where bone turnover was not increased. This effect of interleukin-1 was inhibited by simultaneous treatment with the bisphosphonate ibandronate, which inhibits bone resorption.

Shevrin et al.[81] used prostate cancer cells to induce bone metastases following intravenous injection and occlusion of the inferior vena cava. Pollard et al.[82,83] used rat prostate adenocarcinoma cells in Lobund–Wistar rats to show that these tumors cause a profound local change in bone formation. When this tumor is injected adjacent to a bone surface where the periosteum is often mildly damaged by scratching with a needle tip, the tumor stimulates adjacent new woven bone formation (Fig. 4.10).

TREATMENT APPROACHES FOR METASTATIC OSTEOLYTIC BONE DISEASE

The best form of treatment for metastatic bone disease is ablative therapy for the tumor. Unfortunately, as already indicated, in the vast majority of patients this is not feasible. Most attention at the present time is being focused on drugs which inhibit osteoclast activity such as the bisphosphonates. (These are considered in more detail in Chapters 14–16.) Over the last 20 years there have been many studies examining the effects of bisphosphonates in patients with osteolytic bone metastases, and there is accumulating evidence that bisphosphonates are extremely effective at inhibiting skeletal-related events (pathological fractures, need for radiation, or surgery for osteolytic bone disease, prevention of spinal cord compression due to vertebral collapse, and prevention of episodes of hypercalcemia). The more recent of these studies – most performed with pamidronate used intravenously by infusion every month – have been double-blind, randomized, and controlled, and show a clear benefit for pamidronate used in this way. Pamidronate clearly reduces the number of skeletal-related events and also delays the onset of the first skeletal-related event in breast cancer patients with osteolytic bone metastases.[85] There are varying reports of the effects of pamidronate on tumor mass in soft tissue or bone. Our findings in the model described above in which MDA-MB-231 cells are inoculated into the left ventricle of nude mice suggest that bisphosphonates not only reduce osteolytic bone lesions but also markedly reduce tumor burden in bone.[87]

This is likely due to the decreased production of growth factors in the bone microenvironment by inhibition of bone remodeling.[88] It remains unclear whether this is also associated with effects of bisphosphonates to increase or alter tumor burden in metastatic sites. A recent study by Diel et al.[89] suggests that there may be decreases in tumor burden in both bone and soft tissue sites, but the numbers of patients are relatively small and this study needs confirmation. That bisphosphonates do not have any direct effect on tumor mass has been shown in a number of studies.[90,91] However, they do cause tumor cell apoptosis in vitro,[92,93] and whether these effects are relevant to their decreasing tumor burden in bone still has to be determined. It is hoped that new-generation bisphosphonates which are orally active may be useful not only in the treatment of patients with established metastases, but also in the prevention of the development of new metastases. Although information is not currently available in this regard, it seems likely that inhibitors of osteoclastic bone resorption may be even more effective in the prevention of new metastases than in the treatment of established metastases. Theoretically, inhibition of continued resorption would leave the patient with a residual lytic lesion in bone (although occasional patients may show some sclerosis of the healing lesion). On the other hand, in those patients who have malignancies with a predilection for the skeleton, such as breast cancer, preventative treatment with an inhibitor of osteoclastic bone resorption may prevent the initial development of an osteolytic metastasis.

As indicated earlier, attention should not be focused solely on inhibitors of osteoclasts. Drugs such as laminin antagonists which prevent binding of tumor cells to basement membranes. Inhibitors of proteolytic enzyme disrupt the basement membrane or inhibit tumor cell chemotaxis and also turn out to be useful in the prevention or treatment of established metastases. Laminin antagonists prevent tumor metastasis in an experimental model. Recently, we have used neutralizing antibodies to PTH-rP in order to prevent progression of osteolytic bone lesions in animal models of human metastatic breast cancer.[70] We have also transfected the human tumor cells with inhibitors of the matrix metalloproteinases, namely tissue inhibitor of matrix metalloproteinase-2 (TIMP-2), and shown a decrease in osteolytic bone lesions.[94]

Animal models such as these may have predictive value prior to the initiation of expensive and difficult clinical trials with experimental therapies such as laminin antagonists and inhibitors of proteolytic enzyme digestion.

OSTEOBLASTIC METASTASES

Tumors affect the skeleton not only by causing osteolytic metastases but also occasionally by causing metastases characterized by the formation of new bone around the tumor cell deposits (Figs 4.13 and 4.14). This occurs without prior osteoclastic resorption, and the newly formed bone is laid down directly on trabecular bone surfaces without a preceding resorptive episode.[95] Prostate cancer is the commonest tumor which causes this response. Essentially all patients with prostate cancer will develop osteoblastic bone metastases if they live long enough.[96]

The mechanisms responsible for the osteoblastic metastasis are unknown, but are attracting great interest. From the histomorphometric studies of Charhon et al.,[95] osteoblastic metastases are likely due to soluble factors which are produced by the metastasizing cancer cells and which stimulate bone formation. Osteoblastic metastases may occur at sites of previous resorption, or on quiescent bone surfaces. They may also occur as a consequence of condensation of osteoblastic precursors in the marrow cavity which upon stimulation by the metastatic tumor differentiate to form an osteoblastic nodule. Many investigators have attempted to identify factors produced by prostate cancer cells which have proliferative effects on cells with the osteoblast phenotype *in vitro*. Jacobs and Lawson[97] found that extracts of a well differentiated prostatic carcinoma stimulated ^{3}H thymidine incorporation into fibroblasts. Similar effects were seen with extracts of

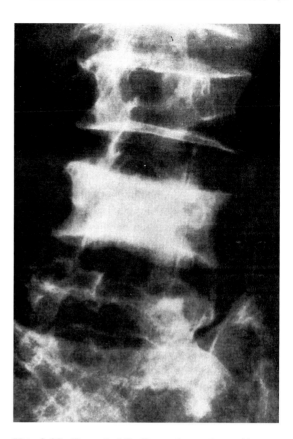

Fig. 4.13 Characteristic X-ray of a patient with an osteoblastic metastasis showing vertebral body sclerosis

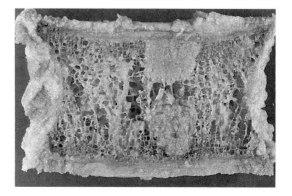

Fig. 4.14 Osteoblastic metastases in a vertebral body caused by solid tumor deposits in the marrow cavity tumor deposits

benign prostatic hyperplasia. Preliminary characterization of this activity showed it to have an apparent molecular weight of greater than 67 kd. In retrospect, this activity may have represented a combination of growth factors now known to be produced by prostate cancer cells, and may not have had any relationship to bone growth stimulatory effects.

Others, including Simpson et al.[98] and Koutsilieris et al.,[99] have described osteoblast stimulating activity produced by prostatic cancer tissue. Simpson et al.[98] took extracts from the human prostate cancer cell line PC3, injected total RNA into xenopus oocytes, and then examined the conditioned media for bone stimulatory activity. These extracts stimulated both mitogenesis and alkaline phosphatase activity in osteosarcoma cells with the osteoblast phenotype. Koutsilieris et al.[99] took extracts of prostate cancer tissue as well as extracts of normal prostatic tissue and also found growth proliferative activity for bone cells.

As noted above, most studies to date which have attempted to identify bone growth regulatory factors produced by prostate cancer cells have utilized well established human prostate cancer cell lines. However, these have not turned out to be satisfactory models. These human cancer cells when inoculated into nude mice cause bone resorption rather than bone formation. This occurs whether the cells are implanted in the peritoneum, intramuscularly, subcutaneously, or adjacent to the calvarium. The reasons these cells do not produce osteoblastic lesions *in vivo* are not clear. However, human prostate carcinoma cells are notoriously difficult to grow *in vitro*, and the established cell lines that are available have changed in some of their characteristics while in culture. For example, PC3 is no longer a hormone-responsive tumor. A better model may be the PA-III model of rat prostate adenocarcinoma. Pollard developed a strain of rats, Lobund–Wistar, that gives a high frequency (10%) of spontaneous prostate adenocarcinoma.[82,83] Several cell lines have been derived from these tumors, and one of these, called PA-III, has been studied extensively in the laboratory and has been found to stimulate new bone formation in Lobund–Wistar rats.[83] We confirmed that when PA-III cells were injected in nude mice near a bone site associated with local damage to the periosteum, the prostate tumors induced a strong local osteoblastic response with extensive new woven bone. This increase in bone formation could not be accounted for by previous bone resorption and, as such, resembles the osteoblastic response to prostate cancer in humans. We have found these PA-III tumor cells express a variety of BMPs, and that transfection of the tumor cells with antisense constructs of the BMP-3 gene reduces their capacity to stimulate an osteoblastic response *in vivo*.[100]

A number of other models of prostate cancer have been utilized. The Mat Ly/Lu variant of the rat Dunning prostate cancer causes bone metastases *in vivo* which are more pronounced when the cells overexpress rat urokinase-type plasminogen activator (uPA).[101] Recently, Gingrich et al.[102] have used transgenic mice in which the transgene is a regulatory element to the rat probasin gene linked to SV40 T antigen and showed the spontaneous development of bone metastases. This TRAMP (for transgenic adenocarcinoma mouse prostate) model is currently being evaluated for insights it may provide into osteoblastic metastasis. It was first described by Greenberg et al.[103]

A number of factors have been suggested as potential mediators of osteoblastic metastasis associated with prostate cancer.

Transforming growth factor β2

TGFβ2 is abundant in PC3 human prostatic cancer cells, and was purified from the human prostate cancer cell line PC3.[104] TGFβ2 stimulates proliferation of osteoblasts *in vitro*, as well as bone formation *in vivo*. It is a powerful stimulator of new bone formation *in vivo*[105] and is a likely candidate as a mediator of osteoblastic metastasis.

Fibroblast growth factor

Prostatic cancer cells express large amounts of both acidic and basic fibroblast growth factors

(FGFs)[106,107] and these are potential mediators of osteoblast proliferation in patients with this disease.[108,109] Both acidic and basic FGFs (also called FGF-I and -II) cause profound stimulation of bone formation *in vivo*.[110,111] Izbicka *et al*.[112] have shown that a human tumor cell line causes bone formation *in vivo* and produces a mitogenic factor for osteoblastic cells which was identified as an extended form of FGF-II.

Plasminogen activator sequence

There have been several reports of purification of mitogenic activity for rat calvarial osteoblastic cells present in the conditioned media of the human prostatic cancer cell line PC3.[113,114] The first 10 amino acids were sequenced and shown to be identical to the serine protease urokinase (uPA). Overexpression of uPA in rat prostate cancer cells leads to bone metastases *in vivo*.[101] An amino terminal fragment of uPA which contains EGF-like repeats has been shown to have mitogenic activity for osteoblasts.[115] The carboxy-terminal proteolytic domain may be responsible for tumor invasiveness or growth factor activation. The expression of proteases in the microenvironment of growth factors such as TGFβ may be very important for their activator in bone.[116,117] Plasmin-sensitive cleavage sites are present in the latent TGFβ binding protein which masks TGFβ activity.

Bone morphogenetic proteins

We have found that both normal and neoplastic prostate tissue express a variety of BMPs. We have examined human and rat neoplastin prostate tissue, and found evidence of BMP-2, 3, 4, and 6 mRNA.[118] In one of these tumors, the bone formation response seems to depend, at least in part, on the amount of BMP-3 expressed (see below).

PTH-rP

Cultured prostatic cancer cells frequently express PTH-rP, which in appropriate doses has an anabolic effect on bone.[119] It is possible that this tumor peptide may be related to the osteoblastic metastases associated with prostate cancers (Laurie McCauley, personal communication). There is no direct data as yet to support this notion.

Prostate-specific antigen (PSA)

This serine protease which is expressed by prostate cancer cells can cleave PTH-rP at the amino terminus[120] and could also potentially activate other growth factors produced by prostate carcinomas. PSA is a serine protease which is produced in excessive amounts by prostate carcinoma cells, and is used as a marker of tumor burden. Whether it has harmful effects is unknown, but one possibility is that its enzymatic action could be responsible for activating anabolic agents such as IGF-I and TGFβ, by cleaving them from their binding proteins, or even by cleaving PTH-rP to an anabolic fragment. It has been shown to cleave PTH-rP into fragments which do not stimulate osteoclastic bone resorption.

Endothelin-1

Endothelin-1 has recently been implicated as an osteoblast stimulant in metastatic prostate cancer.[10] It is a powerful mitogenic factor for osteoblasts[121,122] and is produced in large amounts by the prostatic epithelium.[123] Circulating concentrations are increased in patients with metastatic prostate cancer.[10] However, whether it has more pathophysiologic significance than the numerous other growth regulatory factors for bone cells produced by prostate carcinomas remains unknown.

REFERENCES

1. Wingo PA, Tong T, Bolden S. Cancer statistics. *CA Cancer J Clin* (1995) **45**: 8–30.
2. Mundy GR, Bertolini DR. Bone destruction and hypercalcemia in plasma cell myeloma. *Semin in Oncol* (1986) **13**: 291–9.
3. Mundy GR. *Calcium Homeostasis: Hypercalcemia and Hypocalcemia* (London: Martin Dunitz, 1990).
4. Galasko CSB. Skeletal metastases. *Clin Orthop* (1986) **September:** 18–30.
5. Galasko CSB. *Skeletal Metastases* (London: Butterworth, 1986).
6. Batson OV. The function of the vertebral veins and their role in the spread of metastases. *Ann Surg* (1940) **112**: 138–49.
7. Coman DR, DeLong RP. The role of the vertebral venous system in the metastasis of cancer to the spinal column; experiments with tumour cell suspension in rats and rabbits. *Cancer* (1951) **4**: 610–18.
8. van den Brenk HAS, Burch WM, Kelley H et al. Venous diversion trapping and growth of blood-borne cancer cells en route to the lungs. *Br J Cancer* (1975) **31**: 46–61.
9. Dodds PR, Caride VJ, Lytton B. The role of vertebral veins in the dissemination of prostatic carcinoma. *J Urol* (1981) **126**: 753–5.
10. Nelson JB, Hedican SP, George DJ et al. Identification of endothelin-1 in the pathophysiology of metastatic adenocarcinoma of the prostate. *Nat Med* (1995) **1**: 944.
11. Galasko CSB, Burn JI. Hypercalcemia in patients with advanced mammary cancer. *Br Med J* (1971) **3**: 573–7.
12. Stewart AF, Horst R, Deftos LJ et al. Biochemical evaluation of patients with cancer-associated hypercalcemia: evidence for humoral and non-humoral groups. *N Engl J Med* (1980) **303**: 1377–83.
13. Tuttle KR, Kunau RT, Loveridge N et al. Altered renal calcium handling in hypercalcemia of malignancy. *J Am Soc Nephrol* (1991) **2**: 191–9.
14. Peacock M, Robertson WG, Nordin BEC. Relation between serum and urine calcium with particular reference to parathyroid activity. *Lancet* (1969) **i**: 384–6.
15. Percival RC, Yates AJP, Gray RES et al. Mechanisms of malignant hypercalcemia in carcinoma of the breast. *Br Med J* (1985) **291**: 776–9.
16. Gallacher SJ, Fraser WD, Patel U et al. Breast cancer-associated hypercalcaemia: a reassessment of renal calcium and phosphate handling. *Ann Clin Biochem* (1990) **27**: 551–6.
17. Harinck HI, Bijvoet OL, Plantingh AS et al. Role of bone and kidney in tumor-induced hypercalcemia and its treatment with bisphosphonate and sodium chloride. *Am J Med* (1987) **82**: 1133–42.
18. Liotta LA, Kohn E. Cancer invasion and metastases. *J Am Med Assoc* (1990) **263**: 1123–6.
19. Paget S. The distribution of secondary growths in cancer of the breast. *Lancet* (1889) **i**: 571–3.
20. Zetter BR. The cellular basis of site-specific tumor metastasis. *N Engl J Med* (1990) **322**: 605–12.
21. Weiss L, Orr FW, Honn KV. Interactions between cancer cells and the microvasculature: a rate-regulator for metastasis. *Clin Exp Metastasis* (1989) **7**: 127–67.
22. Liotta LA, Tryggvason K, Garbisa S et al. Metastatic potential correlates with enzymatic degradation of basement membrane collagen. *Nature* (1980) **284**: 67–8.
23. Liotta LA, Mandler R, Murano G et al. Tumor cell autocrine motility factor. *Proc Natl Acad Sci* (1986) **83**: 3302–6.
24. Liotta LA, Steeg PS. Clues to the function of Nm23 and Awd proteins in development, signal transduction, and tumor metastasis provided by studies of dictyostelium discoideum. *J Natl Cancer Inst* (1990) **82**: 1170–2.
25. Albelda SM, Buck CA. Integrins and other cell adhesion molecules. *FASEB J* (1990) **4**: 2868–80.
26. Oka H, Shiozaki H, Kobayashi K et al. Expression of E-cadherin cells adhesion molecules in human breast cancer tissues and its relationship to metastasis. *Cancer Res* (1993) **53**: 1696–701.
27. Hashimoto M, Niwa O, Nitta Y et al. Unstable expression of E-cadherin adhesion molecules in metastatic ovarian tumor cells. *Jpn J Cancer Res* (1989) **80**: 459–63.
28. Mareel MM, Behrens J, Birchmeier W et al. Down-regulation of E-cadherin expression in Madin-Darby canine kidney (MDCK) cells inside tumors of nude mice. *Int J Cancer* (1991) **47**: 922–8.
29. Haynes RO. Integrins: versatility, modulation, and signaling in cell adhesion. *Cell* (1992) **69**: 11–25.
30. Nip J, Shibata H, Loskutoff DJ et al. Human melanoma cells derived from lymphatic metastases use integrins $\alpha_v\beta_3$ to adhere to lymph node vitronectin. *J Clin Invest* (1992) **90**: 1406–13.
31. Seftor REB, Seftor EA, Gehlsen KR et al. Role of

the $\alpha_v\beta_3$ integrin in human melanoma cell invasion. *Proc Natl Acad Sci U S A* (1992) **89**: 1557–61.
32. Nakai M, Mundy GR, Williams PJ *et al*. A synthetic antagonist to laminin inhibits the formation of osteolytic metastases by human melanoma cells in nude mice. *Cancer Res* (1992) **52**: 5395–9.
33. Arguello F, Baggs RB, Frantz CN. A murine model of experimental metastasis to bone and bone marrow. *Cancer Res* (1988) **48**: 6876–81.
34. Takeichi M. Cadherin cell adhesion receptors as a morphogenetic regulator. *Science* (1991) **251**: 1451–4.
35. Behrens J, Mareel MM, van Roy FM *et al*. Dissecting tumor cell invasion: epithelial cells acquire invasive properties after the loss of uvomorulin-mediated cell–cell adhesion. *J Cell Biol* (1989) **108**: 2435–47.
36. Vleminckx K, Vakaet L, Mareel M *et al*. Genetic manipulation of E-cadherin expression by epithelial tumor cells reveals an invasion suppressor role. *Cell* (1991) **66**: 107–19.
37. Sommers CL, Thompson EW, Torri JA *et al*. Cell adhesion molecule uvomorulin expression in human breast cancer cell lines: relationship to morphology and invasive capacities. *Cell Growth Diff* (1991) **2**: 365–71.
38. Mbalaviele G, Dunstan CR, Sasaki A *et al*. E-cadherin expression in human breast cancer cells suppress the development of osteolytic bone metastases in experimental metastasis model. *Cancer Res* (1996) **56**: 4063–70.
39. Carr I, Orr FW. Current reviews: invasion and metastasis. *Can Med Assoc J* (1983) **128**: 1164–7.
40. Heppner G. Tumor heterogeneity. *Cancer Res* (1984) **214**: 2259–65.
41. Poste G. Pathogenesis of metastatic disease: implications for current therapy and for the development of new therapeutic strategies. *Cancer Treat Res* (1986) **70**: 183–99.
42. Fidler IJ, Poste G. The cellular heterogeneity of malignant neoplasms: implications for adjuvant chemotherapy. *Semin Oncol* (1985) **12**: 207–21.
43. Fidler IJ. Tumor heterogeneity and the biology of cancer invasion and metastasis. *Cancer Res* (1978) **38**: 2651–60.
44. Nowell PS. The clonal evolution of tumor cell subpopulations. *Science* (1976) **194**: 23–38.
45. Miller FR. Tumor subpopulation interactions in metastasis. *Invasion Metastasis* (1983) **3**: 234–42.
46. Reedy AL, Fialkow PJ. Multicellular origin of fibrosarcomas in mice induced by the chemical carcinogen 3–methylcholanthrene. *J Exp Med* (1980) **150**: 878–86.
47. Garbisa S, Pozzatti R, Muschel RJ *et al*. Secretion of type IV collagenolytic protease and metastatic phenotype: induction by transfection with c-Ha-ras but not c-Ha-ras plus AD2–Ela. *Cancer Res* (1987) **47**: 1523–8.
48. Slamon DJ, Clark GM, Wong SG *et al*. Human breast cancer: correlation of relapse and survival with amplification of the HER-2/neu oncogene. *Science* (1987) **235**: 177–82.
49. Steeg PS, Bevilacqua G, Kopper L *et al*. Evidence for a novel gene associated with low tumor metastatic potential. *J Natl Cancer Inst* (1988) **80**: 200–4.
50. Ali IU, Lidereau R, Theillet C *et al*. Reduction to homozygosity of genes on chromosome 11 in human breast neoplasia. *Science* (1987) **238**: 185–8.
51. Vogelstein B, Fearon ER, Hamilton SR *et al*. Genetic alterations during colorectal tumor development. *N Engl J Med* (1988) **319**: 525–32.
52. Baker SJ, Fearon ER, Nigro JM *et al*. Chromosome 17 deletions and p53 gene mutations in colorectal carcinomas. *Science* (1989) **244**: 217–21.
53. Warren BA, Vales O. The adhesion of thromboplastic tumor emboli to vessel walls in vivo. *Br J Exp Pathol* (1972) **53**: 301–13.
54. Winterbauer RH, Elfenbein IB, Ball WC. Incidence and clinical significance of tumor embolization to the lungs. *Am J Med* (1968) **45**: 271–90.
55. Hilgard P, Gordon-Smith EL. Microangiopathic hemolytic anemia and experimental tumor-cell emboli. *Br J Haematol* (1974) **26**: 651–9.
56. Auerbach R, Lu WC, Pardon E *et al*. Specificity of adhesion between murine tumor cells and capillary endothelium: an in vitro correlate of preferential metastasis in vivo. *Cancer Res* (1987) **47**: 1492–6.
57. McCarthy JB, Skubitz APN, Palm SL *et al*. Metastasis inhibition of different tumor types by purified laminin fragments and a heparin-binding fragment of fibronectin. *J Natl Cancer Inst* (1988) **80**: 108–16.
58. Wewer UM, Taraboletti G, Sobel ME *et al*. Laminin receptor: role in tumor cell migration. *Cancer Res* (1987) **47**: 5691–8.
59. Basset P, Bellocq JP, Wolf C *et al*. A novel metalloproteinase gene specifically expressed in stromal cells of breast carcinomas. *Nature* (1990) **348**: 699–704.
60. Mundy GR, DeMartino S, Rowe DW. Collagen

and collagen-derived fragments are chemotactic for tumor cells. *J Clin Invest* (1981) **68:** 1102–5.
61. Mundy GR, Poser JW. Chemotactic activity of the gamma-carboxyglutamic acid containing protein in bone. *Calcif Tissue Int* (1983) **35:** 164–8.
62. Orr W, Varani J, Gondek MD et al. Chemotactic responses of tumor cells to products of resorbing bone. *Science* (1979) **203:** 176–9.
63. Orr FW, Varani J, Gondek MD et al. Partial characterization of a bone derived chemotactic factor for tumor cells. *Am J Pathol* (1980) **99:** 43–52.
64. Hauschka PV, Mavrakos AE, Iafrati MD et al. Growth factors in bone matrix. *J Biol Chem* (1986) **261:** 12 665–74.
65. Lemieux PM, Guise TA, Oesterreich S et al. Low cell motility induced by Hsp27 over-expression decreased osteolytic bone metastases formation by human breast cancer cells in vivo. *J Bone Miner Res* (1999) (in press).
66. Boyde A, Maconnachie E, Reid SA et al. Scanning electron microscopy in bone pathology: review of methods. Potential and applications. *Scanning Electron Microscopy* (1986) **IV:** 1537–54.
67. Eilon G, Mundy GR. Direct resorption of bone by human breast cancer cells in vitro. *Nature* (1978) **276:** 726–8.
68. Powell GJ, Southby J, Danks JA et al. Localization of parathyroid hormone-related protein in breast cancer metastases – increased incidence in bone compared with other sites. *Cancer Res* (1991) **51:** 3059–61.
69. Southby J, Kissin MW, Danks JA et al. Immuno-histochemical localization of parathyroid hormone-related protein in breast cancer. *Cancer Res* (1990) **50:** 7710–16.
70. Guise TA, Yin JJ, Taylor SD et al. Evidence for a casual role of parathyroid hormone-related protein in the pathogenesis of human breast cancer-mediated osteolysis. *J Clin Invest* (1996) **98:** 1544–9.
71. Pfeilschifter J, Mundy GR. Modulation of transforming growth factor beta activity in bone cultures by osteotropic hormones. *Proc Natl Acad Sci U S A* (1987) **84:** 2024–8.
72. Yin JJ, Chirgwin JM, Taylor SD et al. Dominant negative blockade of the transforming growth factor β (TGFβ) type II receptor decreases breast cancer-mediated osteolysis. *J Bone Miner Res* (1996) **11 (Suppl 1):** 180 (abst).
73. DeLaMata J, Uy HL, Guise TA et al. Interleukin-6 enhances hypercalcemia and bone resorption mediated by parathyroid hormone-related protein in vivo. *J Clin Invest* (1995) **95:** 2846–52.
74. Uy HL, Mundy GR, Boyce BF et al. Tumor necrosis factor enhances parathyroid hormone related protein (PTH-rP)-induced hypercalcemia and bone resorption without inhibiting bone formation in vivo. *Cancer Res* (1997) **57:** 3194–9.
75. Guise TA, Yoneda T, Yates AJ et al. The combined effect of tumor-produced parathyroid hormone-related protein and transforming growth factor alpha enhance hypercalcemia in vivo and bone resorption in vitro. *J Clin Endocrinol Metab* (1993) **77:** 40–5.
76. Zakalik D, Diep D, Hooks MA et al. Transforming growth factor beta increases stability of parathyroid hormone related protein messenger RNA. *J Bone Miner Res* (1992) **7 (Suppl 1):** 104 (abst).
77. Kuriyama T, Gillespie MT, Glatz JA et al. Transforming growth factor β stimulation of parathyroid hormone-related protein (PTH-rP): a paracrine regulator? *Mol Cell Endocrinol* (1992) **92:** 55–62.
78. Merryman JI, DeWille JW, Werkmeister JR et al. Effects of transforming growth factor β on parathyroid hormone-related protein production and ribonucleic acid expression by a squamous carcinoma cell line in vitro. *Endocrinology* (1994) **134:** 2424–33.
79. Rizzoli R, Bonjour JP. High extracellular calcium increases the production of a parathyroid hormone-like activity by cultured Leydig tumor cells associated with humoral hypercalcemia. *J Bone Miner Res* (1989) **4:** 839–44.
80. Yoneda T, Williams P, Dunstan C et al. Growth of metastatic cancer cells in bone is enhanced by bone derived insulin-like growth factors (IGFs). *J Bone Miner Res* (1995) **10 (Suppl 1):** 269 (abst).
81. Shevrin D, Kukreja SC, Ghosh L et al. Development of skeletal metastasis by human prostate cancer in athymic nude mice. *Clin Exp Metastasis* (1988) **6:** 401–9.
82. Pollard M, Luckert PH. Transplantable metastasizing prostate adenocarcinoma in rats. *J Natl Cancer Inst* (1975) **54:** 643–59.
83. Pollard M, Luckert MS, Scheu J. Effects of diphosphonate and x-rays on bone lesions induced in rats by prostate cancer cells. *Cancer* (1988) **61:** 2027–32.
84. Berenson JR, Lichtenstein A, Porter L et al. Efficacy of pamidronate in reducing the skeletal events in patients with advanced multiple myeloma. *N Engl J Med* (1996) **334:** 488–93.
85. Hortobagyi GN, Theriault RL, Porter L et al.

Efficacy of pamidronate in reducing skeletal complications in patients with breast cancer and lytic bone metastases. *N Engl J Med* (1996) **335**: 1785–91.
86. Lipton A, Theriault RL, Hortobagyi GN *et al.* Long-term treatment with pamidronate reduces skeletal morbidity in women receiving endocrine treatment for advanced breast cancer and lytic bone lesions. *J Clin Oncol* (1999) (in press).
87. Sasaki A, Boyce BF, Story B *et al.* Bisphosphonate risedronate reduces metastatic human breast cancer burden in bone in nude mice. *Cancer Res* (1995) **55**: 3551–7.
88. Mundy GR, Yoneda T. Bisphosphonates as anti-cancer drugs. *N Engl J Med* (1998) **339**: 398–400.
89. Diel IJ, Solomayer EF, Costa SD *et al.* Reduction in new metastases in breast cancer with adjuvant clodronate treatment. *N Engl J Med* (1998) **339**: 357–63.
90. Wingen F, Schmahl D. Distribution of 3-amino-1–hydroxypropane-1, 1–diphosphonic acid in rats and effects on rat osteosarcoma. *Drug Res* (1985) **35**: 1565–71.
91. Krempien B, Wingen F, Eichmann T *et al.* Protective effects of a prophylactic treatment with the bisphosphonate 3-amino-1–hydroxypropane-1, 1–bisphosphonic acid on the development of tumor osteopathies in the rat: experimental studies with the Walker carcinosarcoma 256. *Oncology* (1988) **45**: 41–6.
92. Shipman CM, Rogers MJ, Apperley JF *et al.* Bisphosphonates induce apoptosis in human myeloma cell lines: a novel anti-tumour activity. *Br J Haematol* (1997) **98**: 665–72.
93. Aparicio A, Gardner A, Tu Y *et al.* In vitro cytoreductive effects on multiple myeloma cells induced by bisphosphonates. *Leukemia* (1998) **12**: 220–9.
94. Williams P, Mbalaviele G, Sasaki A *et al.* Multi-step inhibition of breast cancer metastasis to bone. *J Bone Miner Res* (1995) **10 (Suppl 1)**: 121 (abst).
95. Charhon SA, Chapuy MC, Devlin EE *et al.* Histomorphometric analysis of sclerotic bone metastases from prostatic carcinoma special reference to osteomalacia. *Cancer* (1983) **51**: 918–24.
96. Mundy GR (1993) Pathophysiology of skeletal complications of cancer. In Mundy GR, Martin TJ (eds) *Physiology and Pharmacology of Bone. Handbook of Experimental Pharmacology* (Berlin: Springer-Verlag, 1993): 641–71.
97. Jacobs SC, Lawson R. Mitogenic factors in human prostate extracts. *Urology* (1980) **16**: 488–91.
98. Simpson EL, Harrod J, Eilon G *et al.* Identification of a mRNA fraction in human prostatic cancer cells coding for a novel osteoblast stimulating factor. *Endocrinology* (1985) **117**: 1615–20.
99. Koutsilieris M, Rabbani SA, Bennett HP *et al.* Characteristics of prostate-derived growth factors for cells of the osteoblast phenotype. *J Clin Invest* (1987) **80**: 941–6.
100. Harris SE, Boyce B, Feng JQ *et al.* Antisense bone morphogenetic protein 3 (BMP 3) constructions decrease new bone formation in a prostate cancer model. *J Bone Miner Res* (1992) **7 (Suppl 1)**: 92 (abst).
101. Achbarou A, Kaiser S, Tremblay G *et al.* Urokinase overproduction results in increased skeletal metastasis by prostate cancer cells in vivo. *Cancer Res* (1994) **54**: 2372–7.
102. Gingrich JR, Barrios RJ, Morton RA *et al.* Metastatic prostate cancer in a transgenic mouse. *Cancer Res* (1996) **56**: 4096–102.
103. Greenberg NM, DeMayo F, Finegold MJ *et al.* Prostate cancer in a transgenic mouse. *Proc Natl Acad Sci U S A* (1995) **92**: 3439–43.
104. Marquardt H, Lioubin MN, Ikeda T. Complete amino acid sequence of human transforming growth factor type beta 2. *J Biol Chem* (1987) **262**: 12 127–30.
105. Marcelli C, Yates AJP, Mundy GR. In vivo effects of human recombinant transforming growth factor beta on bone turnover in normal mice. *J Bone Miner Res* (1990) **5**: 1087–96.
106. Matuo Y, Nishi N, Matsui S *et al.* Heparin binding affinity of rat prostate growth factor in normal and cancerous prostate: partial purification and characterization of rat prostate growth factor in the Dunning tumor. *Cancer Res* (1987) **47**: 188–92.
107. Mansson PE, Adams P, Kan M *et al.* HBGF1 gene expression in normal rat prostate and two transplantable rat prostate tumors. *Cancer Res* (1989) **49**: 2485–94.
108. Canalis E, Lorenzo J, Burgess WH *et al.* Effects of endothelial cell growth factor on bone remodeling in vitro. *J Clin Invest* (1987) **79**: 52–8.
109. Canalis E, Centrella M, McCarthy T. Effects of basic fibroblast growth factor on bone formation in vitro. *J Clin Invest* (1988) **81**: 1572–7.
110. Mayahara H, Ito T, Nagai H *et al.* In vivo stimulation of endosteal bone formation by basic fibroblast growth factor in rats. *Growth Factors* (1993) **9**: 73–80.

111. Dunstan CR, Garrett IR, Adams R et al. Systemic fibroblast growth factor (FGF-1) prevents bone loss, increases new bone formation, and restores trabecular microarchitecture in ovariectomized rats. *J Bone Miner Res* (1995) **10 (Suppl 1):** 279 (abst).

112. Izbicka E, Dunstan C, Esparza J et al. Human amniotic tumor which induces new bone formation in vivo produces a growth regulatory activity in vitro for osteoblasts identified as an extended form of basic fibroblast growth factor (bFGF). *Cancer Res* (1996) **56:** 633–6.

113. Rabbani SA, Desjardins J, Bell AW et al. An amino-terminal fragment of urokinase isolated from a prostate cancer cell line (PC-3) is mitogenic for osteoblast-like cells. *Biochem Biophys Res Commun* (1990) **173:** 1058–64.

114. Rabbani SA, Desjardins J, Bell AW et al. Identification of a new osteoblast mitogen from a human prostate cancer cell line, PC-3. *J Bone Miner Res* (1990) **5 (Suppl):** 549 (abst).

115. Rabbani SA, Mazar AP, Bernier SM et al. Structural requirements for the growth factor activity of the amino-terminal domain of urokinase. *J Biol Chem* (1992) **267:** 14 151–6.

116. Dallas SL, Park-Snyder S, Miyazono K et al. Characterization and autoregulation of latent TGFβ complexes in osteoblast-like cell lines: production of a latent complex lacking the latent TGFβ-binding protein (LTBP). *J Biol Chem* (1994) **269:** 6815–22.

117. Dallas SL, Miyazono K, Skerry TM et al. Dual role for the latent transforming growth factor-beta binding protein in storage of latent TGF-beta in the extracellular matrix and as a structural matrix protein. *J Cell Biol* (1995) **131:** 539–49.

118. Harris SE, Bonewald LF, Harris MA et al. Effects of transforming growth factor beta on bone nodule formation and expression of bone morphogenic protein 2, osteocalcin, osteopontin, alkaline phosphatase, and type 1 collagen mRNA in long-term cultures of fetal rat calvarial osteoblasts. *J Bone Miner Res* (1994) **9:** 855–63.

119. Stewart AF. PTHrP (1-36) as a skeletal anabolic agent for the treatment of osteoporosis. *Bone* (1996) **19:** 303–6.

120. Cramer SD, Chen Z, Peehl DM. Prostate specific antigen cleaves parathyroid hormone-related protein in the PTH-like domain: inactivation of PTH-rP stimulated cAMP accumulation in mouse osteoblasts. *J Urol* (1996) **156:** 526–31.

121. Takuwa Y, Ohue Y, Takuwa N et al. Endothelin-1 activates phopholipase C and mobilizes Ca2+ from extra- and intracellular pools in osteoblastic cells. *Am J Physiol* (1989) **257:** E797–803.

122. Takuwa Y, Masaki T, Yamashita K. The effects of the endothelin family peptides on cultured osteoblastic cells from rat calvariae. *Biochem Biophys Res Commun* (1990) **170:** 998–1005.

123. Langenstroer P, Tang R, Shapiro E et al. Endothelin-1 in the human prostate: tissue levels, source of production and isometric tension studies. *J Urol* (1993) **150:** 495–9.

124. Tofe AJ, Francis MD, Harvey WJ. Correlation of neoplasms with incidence and localization of skeletal metastases. An analysis of 1355 diphosphonate bone scans. *J Nucl Med* (1975) **16:** 986–9.

5

Bone metastases – morphology

Toru Hiraga, Gregory R Mundy and Toshiyuki Yoneda

Introduction • Morphology of bone metastasis • Effects of bisphosphonates on bone metastasis • Conclusion

INTRODUCTION

Bone metabolism is regulated by a variety of systemic and local factors which control the functions of bone cells including osteoblasts, osteoclasts, and osteocytes. In normal conditions, bone continually remodels through coupling between osteoblasts and osteoclasts to maintain dynamic homeostasis. However, once cancer colonizes bone, the coupling process is dramatically disrupted and prominent characteristic morphological changes result. These changes are mainly caused by cytokines and growth factors produced by metastatic cancer cells. Altered cell–cell and cell–extracellular matrix interactions between metastatic cancer cells and host cells or matrix also account for these morphological changes.

This chapter will focus on the morphological characteristics of bone metastasis using materials obtained in an animal experimental model of bone metastasis and patients with bone metastases. In addition, the inhibitory effects of bisphosphonates on bone metastases will also be reviewed morphologically.

MORPHOLOGY OF BONE METASTASIS

Histopathological classification of bone metastasis

Histopathologically, bone metastasis can be classified into four types, namely, osteolytic, osteoblastic, mixed, or intertrabecular type.[1,2] The osteolytic type, which is characterized by extensive destruction of the bony trabeculae, occurs most frequently and induces serious clinical problems such as bone pain, hypercalcemia, and pathological fractures. Amongst tumors that are associated with osteolytic lesions, breast cancer is the most common.[3] Although still controversial, the most widely accepted notion is that osteoclasts play a major role in tumor-associated osteolysis. In our previous histological study[2] using human surgical specimens of untreated bone metastases, the major part of the original bony architecture had been destroyed and the residual bone surrounding or in the metastatic lesions had scalloped surfaces. Although the reactions of bone cells were somewhat different from case to case, numerous multinucleated osteoclasts were observed along the residual bone surface in all cases irrespective of the histological pattern of primary tumors. Mononuclear osteoclast precursor cells were also observed in these lesions.

The osteoblastic type, which is characterized by prominent new bone formation, occurs most commonly in prostate cancer.[3] This type is further classified into two subtypes. One is represented by reactive bone formation, which occurs subsequent to preceding bone resorption.[4] In this type, bone formation frequently occurs on one side of trabecular bone with bone resorption occurring on the opposite side. We have reported that A375 (human melanoma cell line)[5] and HARA (human lung squamous cell carcinoma cell line)[2,6] develop reactive bone formation around tumor nests. The mechanism of reactive bone formation might involve growth factors such as the insulin-like growth factors (IGFs), transforming growth factor β (TGF-β), platelet-derived growth factor (PGDF), fibroblast growth factors (FGFs), and bone morphogenetic proteins (BMPs) that are stored in bone and released during bone resorption.[7] These factors are known to stimulate bone formation and tumor cell proliferation. Nemoto et al.[8] reported that the extent of reactive bone formation appears to correlate inversely with the rate of tumor growth. It seems likely that the reactive bone formation occurs when tumor cells grow slowly at the metastatic sites.

The other type of bone formation response is represented by direct stimulation of osteoblasts by tumor cells, leading to bone formation without evidence for preceding bone resorption. In this type, soluble factors produced by tumor cells, such as TGF-β, IGFs, FGFs, BMPs, urokinase-type plasminogen activator (uPA), and endothelin-1 (ET-1), have been implicated in the pathogenesis.[3]

The mixed type shows transitional or mixed features of the osteoblastic and osteolytic type. It is generally recognized that tumor-induced bone formation and resorption are not coupled but closely related. According to Fornasier and Horne,[9] who examined 140 cases with vertebral metastases at autopsy, the majority of bone metastases showed a combination of both lytic and sclerotic features. The mechanism by which mixed-type metastases are formed is unknown. One likely mechanism is that tumor cells produce both osteolytic and osteoblastic factors. Alternatively, it is also possible that the reactive bone formation results from an excessive response to preceding or conjunctive bone resorption.

The intertrabecular type of bone metastasis is characterized by the infiltration of tumor cells in the bone marrow space without significant substantial changes of trabecular bone.[1] Some oncologists differentiate bone metastasis (with bone destruction) from bone marrow metastasis (with no bone destruction).[10] According to their classification, the intertrabecular type is categorized as bone marrow metastasis. The mechanism underlying the development of this type of metastases has not been extensively examined. Yamaguchi et al.[1] reported that 255 out of 734 metastatic lesions of vertebral bodies were of this intertrabecular type. The major clinical problem in the intertrabecular type of bone metastases is the difficulty of radiographical detection. Detection rates on roentgenogram or bone scan were less than 10%.

Animal experimental model

One approach to study the morphological features of bone metastasis in a well controlled and systematic manner is to develop reproducible animal models of bone metastasis. In earlier studies of experimental bone metastasis, tumor cells were injected adjacent to bone[8] or directly into the bone marrow cavity[11] to establish tumor growth in bone, but these models represent only the final stage of bone metastasis and, thus, are obviously different from the natural course of bone metastasis. Recently, the intravascular approach comprising intra-arterial,[12] intravenous,[13] and intracardiac[5,14–17] injections has become widely used. One evident disadvantage of these models is that they do not have several critical steps that occur before cancer cells enter the circulation because cells

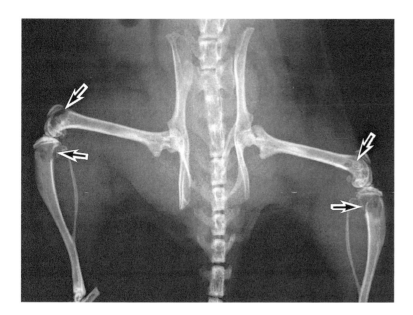

Fig. 5.1 Radiograph of osteolytic lesions developed by MDA-231 human breast cancer. Distinct radiolucent lesions (arrows) are observed.

are directly introduced into the blood stream. In our experiments, the cardiac injection model, which was initially described by Arguello *et al.* in 1988 using B16 melanoma cells,[14] is used. In this model bone metastases reproducibly develop and thus morphological studies are readily performed. The model is also useful in evaluating the effects of drugs such as bisphosphonates on bone metastases and developing potential therapeutic agents.[15–17]

Of the four types of bone metastases described above, the osteolytic type is the most common in animal models (as it is in human disease). Osteolytic metastases can be easily detected by radiographs as well circumscribed radiolucent lesions (Fig. 5.1). On the other hand, there are only a very limited number of models available for the study of the osteoblastic type. Nemoto[8] and Izbicka *et al.*[18] reported tumor-induced bone formation by inoculations of tumor cells on calvariae. These authors suggest the involvement of osteoblastic cytokines produced by tumor cells in the development of osteoblastic bone lesions. The intertrabecular type of bone metastasis has been also rarely described. We found that B16/F1 mouse melanoma cells formed intertrabecular type bone metastases.[2] To study the mechanism underlying these diverse reactions of bone cells to cancer metastasis, reliable animal models for each of the respective types of bone metastasis are needed.

Osteoclastogenesis induced by tumor

There is now general agreement that osteoclasts play a major role in tumor-associated bone destruction. However, the mechanisms responsible for osteoclastogenesis induced by metastatic tumors still remain largely unclear.

In the case of A375 cells, even 1 week after cell inoculation, small tumor nests with well vascularized stroma and resorption of trabecular bone are observed histologically.[2] When stained with tartrate-resistant acid phosphatase (TRAPase), a marker enzyme of the osteoclastic cell lineage, numerous TRAPase-positive cells are observed surrounding A375 tumor. The findings suggest that even at early stages of metastasis, osteoclastogenesis had already been stimulated by A375 tumor. At 5 weeks, the bone marrow was almost completely replaced by metastatic A375 tumor cells.[5] Many TRAPase-positive multinucleated osteoclasts are seen along the endosteal bone surface with formation of Howship's lacunae and TRAPase-positive cement line (Fig. 5.2). The number of osteoclasts is aberrantly increased in

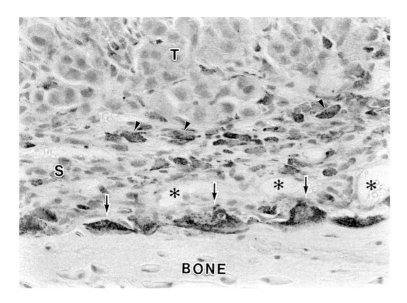

Fig. 5.2 Histological view of a metastatic lesion developed by A375 human melanoma. Many TRAPase-positive multinucleated cells (arrows) are seen along the bone surface with formation of resorption lacunae and TRAPase-positive cement line. Between the tumor (T) and bone surface, a well vascularized stromal cell layer (S) is observed. TRAPase-positive mononuclear cells (arrow heads) are also present in stromal cell layer. (* = blood vessel; TRAPase staining.)

metastatic lesions compared with that in those sites where no metastases formed. Between tumor nests and bone surfaces, well vascularized stromal cell layers were occasionally observed and TRAPase-positive mononuclear cells were present in these stromal cells. TRAPase-positive mononuclear cells were also present in the tumor nests distant from the bone surfaces. Autoradiographic studies using ^{125}I-calcitonin exhibited specific binding of calcitonin to these mononuclear cells,[2] which is one of the characteristic features of the osteoclastic cell lineage.[19] In addition, ultrastructural examination showed that these cells were round or ovoid in shape and characterized by irregularly shaped nuclei, numerous mitochondria, and Golgi apparatus distributed around the nuclei. These findings, which include 1) positive for TRAPase staining, 2) presence of calcitonin receptors, and 3) characteristic ultrastructure, suggest that these TRAPase-positive cells are osteoclast precursor cells and that tumor cells promoted the differentiation and activation of osteoclasts.

Stromal cells and extracellular matrix (ECM) as well as tumor cells themselves also play important roles in the biological behavior of tumors. Similar events also occur at the sites of bone metastases. Ultrastructurally, although osteoclast precursors are occasionally in direct contact with tumor cells, suggesting that tumor cells directly induce the differentiation of osteoclasts, stromal cells or ECM usually exist between tumor cells and osteoclast precursor cells. It has been suggested that direct contact of osteoblasts or stromal cells with hematopoietic cells is necessary for osteoclast differentiation.[20,21] Our findings are consistent with the notion that the interactions between stromal cells and osteoclast precursor cells are also important in the process of osteoclast formation.

However, the nature of these stromal cells is not clear at the present time. Bone marrow stroma is composed of fibroblasts, endothelial cells, macrophages, and reticular-like cells.[22] Stromal cells present in bone metastases are probably derived from bone marrow stromal cells. From the morphological point of view, stromal cells represent mesenchymal fibroblast-like cells, and endothelial cells and macrophages surrounding tumor cells are not included. In our previous study,[2] stromal cells in the metastatic bony lesions were positive for alkaline phosphatase (ALPase). In bone, osteoblasts and preosteoblasts are positive for ALPase.[23] Bone marrow stromal cells also have been reported to express ALPase activity when cultured under the appropriate conditions.[24] These ALPase-positive stromal cells were in contact with TRAPase-positive mononuclear cells present in tumor cells that were isolated from the bone surfaces.[2]

To study the role of ECM in osteoclastogenesis, distribution of heparan-sulfate proteoglycan (HSPG) and fibronectin (FN) was examined using immunohistochemical techniques in the model of A375 cells.[5] HSPG was observed in the stroma present around tumor nests, but not in tumor cells. TRAPase-positive cells were embedded in the HSPG-positive stroma. HSPG was also positive in the stroma distant from bone surface. HSPG is a ubiquitous component of stroma, which retains heparin-binding growth factors such as FGF and GM-CSF,[25,26] and protects these growth factors from degradation and inactivation.[27] It is also reported that HSPG binds with a bone resorption activating factor released from osteoblasts.[28] FN showed a pattern of localization essentially similar to that of HSPG. In addition, FN, which has heparin-binding sites, may also be bound to heparin sulfate chains of HSPG. The finding that many osteoclast precursor cells were observed in the stroma rich in HSPG and FN may suggest that these ECMs play an important role in providing a microenvironment favorable for osteoclast differentiation and activation. Although the origin of HSPG and FN is unknown, dense localization of these ECMs around tumor nests leads us to suggest that tumor cells contribute to the deposition of these extracellular matrix components.

A number of cytokines are known to be stimulators of osteoclastic bone resorption. At the sites of bone metastases, parathyroid hormone-related protein (PTH-rP) is the most well-known cytokine.[6,29] When MDA-231 (human breast cancer cell line) or HARA, both of which produce PTH-rP, were tested in the cardiac injection model, they showed extensive osteoclastic bone resorption. However, S375 cells, which do not produce PTH-rP, also form osteolytic lesions in a similar manner to MDA-231 and HARA. In bone metastases caused by A375 cells, expression of interleukin-6 (IL-6), prostaglandin E2 (PGE2), and transforming growth factor α (TGF-α) has been shown by immunohistochemistry, suggesting these factors might play a role in osteoclast differentiation and activation.[5] Therefore, it is likely that PTH-rP plays a major role in tumor-induced bone resorption in cancers such as breast cancer, but other cytokines are involved in other tumors.

Angiogenesis is essential for the development and remodeling of tissues. It is also a critical factor to the growth, progression, and metastasis of malignant tumors. To stimulate angiogenesis, tumor cells produce angiogenetic cytokines. For example, several breast cancer cell lines and primary human breast tumors express vascular growth factors including vascular endothelial growth factor (VEGF), placenta growth factor, pleiotrophin, TGF-β1, acidic and basic fibroblast growth factor (FGF), and platelet-derived endothelial cell growth factor.[30] In bone, angiogenesis is probably important for bone formation, remodeling, and possibly osteoclastgenesis. At the metastatic sites in bone, tumor growth is always accompanied by angiogenesis. Harada et al.[31] reported that VEGF, a secreted endothelial cell-specific mitogen, was produced by osteoblasts, implicating VEGF in bone metabolism. An immunohistochemical study has shown that VEGF was found in tumor cells in all cases of bone metastases in cancer patients.[32]

Direct bone resorption by tumor cells

As to whether tumor cells directly resorb bone is still controversial. Osteocytes,[33] monocytes,[34] macrophages,[35] and some tumor cells[36–38] in addition to osteoclasts have been reported to resorb bone. According to Galasko,[36] there are two mechanisms of bone destruction by tumors. The first mechanism is explained by osteoclastic bone destruction and responsible for the early phase of bone metastasis; the second mechanism involves nonosteoclastic bone destruction that occurs at a later phase of bone metastasis. Eilon et al.[37] described direct bone resorption by MCF-7 human breast cancer cells using organ cultures of devitalized bone. Recently, Sanchez-Sweatman et al.[38] showed some lines of evidence for tumor-mediated osteolysis by B16/F1 melanoma cells *in vitro* and *in vivo*. *In vivo* they found that B16/F1 cells were in direct contact

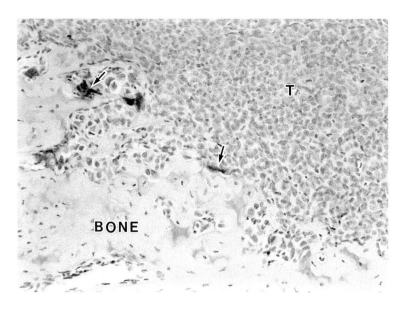

Fig. 5.3 Histological view of a metastatic lesion developed by MDA-231 human breast cancer treated with ibandronate. Number of TRAPase-positive cells (arrows) are markedly decreased. (T = tumor; TRAPase staining.)

with resorbing bone surfaces, and the number of osteoclasts and osteoblasts was reduced dramatically in the affected bones. Their *in vitro* study using scanning electron microscopy displayed pit formation on bone surfaces by B16/F1 cells. It was also shown that B16/F1 cells produce matrix metalloproteinases (MMPs). From these findings, these authors suggest that direct bone resorption is partially mediated by MMPs.[14]

In our animal experiments using A375 cells,[5] many osteoclasts were usually observed at the sites of osteolysis, suggesting that they are involved in tumor-induced bone resorption. At the tumor and bone interface, osteoclasts, osteoblasts, bone lining cells, and/or stromal cells were usually present, and tumor cells rarely contacted bone directly. Even when tumor cells were juxtaposed to bone surfaces with a scalloped appearance and osteoclasts were not identified on sections stained with haematoxylin and eosin, TRAPase staining clearly demonstrated the presence of osteoclasts. These osteoclasts were small and flat and the TRAPase activity was weak compared to that of representative osteoclasts. Obviously, they were not actively resorbing bone. The presence of these cells, however, may indicate that they had once been involved in bone resorption. In our hands, using the heart injection model, B16/F1 cells formed the intertrabecular type of bone metastasis.[2] Tumor cells grew and invaded into intertrabecular spaces without causing trabecular bone resorption. TRAPase-positive cells were observed on bone surfaces, but their number was not increased. We did not observe direct bone resorption by B16/F1 cells ultrastructurally (unpublished data).

Because tumor cells clearly have the capacity to resorb bone directly, it is difficult to exclude the possibility of direct bone resorption by tumor cells *in vivo*, and even more difficult to assess its relative importance compared with osteoclastic bone resorption. Nonetheless, bone resorption is always associated with the occurrence of osteoclasts at bone metastatic sites in all tumors we have studied. To prove a major role for direct bone resorption by tumor cells *in vivo*, more extensive ultrastructural studies may be required.

EFFECTS OF BISPHOSPHONATES ON BONE METASTASIS

The primary effect of bisphosphonates is the inhibition of osteoclastic bone resorption. Some bisphosphonates have been developed and used in the treatment of hyper-resorptive bone diseases, such as Paget's disease, myeloma,

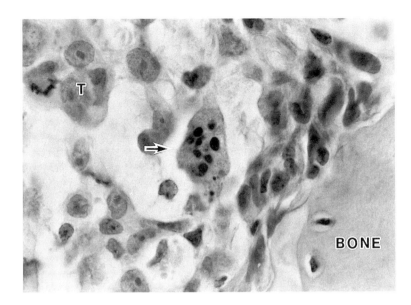

Fig. 5.4 An apoptotic osteoclast (arrow) in a metastatic lesion developed by MDA-231 human breast cancer treated with ibandronate. The morphological features of apoptosis (chromatin condensation and nuclear fragmentation) are clearly represented. (T = tumor; hematoxylin and eosin staining.)

hypercalcemia, osteoporosis, and bone metastasis. There is unanimous agreement that the ultimate cellular target of bisphosphonate action is the osteoclast, although it is possible that the inhibitory effects on osteoclasts may be mediated by intermediary cells. According to Fleisch,[39] bisphosphonates reduce osteoclastic bone resorption through: 1) inhibition of osteoclast recruitment; 2) inhibition of osteoclastic adhesion to the mineralized matrix; 3) shortening of the osteoclast life-span; and 4) inhibition of osteoclast activity. At the molecular level, it has been proposed that bisphosphonates are potent inhibitors of the vacuolar H^+-ATPase[40] and protein-tyrosine phosphatase (PTP) activity in osteoclasts.[41] Recently, Luckman et al.[42] reported that nitrogen-containing bisphosphonates inhibited the mevalonate pathway which is involved in cholesterol biosynthesis. This may be a potential molecular target of bisphosphonates. But the detailed mechanisms of action are yet to be elucidated. Furthermore, the mode of action may differ among bisphosphonates.

Animal experiments

Administration of bisphosphonates initially increased the number of multinucleated osteoclasts on bone surface, followed by a subsequent decrease in osteoclast number.[39] The initial increase in osteoclast number may be a reaction to compensate for the decrease in osteoclast activity. At the sites of bone metastases in animal experiments, the number of osteoclasts was decreased regardless of the dose and duration of bisphosphonate treatment[15–17] (Fig. 5.3). Even 3 days after a single injection of YM175, there was a decrease in osteoclast number.[2,16]

Bisphosphonates also cause various morphological changes which indicate impaired activity of osteoclasts.[16,43] After treatment with bisphosphonates, osteoclasts become round in shape and lose cell polarity. Changes in the cytoskeleton, especially actin and vinculin, are likely responsible for these changes.[44] Some osteoclasts become detached from bone surfaces and occasionally vacuolated. Histochemically, most osteoclasts are only weakly and/or homogeneously stained with TRAPase. Ultrastructurally, they are round and devoid of ruffled borders and clear zones. Cytoplasmic vacuoles frequently accumulate in the cytosol, indicating degeneration of osteoclasts. Osteoclast apoptosis is prominent, suggesting that bisphosphonates cause irreversible damage to osteoclasts and thus shorten their life-span[45] (Fig. 5.4). In addition to these effects on mature osteoclasts, inhibition of the recruitment of osteoclasts is also an important mechanism of action of bisphosphonates. Several bisphosphonates have been reported to inhibit osteoclast differentiation.[39] At sites of bone metastases, there is an obvious decrease in the number of osteoclast precursor cells. In the case of A375 cells,[16] a marked reduction in the stromal cell number is also observed. Although the biological significance of the effects of bisphosphonates on stromal cells is currently unknown, this decrease in stromal cell number may be one of the causes of the decrease in osteoclast precursor cells. As described, the decrease in osteoclast number appears to be due to increased apoptosis and inhibition of osteoclast recruitment.

The effects of bisphosphonates on tumor cells are unclear. Sasaki et al. reported that continuous treatment with risedronate[15] and YH529[17] decreased tumor burden. However, a single injection of YM175[16] did not cause evident morphological changes in tumor cells. One possibility is that continuous treatment of bisphosphonates might increase trabecular bone area which in turn prevents tumor cells from proliferating due to the limited space available in bone. Another possibility is an impairment of osteoclast activity might decrease release of growth factors stored in bone matrix which are essential for stimulation to tumor cell growth in bone. In addition, recent reports have described direct effects of bisphosphonates on tumor cells. Shipman et al.[46] and Aparicio et al.[47] reported that pamidronate, YM175, and zoledronate induced apoptosis in myeloma cells, although the doses of these bisphosphonates were pharmacological. Furthermore, Diel et al.[48] have shown that adjuvant treatment of clodronate together with conventional chemotherapy reduced the incidence of not only bone metastases but also visceral metastases in breast cancer patients, resulting in prolonged survival of these patients.

Human specimens

Over two decades have passed since bisphosphonates were used for the treatment of malignant bone diseases. However, there are few reports describing the morphological changes induced by these drugs in clinical samples. Because patients with bone metastases are usually treated with various chemotherapeutic agents and/or irradiation, it is difficult to study the sole effects of bisphosphonates.

We reported the effects of pamidronate on bone metastasis in a patient with a squamous cell carcinoma of the tongue.[49] The morphological changes caused by pamidronate were essentially similar to those seen in animal experiments. The bone marrow space was occupied by tumor cells and bone surfaces showed a scalloped appearance. Essentially similar findings were obtained in patients without bisphosphonate treatment, but multinucleated giant cells were rarely seen on the bone surfaces with bisphosphonate treatment. Histochemical and ultrastructural observations of osteoclasts and their precursor cells were also similar to the results of animal experiments.

When the effects of bisphosphonates on bone metastases are examined in patients, it is impossible to estimate the bone resorbing activity of tumor cells before bisphosphonate treatment. Therefore, in our experiments, tumor cells obtained from a metastatic submandibular lymph node of a patient were established in culture and injected in the left ventricle of nude mice. In a metastatic lesion which developed in a vertebra, most of the original bone was replaced by tumor cells and the remaining bone underwent osteoclastic resorption. Many osteoclasts and their precursor cells were observed, which suggests the tumor cells have the capacity to induce osteoclast formation and activation. Thus, animal models of bone metastasis may be useful in evaluating the capacity of human tumor cells to stimulate osteoclastogenesis and bone resorption *in vivo*.

CONCLUSION

Bone is one of the most common sites of cancer metastasis. Despite its clinical importance, morphological observations which should serve to determine the mechanisms responsible for bone metastasis have not been extensive. This has been partly due to the lack of adequate experimental models. However, the recent development of improved animal models such as those described here should allow us to study bone metastases *in vivo* in detail morphologically. The combination of conventional histological techniques together with modern techniques such as immunohistochemistry and *in situ* hybridization will be required to further our understanding of the mechanisms underlying bone metastases at molecular levels.

REFERENCES

1. Yamaguchi T, Tamai K, Yamato M *et al.* Intertrabecular pattern of tumor metastatic to bone. *Cancer* (1996) **78**: 1388–94.
2. Hiraga T, Tanaka S, Ikegame M *et al.* Morphology of bone metastasis. *Eur J Cancer* (1998) **34**: 230–9.
3. Guise TA, Mundy GR. Cancer and bone. *Endocrine Rev* (1998) **19**: 18–54.
4. Galasko CSB. Mechanism of lytic and blastic metastatic disease of bone. *Clin Orthop Relat Res* (1982) **169**: 20–7.
5. Hiraga T, Nakajima T, Ozawa H. Bone resorption by a metastatic human melanoma cell line. *Bone* (1995) **16**: 349–56.
6. Iguchi H, Tanaka S, Ozawa Y *et al.* An experimental model of bone metastasis by human lung cancer cells: the role of parathyroid hormone-related protein in bone metastasis. *Cancer Res* (1996) **56**: 4040–3.
7. Yoneda T, Sasaki A, Mundy GR. Osteolytic bone metastasis in breast cancer. *Breast Cancer Res Treat* (1994) **32**: 73–84.
8. Nemoto R. New bone formation and cancer implants; relationship to tumour proliferative activity. *Br J Cancer* (1991) **63**: 348–50.
9. Fornasier VL, Horne JG. Metastases to the vertebral column. *Cancer* (1975) **36**: 590–4.
10. McCarthy EF, Frassica FJ. Metastatic carcinoma in bone. In McCarthy EF, Frassica FJ (eds) *Pathology of Bone and Joint Disorders with Clinical and Radiographic Correlation* (Philadelphia, PA: WB Saunders, 1998): 175–83.
11. Krempien B, Wingen F, Eichmann T *et al.* Protective effects of a prophylactic treatment with the bisphosphonate 3-amino-1-hydroxypropane-1,1-bisphosphonic acid on the development of tumor osteopathies in the rat: experimental studies with the Walker carcinosarcoma 256. *Oncology* (1988) **45**: 41–6.
12. Powles TJ, Clark SA, Easty DM *et al.* The inhibition by aspirin and indomethacin of osteolytic tumor deposits and hypercalcemia in rats with Walker tumor, and its possible application to human breast cancer. *Br J Cancer* (1973) **28**: 316–21.
13. Iwakawa M, Ando K, Ohkawa H *et al.* A murine model for bone marrow metastasis established by an i.v. injection of C-1300 neuroblastoma in A/J mice. *Clin Exp Metastasis* (1994) **12**: 231–7.
14. Arguello F, Baggs RB, Frantz CN. A murine model of experimental metastasis to bone and bone marrow. *Cancer Res* (1988) **48**: 6876–81.
15. Sasaki A, Boyce BF, Story B *et al.* Bisphosphonate risedronate reduces metastatic human breast cancer burden in bone in nude mice. *Cancer Res* (1995) **55**: 3551–7.
16. Hiraga T, Tanaka S, Yamamoto M *et al.* Inhibitory effects of bisphosphonate (YM175) on bone resorption induced by a metastatic bone tumor. *Bone* (1996) **18**: 1–8.
17. Sasaki A, Kitamura K, Alcalde RE *et al.* Effect of a newly developed bisphosphonate, YH529, on osteolytic bone metastases in nude mice. *Int J Cancer* (1998) **77**: 279–85.
18. Izbicka E, Dunstan CR, Horn D *et al.* Effects of human tumor cell lines on local new bone formation in vivo. *Calcif Tissue Int* (1997) **60**: 210–15.
19. Hattersley G, Chambers TJ. Calcitonin receptors as markers for osteoclastic differentiation: correlation between generation of bone-resorptive cells and cells that express calcitonin receptors in mouse bone marrow cultures. *Endocrinology* (1989) **125**: 1606–12.
20. Udagawa N, Takahashi N, Akatsu T et al. The bone marrow-derived stromal cell line MC3T3-G2/PA6 and ST2 support osteoclast-like cell differentiation in co-cultures with mouse spleen cells. *Endocrinology* (1989) **125**: 1805–13.
21. Caligaris-Cappis F, Bergui L, Gregoretti MG *et al.* Role of bone marrow stromal cells in the growth of human multiple myeloma. *Blood* (1991) **77**: 2688–93.
22. Takahashi S, Reddy SV, Dallas M *et al.* Development and characterization of a human marrow stromal cell line that enhances osteoclast-like cell formation. *Endocrinology* (1995) **136**: 1441–9.
23. Hoshi K, Amizuka N, Oda K *et al.* Immuno-

localization of tissue non-specific alkaline phosphatase in mice. *Histochem Cell Biol* (1997) **107**: 183–91.
24. Majors AK, Boehm CA, Nitto H *et al.* Characterization of human bone marrow stromal cells with respect to osteoblastic differentiation. *J Orthop Res* (1997) **15**: 546–57.
25. Globus RK, Plouet J, Gospodarowicz D. Cultured bovine bone cells synthesize basic fibroblast growth factor and store it in their extracellular matrix. *Endocrinology* (1989) **124**: 1539–47.
26. Klagsbrun M. The affinity of fibroblast growth factor (FGFs) for heparin; FGF-heparin sulfate interaction in cells and extracellular matrix. *Curr Opin Cell Biol* (1990) **2**: 857–63.
27. Saksela O, Moscatelli D, Sommer A *et al.* Endothelial cell-derived heparin sulfate binds basic growth factor and protects it from proteolytic degradation. *J Cell Biol* (1988) **107**: 743–51.
28. Fuller K, Gallagher AC, Chambers TJ. Osteoclast resorption-stimulating activity is associated with the osteoclast cell surface and/or the extracellular matrix. *Biochem Biophys Res Commun* (1991) **181**: 67–73.
29. Guise TA, Yin JJ, Taylor SD *et al.* Evidence for a causal role of parathyroid hormone-related protein in the pathogenesis of human breast cancer-mediated osteolysis. *J Clin Invest* (1996) **98**: 1544–9.
30. Harris AL, Zhang H, Monghaddam A *et al.* Breast cancer angiogenesis – new approaches to therapy via antiangiogenesis, hypoxic activated drugs, and vascualr targeting. *Breast Cancer Res Treat* (1996) **38**: 97–108.
31. Harada S, Rodan SB, Rodan GA. Expression and regulation of vascular endothelial growth factor in osteoblasts. *Clin Orthop Relat Res* (1995) **313**: 76–80.
32. Hiraga T, Shiraishi S, Nakajima T *et al.* Vascular endothelial growth factor regulates bone metabolism in human bone metastasis. *J Bone Miner Res* (1996) **11 (Suppl 1)**: S480 (abst).
33. Belanger LF. Osteocytic osteolysis. *Calcif Tissue Res* (1969) **4**: 1–12.
34. Mundy GR, Altman AJ, Gondek MD *et al.* Direct resorption of bone by human monocytes. *Science* (1977) **196**: 1109–11.
35. Athanasou NA, Quinn JMW. Human tumor-associated macrophages are capable of bone resorption. *Br J Cancer* (1992) **65**: 523–6.
36. Galasko CSB. Mechanisms of bone destruction in the development of skeletal metastasis. *Nature* (1976) **263**: 507–8.
37. Eilon G, Mundy GR. Direct resorption of bone by human breast cancer cells in vitro. *Nature* (1978) **276**: 726–8.
38. Sanchez-Sweatman OH, Lee J, Orr FW *et al.* Direct osteolysis induced by metastatic murine melanoma cells: role of matrix metalloproteinases. *Eur J Cancer* (1997) **33**: 918–25.
39. Fleisch H. Bisphosphonates: mechanism of action. *Endocrine Rev* (1998) **19**: 80–100.
40. David P, Nguyen H, Barbier A *et al.* The bisphosphonate tiludronate is a potent inhibitor of the osteoclast vacuolar H^+-ATPase. *J Bone Miner Res* (1996) **11**: 1498–507.
41. Skorey K, Ly HD, Hammond M *et al.* How does alendronate inhibit protein-tyrosine phosphatase? *J Biol Chem* (1997) **272**: 22 472–80.
42. Luckman SP, Hughes DE, Coxon FP *et al.* Nitrogen-containing bisphosphonates inhibit the mevalonate pathway and prevent post-transitional prenylation of GTP-binding protein, including Ras. *J Bone Miner Res* (1998) **13**: 581–9.
43. Sato M, Grasser W, Endo N *et al.* Bisphosphonate action: alendronate localization in rat bone and effects on osteoclast ultrastructure. *J Clin Invest* (1991) **88**: 2095–105.
44. Selander K, Lehenkari P, Vaananen HK. The effects of bisphosphonates on the resorption cycle of isolated osteoclasts. *Calcif Tissue Int* (1995) **55**: 368–75.
45. Hughes DE, Wright KR, Uy HL *et al.* Bisphosphonates promote apoptosis in murine osteoclasts in vitro and in vivo. *J Bone Miner Res* (1995) **10**: 1478–87.
46. Shipman CM, Rogers MJ, Apperley JF *et al.* Bisphosphonates induce apoptosis in human myeloma cell lines: a novel anti tumor activity. *Br J Haematol* (1997) **98**: 665–72.
47. Aparicio A, Gardner A, Tu Y *et al.* In vitro cytoreductive effects on multiple myeloma cells induced by bisphosphonates. *Leukemia* (1998) **12**: 220–9.
48. Diel IJ, Solomayer E-F, Costa SD *et al.* Reduction in new metastases in breast cancer with adjuvant clodronate treatment. *N Engl J Med* (1998) **339**: 357–63.
49. Hiraga T, Takada M, Nakajima T *et al.* Effects of bisphosphonate (pamidronate) on bone resorption resulting from metastases of a human squamous cell carcinoma. Report of an autopsy case and evaluation of bone resorbing activity by animal experimental model. *J Oral Maxillofac Surg* (1996) **54**: 1327–33.

6

Hypercalcemia

Vivian Grill and T John Martin

Clinical features • Differential diagnosis • Hypercalcemia in cancer • Treatment • Significance of PTHrP as a predictor of response to treatment of hypercalcemia of malignancy with bisphosphonates • Summary and perspective

The blood level of calcium is maintained within very narrow limits in healthy people. This is achieved through the actions of parathyroid hormone (PTH) on the skeleton to promote bone resorption and on the kidney to restrict calcium excretion, with dietary calcium provided mainly through the action of 1,25 dihydroxyvitamin D in promoting intestinal calcium absorption. The bone action of PTH makes use of several locally produced cytokines whose production is influenced by the hormone and which enhance bone resorption. The calcium ion is an essential regulator of many body processes, including muscle contraction, neuronal excitation, and many secretory mechanisms. Its physiological importance is such that it is not surprising that profound effects result when its homeostatic controls are breached.

CLINICAL FEATURES

Many patients with cancer develop the metabolic complication of hypercalcemia. This occurs especially commonly with squamous cell carcinoma of the lung, breast cancer, renal cortical carcinoma, and a number of hematological malignancies. Indeed malignancy is the most frequent cause of hypercalcemia in a general hospital patient population, whereas primary hyperparathyroidism is a more common cause of elevated blood calcium in the community at large.

Hypercalcemia may present with symptoms referrable to almost any organ system.[1] The severity of the symptoms in the individual patient depends on the level of the plasma calcium, on how rapidly it rose, and on the general medical condition of the patient. The clinical features of hypercalcemia are the same regardless of the etiology, although patients with malignant disease and hypercalcemia usually have a significant tumor burden, sometimes with widespread metastases and are often symptomatic from the disease process itself. Because symptoms are nonspecific they may be confused with features of malignant disease. It is important to recognize those symptoms and signs which may be caused by hypercalcemia because hypercalcemia is reversible with appropriate treatment, and its progression can be prevented if it is recognized early.

Table 6.1 summarizes the main features of hypercalcemia, illustrating the substantial involvement of several major organ systems which is evident in those patients who are severely affected. It is important to note that a mild elevation of plasma calcium can manifest

Table 6.1 Symptoms and signs of hypercalcemia

Renal
    polyuria and thirst
    dehydration
Gastrointestinal
    nausea and anorexia
    vomiting
    constipation
    abdominal pain
Neurological
    headache
    confusion
    psychosis
    drowsiness
    coma

itself with quite subtle clinical features. This is particularly to be remembered in patients with cancer, in whom such symptoms can so readily be ascribed to the cancer itself.

Major renal manifestations of hypercalcemia are polyuria and polydipsia, which occur because hypercalcemia interferes with antidiuretic hormone action at the distal nephron, causing a syndrome like diabetes insipidus. The resulting dehydration further exacerbates the hypercalcemia. In patients with hypercalcemia it is important to seek a history of thirst and polyuria, symptoms which are often not volunteered. Particularly in elderly subjects, nocturia is common, and the clinician needs to be alert to the significance of a requirement for fluid at the time of nocturnal voiding.

The gastrointestinal symptoms of hypercalcemia are constipation, nausea and vomiting, and abdominal pain, with severe anorexia, nausea, and vomiting as early and frequent features in the hypercalcemia associated with malignancy. It is obvious that a selection of these symptoms can be associated with many diseases. This is a particular problem in patients with cancer, where it is easy to ascribe any of these gastrointestinal symptoms to the underlying disease, or to cytotoxic or radiation therapy.

Neurological manifestations of hypercalcemia occur in over 50% of patients. They consist of cognitive and behavioural changes, alteration in the level of consciousness, and neuromuscular disturbances. The most subtle symptom is frequently some difficulty in concentrating on a common task, e.g. reading, calculation. This is usually not volunteered and the history needs to be elicited by someone aware of the possibility. Mild mental disturbances consist of fatigue, distractability, and a neurasthenic personality change which is often characterized by lack of initiative and depression. Severe psychiatric symptoms may resemble mania, schizophrenia, acute confusion, and even catatonic stupor. A common sequence of events is of a patient with moderate hypercalcemia whose fluid intake decreases because of some mental confusion, perhaps compounded by anorexia and nausea. The further fluid depletion results in more severe hypercalcemia, with progression to drowsiness and coma.

DIFFERENTIAL DIAGNOSIS

Although there are a number of possible causes of hypercalcemia which need to be recalled (Table 6.2), the major decision necessary in patients with cancer is whether the high calcium is due to the cancer or to primary hyperparathyroidism. The latter is such a common condition, and so readily treatable, that it needs to be excluded in all hypercalcemic subjects, even in the presence of coexistent malignancy. Hypercalcemia in cancer can occur even when the cancer is clinically occult. A number of laboratory tests are helpful to establish the cause of hypercalcemia. Plasma phosphate is usually below the normal range in primary hyperparathyroidism and in humoral hypercalcemia of malignancy (HHM) because of the phosphaturic effects of PTH and PTHrP (Table 6.3). If renal function is significantly impaired, this lowering of phosphate is not seen. In distinguishing between primary hyperparathy-

Table 6.2 Causes of hypercalcemia

Primary hyperparathyroidism
    adenoma
    hyperplasia
    carcinoma
    MEN I and II

Malignant disease
    solid tumors with bone metastases
    humoral hypercalcemia of malignancy
    hematological malignancy

Sarcoidosis and other granulomatous disorders

Endocrine causes
    thyrotoxicosis
    Addison's disease
    pheochromocytoma

Immobilization

Drug induced
    vitamin D
    vitamin A
    lithium
    theophylline
    thiazides

Milk-alkali syndrome

Familial hypocalciuric hypercalcemia

Table 6.3 Biochemical features of primary hyperparathyroidism and humoral hypercalcemia of malignancy (HHM)

	HHM	Primary hyperparathyroidism
Plasma calcium	high	high
Plasma phosphorus	low	low
Nephrogenous cAMP	high	high
Plasma chloride	low	high
Plasma bicarbonate	high	low

roidism and HHM, plasma bicarbonate and chloride can provide useful information since a mild hyperchloremic acidosis often accompanies primary hyperparathyroidism, whereas a mild hypokalemic, hypochloremic alkalosis can accompany the humoral hypercalcemia of malignancy syndrome.

Plasma assay for PTH has reached a level of sensitivity that makes it the single most important measurement in the differential diagnosis of hypercalcemia. There are now widely available two-site assays which detect full-length PTH. A nonsuppressed level in the presence of an elevated plasma calcium concentration points to primary hyperparathyroidism as the diagnosis. The sensitivity of the two-site assays is such that in nonparathyroid hypercalcemia the PTH level is usually suppressed below the normal range.

Although there is no existing assay which convincingly measures PTHrP in the plasma of normal adults, assays detect PTHrP in 90–100% of patients with the humoral hypercalcemia of malignancy, and in 50–70% of subjects with breast cancer-associated hypercalcemia. The use of this assay is often to confirm a diagnosis which is suspected, or to monitor cancer treatment. However, the PTHrP levels are so invariably elevated in patients with HHM that, in a given patient suspected on clinical grounds to have HHM, failure to detect PTHrP would raise the possibility of primary hyperparathyroidism coexistent with the cancer. More detailed discussion of the PTHrP assay will follow.

HYPERCALCEMIA IN CANCER

Because the pathophysiology of hypercalcemia is heterogeneous, it has been traditionally considered as three separate syndromes in cancer: 1) humoral hypercalcemia of malignancy; 2) hypercalcemia associated with localized osteolysis due to bone metastases; and 3) hypercalcemia associated with myeloma and other hematological malignancies.

Our understanding of the ways in which various tumors induce hypercalcemia has increased rapidly in the last few years with the identification of several tumor-derived factors that elevate plasma calcium. The division into these three syndrome classes is now less clear-cut than it was, and the following discussion attempts to clarify this.

Humoral hypercalcemia of malignancy

The term 'humoral hypercalcemia of malignancy' (HHM) was introduced[2] to describe patients with certain cancers in whom the blood calcium is elevated in the absence of skeletal metastases. The most common cause of this is squamous cell carcinoma of the lung. Squamous cell cancers at other sites, including skin, oesophagus, and head and neck, and also renal cortical carcinoma, primary liver cancer, breast cancer, pancreatic cancer, bladder and prostatic carcinoma, and melanoma, may all be associated with humoral hypercalcemia. In the absence of secondary lesions, removal of the primary tumor results in resolution of the hypercalcemia.[3] Tumor factors are secreted that act on the skeleton generally to increase bone resorption, and on the kidney to reduce calcium excretion and increase phosphorus excretion.[2] Nephrogenous cyclic AMP excretion is also increased,[4-6] and there is often a mild hypokalemic, hypochloremic alkalosis.

The degree of hypercalcemia can remain constant for many months; sometimes it progresses steadily and sometimes apparently stable hypercalcemia can progress rapidly to severe and even life-threatening forms. This may occur without any obvious explanation, or be associated with rapid progression of tumor. Alternatively, it may be a consequence of dehydration in the patient in association with treatment or coexistent infection. As pointed out earlier, the symptoms of hypercalcemia are convincing enough as a group, but when they occur singly or in various combinations, the diagnosis need not be so obvious. Thus, for example, the clinician must resist the temptation to ascribe nausea or headache to the cancer or its treatment, and be very aware of the possibility of development of symptomatic hypercalcemia.

It is clear that patients with HHM resemble those with primary hyperparathyroidism in their main biochemical features, a similarity which has been recognized for many years. In 1941, in discussing a case of hypercalcemia and hypophosphatemia in a patient with renal cortical carcinoma, Fuller Albright proposed that the hypercalcemia might be due to production by the cancer of PTH.[7] In succeeding years this idea gained acceptance, and the term 'ectopic PTH syndrome' was widely used to apply to patients with cancer who had a high plasma calcium, low phosphorus, and minimal or no bony metastases. Support for this came in 1966 when Berson and Yalow published results with the first radioimmunoassay for PTH, in which they found significant elevations of the PTH level in a number of unselected patients with lung cancer.[8] Over the next several years until the early 1970s, several reports were published of measurable PTH (by radioimmunoassay) in extracts of cancer from such patients.[1,2] There was one report of an arteriovenous gradient across a tumor bed, indicating release of PTH from tumor,[9] and production of immunoreactive PTH was shown by a cell culture established from a renal cortical carcinoma of a hypercalcemic patient.[10] However, throughout this time it was evident that the radioimmunoassay of PTH presented technical problems, and in none of the above instances were circulating levels of PTH convincingly very high – certainly not at the levels frequently found with corresponding degrees of elevation of plasma calcium in patients with primary hyperparathyroidism. Three groups of workers in the early 1970s published results indicating that the circulating immunoreactive PTH in the cancer patients differed from 'authentic' PTH.[11-13] The levels in plasma were in these cases lower than in primary hyperparathyroidism; in one series the cancer immunoreactivity was significantly nonparallel to PTH standards[12] and in another it was of higher molecular weight than PTH.[13]

Thus the early 1970s saw some doubt arising that PTH itself was a major contributor to the

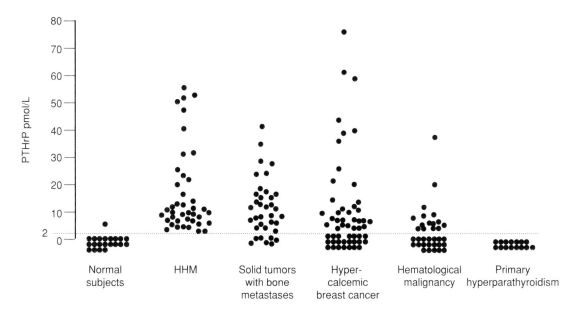

Fig. 6.1 Circulating PTHrP levels by N-terminal radioimmunoassay in different clinical groups

clinical and biochemical features of this cancer syndrome. This doubt became more firmly based when Powell and colleagues[3] showed in studies of several patients with humoral hypercalcemia that PTH could not be detected in plasma or in tumor extracts, despite their use of a wide range of PTH anti-sera directed against different parts of the molecule.

The more comprehensive clinical and biochemical investigations that followed[4-6] indicated that the manifestations of HHM were mediated via PTH receptors in kidney and bone.[1] These clinical observations have now been explained, with the isolation, cDNA cloning and expression of PTHrP.[14-16] The amino acid sequence of PTHrP bears 60% homology with that of PTH over the first 13 amino acids, and the PTH-like biological activity of PTHrP is contained within the first 34 amino acids. Beyond this region the two molecules have unique sequences.

PTHrP resembles PTH in its actions on bone and kidney, it stimulates cAMP production only in PTH target tissues, and this action is prevented by antagonists of PTH.[15] PTHrP is immunologically distinct from PTH since antisera against PTH which completely inhibit the biological effects of PTH have no effect on the activity of PTHrP.[17] The limited homology at the amino terminal region of the mature protein between PTHrP and PTH seemed sufficient to account for the similar actions of PTHrP and PTH, and indeed the amino terminal region of PTHrP interacts with the PTH receptor.[17]

PTHrP has been detected immunohistochemically and by Northern blotting in many tumors which give rise to HHM. It has also been detected in parathyroid adenomata, breast tumors from normocalcemic patients,[18] hypertrophic breast tissue, and in a percentage of hypercalcemic patients with human lymphotropic virus Type I (HTLV-I) associated lymphomas. In normal subjects PTHrP can be identified in high turnover epithelial tissues in skin and lactating breast (and breast milk).[19] It is also present in many early fetal tissues including fetal epithelia, muscle, bone, kidney, parathyroids, and placenta, and also in embryonal carcinoma cells suggesting a possible role in developmental processes.

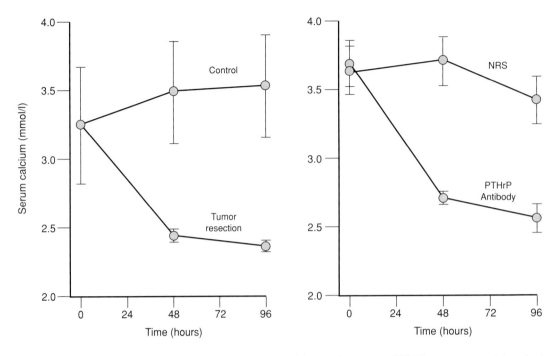

Fig. 6.2 Effect of tumor resection or injection of neutralizing anti-serum to PTHrP on serum calcium in tumor-bearing athymic mice. NRS: normal rabbit serum. (Modified from ref. 20 with permission.)

Radioimmunoassays are currently not sensitive enough to identify PTHrP convincingly in the plasma of normal subjects, but elevated levels of PTHrP are detected in a high proportion of patients with hypercalcemia in cancer[20] (Fig. 6.1). Furthermore, antibodies to N-terminal PTHrP can reduce the hypercalcemia and prevent the bone abnormalities in an immunodeficient mouse model of HHM.[21,22] Indeed in the latter model, treatment with neutralizing antibodies was as effective in reducing the plasma calcium level as was surgical removal of the tumor (Fig. 6.2).

There are some discrepancies between the features of HHM and hyperparathyroidism which may relate either to interactions with other tumor factors which may be cosecreted with PTHrP, or possibly to actions mediated via regions of the PTHrP molecule beyond the first 34 amino acids. An example is the hypokalemic alkalosis seen in hypercalcemia of cancer, whereas mild hyperchloremic acidosis is more commonly noted in primary hyperparathyroidism (Table 6.1). As a possible explanation for this difference, altered renal handling of bicarbonate by the rat kidney perfused with PTHrP (1-141) has been found as compared to PTHrP (1-34).[23] Prolonged infusion with PTHrP (1-141) resulted in restricted bicarbonate excretion, after the initial increased excretion noted in response to shorter forms of PTHrP and to PTH itself.

There seems little doubt that PTHrP is the major, if not the sole, mediator of hypercalcemia in patients with the HHM syndrome. However it is still possible that in some cases other bone resorbing factors (interleukin-1, tumor necrosis factor, TGFα) could contribute to the development of hypercalcemia on a humoral basis.

Although the assay data to the present time (Fig. 6.1) have provided very useful information, clearly more sensitive assays are needed. Even with the present systems the detection of elevated levels of PTHrP in the plasma of patients with hypercalcemia is strongly suggestive of the diagnosis of malignancy, but there are some exceptions to this. We have reported cases of hypercalcemia in sarcoidosis associated with elevated circulating levels of PTHrP.[24] PTHrP was identified in the cytoplasm of sarcoid macrophages in the granulomata in these cases by immunohistochemistry. PTHrP protein and gene expression were also identified in the cytoplasm of sarcoid macrophages in a significant proportion of a series of lymph node biopsies, suggesting that PTHrP may play an important role in the abnormal calcium metabolism in this disease.[24]

Hypercalcemia associated with bone metastases

Despite many improvements in early cancer detection and more effective treatment, metastatic disease remains the leading cause of cancer-related deaths. Bone is the most common site of metastasis in breast cancer and 25% of early-stage patients will develop this complication. This figure increases to 75% in patients with advanced disease. Currently there is no single, accurate predictor to identify which patients will develop this complication. In the clinical follow-up of patients with breast cancer especially, bone scanning at regular intervals is important in the detection of bone metastases. Recognition of the symptoms of early hypercalcemia is of the utmost importance, since progression to severe hypercalcemia can be prevented by appropriate measures, including increased fluid intake and anti-tumor therapy.

Although for many years it was considered that the main mechanism of hypercalcemia in patients with breast cancer was the release of calcium from bone by osteolytic deposits,[1] there is now evidence for a humoral contribution in these patients also. The extent of metastatic bone disease correlates poorly with both the occurrence and the degree of hypercalcemia in malignancy.[25] In 80–90% of cases of unselected solid tumor patients with hypercalcemia, irrespective of whether bone metastases are present, there is evidence of an underlying humoral mechanism.[25] The putative humoral mediator produces hypercalcemia both by stimulating generalized osteolysis and, in most cases, by impairing the renal excretion of the resultant increase in filtered calcium load. A reduced renal phosphate threshold and increased tubular calcium reabsorption were observed in hypercalcemic patients when compared with their normocalcemic counterparts, emphasizing the importance of renal mechanisms in mediating the hypercalcemia.

PTHrP has been purified from a breast cancer[26] and we have found evidence by immunohistology for the presence of PTHrP in 60% of an unselected series of breast cancers.[18] Furthermore, PTHrP is produced by the lactating breast, and elevated plasma PTHrP levels were found in nursing mothers.[27]

We have also found an increased incidence of positive localization of PTHrP by immunohistochemistry in breast cancer metastases to bone compared to other sites.[28] All these observations focus on a likely role for PTHrP in malignant breast disease. One possibility we proposed is that PTHrP production might contribute to the ability of breast cancers to erode bone and establish there as metastases. The clinical observations have been extended by using a mouse model of bone metastases in which inoculation of a human cancer cell line into the left ventricle of the mouse reliably produces osteolytic metastases. When the malignant cells were engineered to overexpress PTHrP (by transfection with the cDNA for preproPTHrP), an increase in the number of osteolytic metastases was observed.[29] These data strongly suggest that PTHrP expression by breast cancer cells enhances their metastatic potential to bone.

In some normocalcemic patients with malignancy, PTHrP levels close to the detection limit of various assays have been reported. We have shown by immunohistology that PTHrP is present in 100% of a series of squamous cell cancers of various origins.[30] This suggests that further sensitivity is needed for PTHrP assays to be applied to the early identification of those patients with cancer, in whom circulating

PTHrP levels are rising, and who are therefore at risk of the development of hypercalcemia.

Hematological malignancies

Hypercalcemia occurs in approximately one third of all patients with multiple myeloma,[1] a disease resulting from uncontrolled clonal proliferation of plasma cells. Hypercalcemia is very common in HTLV-1 associated T-cell leukemia/lymphoma.[31] It occurs to a far lesser extent in non-Hodgkin's lymphoma (NHL),[32] usually in the intermediate and high-grade rather than the low-grade categories defined by the International Working Formulation Criteria. It is uncommon in other hematological malignancies, but has been reported as a sporadic complication of chronic lymphatic leukemia, Hodgkin's disease, and myeloid blast crisis of chronic myeloid leukemia.

In one study of 165 unselected patients consecutively hospitalized in a clinical hematology unit with either myeloproliferative disorders or myeloid and lymphoplasmacytic neoplastic conditions, we detected hypercalcemia in 10.9% of the patients.[33] Hypercalcemia was due to coincidental primary hyperparathyroidism in 18% of the hypercalcemic patients, emphasizing the importance of considering that primary hyperparathyroidism can be the cause of the hypercalcemia in patients with hematological or other malignancies. In the cases where the hypercalcemia was due to the hematological malignancy it occurred in 32% of patients with multiple myeloma, and in 12% of those with NHL. The association of hypercalcemia with lymphoplasmacytic neoplasia was stronger than with myeloid neoplasia or myeloproliferative disorders, since the single instance of an association with a myeloid disorder was myeloid blast crisis of chronic myeloid leukemia.

In multiple myeloma, hypercalcemia is almost invariably associated with widespread bone involvement, as well as some irreversible impairment of renal function, which reduces the ability of the kidney to clear the excess calcium load due to increased bone resorption. Bone involvement in myeloma is characterized by extensive bone destruction accompanied by pain and susceptibility to fracture. Skeletal X-rays reveal abnormalities in 79% of patients.[34] These consist of osteoporosis, lytic lesions, and fractures, with over half the patients having a combination of all three. The characteristic skeletal lesions of myeloma are the punched-out lytic areas which are sharply circumscribed. The vertebrae, skull, thoracic cage, pelvis, and proximal portions of humerus and femur are the most common sites of bone involvement in multiple myeloma. Pathological fractures are common and should always suggest the possibility of myeloma. In contrast to patients with metastatic carcinoma, the vertebral pedicles are rarely involved in myeloma. Quantitative histological evaluation of myeloma-induced bone changes reveals increased osteoclastic resorption surfaces and increased numbers of osteoclasts in areas of bone invaded by plasma cells. Reduced thickness of osteoid seams and a low calcification rate are consistent with reduced osteoblastic activity.[35] This is reflected by significantly reduced levels of osteocalcin which are low in advanced disease.[36] This suggests an uncoupling of bone resorption and bone formation and explains the negative isotopic bone scan observed in multiple myeloma. Histomorphometric parameters are not changed by chemotherapy,[35] highlighting the requirement for specific inhibitors of osteoclastic bone resorption in the treatment of the hypercalcemia and the skeletal complications of this disease. Histological examination of the lytic lesions in multiple myeloma has shown increased bone resorption by osteoclasts in areas near myeloma cells.[37] This observation suggests that myeloma cells secrete factors which stimulate osteoclasts. A number of cytokines previously described by the generic name 'osteoclast-activating factor'[38] have now been identified: interleukin-1, TNFα (cachectin), and TNFβ (lymphotoxin). It is not yet certain whether one or more of these cytokines are responsible for the stimulation of osteoclastic bone resorption in multiple myeloma. One study found that most, but not all, of the bone resorbing activity from a human myeloma cell line could be suppressed by neutralizing antibodies to lymphotoxin,[39] but other investigators have attributed the bone resorbing activity of myeloma cells to interleukin-1.[40] Other cytokines may also be involved. In our series of consecutive hypercalcemic patients admitted to hospital with hematological malignancies, elevated plasma levels of PTHrP were measured in one third of patients with multiple myeloma.[33] We have also demonstrated PTHrP gene transcripts and protein in the bone marrow plasma cells from a hypercalcemic patient with elevated plasma PTHrP levels indicating PTHrP production by the myeloma cells.[41] It seems likely that PTHrP is another cytokine contributing to the hypercalcemia and the skeletal complications of this disease. It is possible that PTHrP has a role as local mediator of increased bone resorption in multiple myeloma, and that it is at times produced in sufficient quantities to reach the circulation and produce an endocrine effect. Such a process could contribute to the osteoporosis in multiple myeloma as well as to the hypercalcemia.

A subset of patients have nonsecretory myeloma and do not exhibit either fragments or intact monoclonal immunoglobulins in their circulation. Although it is rare, accounting for approximately 1% of patients with multiple myeloma, bone loss and hypercalcemia may be the presenting features and therefore this diagnosis must be considered in a patient in whom no other cause for the hypercalcemia has been found. In patients with nonsecretory myeloma, clinical and laboratory findings related to renal tubular complications, plasma expansion, or hyperviscosity do not occur, and the diagnosis under these circumstances is obscured until suggested by skeletal pain, pathologic fractures, or bony disruption.

Hypercalcemia in patients with lymphoma, although most often associated with bone involvement and related to direct tumor invasion of bone, can also occur in the absence of lytic lesions in bone, consistent with a humoral mechanism. A number of case reports have identified patients with hypercalcemia with no lytic bone lesions in both Hodgkin's and non-Hodgkin's lymphoma, which was associated with elevated levels of 1,25 (OH)$_2$D in plasma.[42,43] These patients also had suppressed immunoreactive PTH levels. The development of RIAs that measure PTHrP in plasma has also resulted in the finding of elevated PTHrP levels in a proportion of patients with hematological malignancies and hypercalcemia (Fig. 6.1). We have detected circulating levels of PTHrP of the order of those associated with HHM in cases of NHL of B-cell lineage.[33] Immunohistochemical staining demonstrated intracellular PTHrP in some of the neoplastic cells from a lymph node section in one of the cases.

A particular diagnostic subgroup of patients with adult T-cell lymphoma has a very high incidence of hypercalcemia, varying from 26% to 100% in different reports. This disease is strongly associated with a retrovirus, human T-cell lymphotrophic virus Type 1 (HTLV-1). Hypercalcemia in these patients is associated with elevated nephrogenous cyclic adenosine monophosphate (NcAMP) levels and low–normal PTH levels,[44] in the absence of lytic lesions in bone, features like those seen in HHM. Conditioned media from cultures of human T-cell lymphotrophic virus Type 1-infected cells were shown to contain a PTH-like biological activity with all the expected properties of PTHrP.[44] Expression of PTHrP within HTLV-1 infected T-cells in culture was demonstrated[45] and circulating levels were detected in hypercalcemic patients with this disease.[46]

TREATMENT

Severe symptomatic hypercalcemia is a metabolic emergency requiring immediate treatment. Continuous administration of intravenous isotonic saline (0.9% NaCl solution) will result in a modest decrease in the plasma calcium concentration due to a dilutional effect and enhanced calciuresis, and is the first step in the management of severe hypercalcemia. The rate of administration is based on the severity of the hypercalcemia, the degree of dehydration, and the ability of the patient's cardiovascular system to tolerate volume expansion. Clinical improvement usually occurs after rehydration over 24–48 hours, but normalization of plasma calcium rarely occurs except in very mild hypercalcemia, and other treatments are needed.

Although frusemide and ethacrynic acid inhibit calcium and sodium reabsorption in the ascending limb of the loop of Henle, loop diuretics should not be used routinely since they may exacerbate fluid loss and dehydration with consequent increase in hypercalcemia. Intensive administration of frusemide in very large doses of 80–100 mg every 2 hours is effective[47] in lowering plasma calcium but requires an intensive care unit to monitor electrolytes and central venous pressures at frequent intervals. This form of treatment can be dangerous in patients with myocardial dysfunction and is not necessary today with the availability of potent antiresorptive agents.

Calcitonin administered subcutaneously or intramuscularly in doses of 4–8 U/kg body weight every 6–12 hours can rapidly lower the plasma calcium, but the effect is brief with most patients showing only a transient response. This escape phenomenon may be combated with concomitant administration of glucocorticoids.[48] However, the present role of calcitonin in the treatment of hypercalcemia is that of an adjunctive drug in patients with severe hypercalcemia while waiting for the effect of slower-acting agents with longer duration of action, such as the bisphosphonates.

The bisphosphonates are a class of drugs developed over the past three decades for use in various diseases of bone and calcium metabolism.[49] Several are commercially available today and the availability and indications for which they are registered vary from country to country. Bisphosphonates are potent inhibitors of bone resorption. Mechanisms other than their well-known physicochemical property of inhibition of crystal dissolution result in inhibition of the activity of the osteoclast. This effect appears to be at least in part mediated by an inhibitor of osteoclast survival or recruitment[50] secreted by osteoblasts in response to bisphosphonates.

Bisphosphonates are very poorly absorbed from the gut. They have a very short plasma half-life, depositing rapidly into bone in areas both of bone formation and destruction. Renal clearance is very high and skeletal retention is very long, possibly life-long. Bisphosphonates have been used in a variety of schedules and dosages. Pamidronate disodium (APD) has been used successfully in the treatment of hypercalcemia associated with cancer. Pamidronate disodium given intravenously as a single dose of 15–90 mg according to the severity of the hypercalcemia can result in normalization of plasma calcium in the majority of patients. The duration of the response is variable lasting up to 3 or 4 weeks. The most important adverse effect of bisphosphonates is their potential nephrotoxicity mediated by the precipitation of bisphosphonate–calcium complexes in the kidney. This can be prevented by administering the drug by slow intravenous infusion over one to several hours depending on the dose given. A transient febrile reaction may occur within 24 hours.

Mithramycin, an inhibitor of DNA-directed RNA synthesis, exerts a hypocalcemic effect by damaging the osteoclast.[51] Doses of 1.5–2.0 mg given as intravenous infusion over 4 hours result in lowering of plasma calcium after 24–48 hours. Its administration can be complicated by nausea, vomiting, thrombocytopenia and hepatic, renal, and neurotoxicity. It should only be considered if treatment with maximally tolerated doses of bisphosphonates fails to normalize the plasma calcium.[52] Clinical experience with gallium nitrate, another inhibitor of bone resorption, is still limited. It is administered by continuous intravenous infusion for 5 days in a dose of 200 mg/m twice daily. Nephrotoxicity is a potential adverse effect.

SIGNIFICANCE OF PTHrP AS A PREDICTOR OF RESPONSE TO TREATMENT OF HYPERCALCEMIA OF MALIGNANCY WITH BISPHOSPHONATES

PTHrP has potent effects on the renal tubule and on bone resorption. These actions are detected by a rise in the tubular calcium threshold and nephrogenous cAMP and a fall in the tubular phosphate threshold. Despite PTHrP having a dual action on bone and kidney, the agents available for the treatment of hypercalcemia in

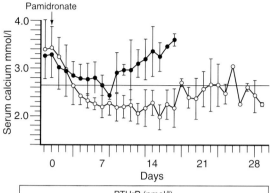

Fig. 6.3 PTHrP and calcium concentrations in poor and good responders to treatment of tumor-induced hypercalcemia with pamidronate. (Modified from ref. 52, with permission.)

cancer are primarily aimed at reducing bone resorption and no agent has a substantial effect on calcium excretion. The bisphosphonates, as powerful inhibitors of bone resorption, all fall into this category, having no effect on the renal tubular handling of calcium. Calcitonin and perhaps mithramycin have a weak calciuric effect but the main effect of these agents is inhibition of bone resorption. A poor response to pamidronate disodium occurs in cases of hypercalcemia of malignancy that have evidence of renal tubular stimulation as indicated by a low tubular threshold for phosphate or high threshold for calcium.[53] It is therefore not surprising that in a study of patients with tumor-induced hypercalcemia, the PTHrP level was the best determinant for the calcemic response to pamidronate, with high levels correlating with poor response and *vice versa*[54] (Fig. 6.3). Other parameters which indirectly indicated the presence of a humoral factor also correlated with response. The presence of bone metastases on the other hand predicted a good response to treatment. This study established that plasma PTHrP levels correlate inversely with the duration of response to pamidronate in patients with solid tumors causing hypercalcemia. Duration of response rather than the acute fall in calcium level may be a more clinically relevant definition of response and may give a better indication of the activity of anti-hypercalcemia agents. It is possible that high circulating PTHrP levels may have a more potent effect on bone resorption than locally released factors from skeletal deposits, thus explaining the poor response associated with high plasma levels of PTHrP. However, effective inhibition of bone resorption by pamidronate was demonstrated in patients who were poor responders, whereas complete correction of the tubular defect did not occur in these patients. This implies that the failure to inhibit the renal mechanism of hypercalcemia is the major cause of a poor response. A high PTHrP level predicts a poor response which may relate to the failure to correct the renal component of hypercalcemia induced by this hormone. Currently, the prediction of a poor response will not change clinical practice because agents are not available that conveniently increase calcium excretion. The development of drugs that inhibit the tubular reabsorption of calcium,[55] specific inhibitors of PTH or PTHrP action,[56] antibodies to PTHrP,[19] or inhibitors of PTHrP production may allow better control of hypercalcemia in these patients when used in combination with the available inhibitors of osteolysis. Of particular interest in this category may be the new analogs of vitamin D which have low calcemic activity yet retain the property of inhibition of PTH gene expression. The first reported analog of this type was 22-oxa-1,25(OH)$_2$D, or 22-oxacalcitriol (OCT),[57] which has been shown to inhibit expression of the PTH gene *in vitro* and *in vivo*,[58] and is currently under investigation in the treatment of secondary hyperparathyroidism associated with chronic renal failure. Since 1,25(OH)$_2$D is known to inhibit PTHrP gene expression,[59] it is conceivable that 1,25(OH)$_2$D analogs may have the same effect and hence offer a valuable option in addition to bisphosphonates in the treatment of PTHrP-mediated hypercalcemia.

SUMMARY AND PERSPECTIVE

The discovery of PTHrP has provided an explanation for much of the pathogenesis of the hypercalcemia of cancer, contributing to the humoral syndrome certainly but also to the hypercalcemia accompanying bony metastases and hematological malignancies. It is useful to keep in mind, however, that even in HHM there may in many instances be contributions from other bone resorbing factors. That is certainly so in metastatic bone disease and hematological cancers, where other bone resorbing cytokines (e.g. IL-11, IL-6) could be significant contributors.

Whatever the contributing cytokines and hormones, it is clear that increased osteoclast formation is a prime pathogenetic mechanism in the hypercalcemia of cancer, whether this be a generalized increase, as in the case of HHM, or localized at sites of tumor invasion of bone, where enhanced osteoclast formation facilitates the growth of tumor in bone. Recent discoveries of mechanisms involved in osteoclast formation may provide further insights into these processes. Osteoprotegerin (OPG) is a secreted member of the TNF receptor family which is produced by osteoblastic stromal cells and profoundly inhibits osteoclast formation at a late stage of their development.[60,61] The ligand for OPG is a cell surface molecule of the stromal cell which is a member of the TNF superfamily.[62,63] Given the name osteoclast differentiation factor (ODF), this molecule is a powerful inducer of osteoclast formation by acting directly on hemopoietic cells in the presence of M CSF and without accompanying stromal cells.[62,64] ODF was discovered independently as a T-cell molecule and given the name TRANCE[65] and, interestingly, activated T-cells when co-cultured with spleen cells generate authentic, functional osteoclasts.[66] Furthermore, breast cancer cell lines have been found to produce OPG,[67] raising the possibility of local production of OPG influencing tumor interaction with bone. Certainly it is likely that tumor-derived cytokines can influence production of ODF in bone to favor osteoclast formation, and some experimental evidence for this has been obtained.[67]

REFERENCES

1. Mundy GR, Martin TJ. The hypercalcemia of malignancy: pathogenesis and treatment. *Metabolism* (1982) **31**: 1247–77.
2. Martin TJ, Atkins D. Biochemical regulators of bone resorption and their significance in cancer. *Essays Med Biochem* (1979) **4**: 49–82.
3. Powell D, Singer FR, Murray TM, Minkin C, Potts JT. Non-parathyroid humoral hypercalcemia in patients with neoplastic disease. *N Engl J Med* (1973) **289**: 176–81.
4. Kukreja SC, Shermerdiak WP, Lad TE, Johnson PA. Elevated nephrogenous cyclic AMP with normal serum parathyroid hormone levels in patients with lung cancer. *J Clin Endocrinol Metab* (1980) **51**: 167–9.
5. Stewart AF, Horst R, Deftos LJ, Cadman EC, Lang R, Broadus AE. Biochemical evaluation of patients with cancer-associated hypercalcemia. Evidence for humoral and non-humoral groups. *N Engl J Med* (1980) **303**: 1377–81.
6. Rude RK, Sharp CF Jr, Fredericks RS *et al.* Urinary and nephrogenous adenosine 3'5'-monophosphate in the hypercalcemia of malignancy. *J Clin Invest* (1981) **52**: 765–71.
7. Fuller Albright. Case records of the Massachusetts General Hospital (Case 27401). *N Engl J Med* (1941) **225**: 789–91.
8. Berson AS, Yalow RS. Parathyroid hormone in plasma in adenomatous hyperparathyroidism, uremia and bronchogenic sarcoma. *Science* (1966) **154**: 907–9.
9. Knill-Jones RP, Buckle RM, Parsons V, Caine RY, Williams R. Hypercalcaemia and increased parathyroid hormone activity in a primary hepatoma. Studies before and after hepatic transplantation. *New Engl J Med* (1970) **282**: 704–8.
10. Greenberg PB, Martin TJ, Sutcliffe HS. Synthesis and release of parathyroid hormone by a renal carcinoma in cell culture. *Clin Sci* (1973) **45**: 183–7.
11. Riggs BL, Arnaud CD, Reynolds JC, Smith LH. Immunological differentiation of primary hyper-

parathyroidism from hyperparathyroidism due to non-parathyroid cancer. *J Clin Invest* (1971) **50**: 2079–83.
12. Roof BS, Carpenter B, Fink DJ, Gordan GS. Some thoughts on the nature of ectopic parathyroid hormones. *Am J Med* (1971) **50**: 686–91.
13. Benson RC, Riggs BL, Pickard BM, Arnaud CD. Immunoreactive forms of circulating parathyroid hormone in primary and ectopic hyperparathyroidism. *J Clin Invest* (1974) **54**: 175–81.
14. Moseley JM, Kubota M, Diefenbach-Jagger H et al. Parathyroid hormone-related protein purified from a human lung cancer cell line. *Proc Natl Acad Sci U S A* (1987) **84**: 5048–52.
15. Suva LJ, Winslow GA, Wettenhall REH et al. A parathyroid hormone-related protein implicated in malignant hypercalcemia: cloning and expression. *Science* (1987) **237**: 893–6.
16. Mangin M, Webb AC, Dreyer BE et al. Identification of a cDNA encoding a parathyroid hormone-like peptide from a human tumor associated with humoral hypercalcemia of malignancy. *Proc Natl Acad Sci U S A* (1988) **85**: 597–601.
17. Martin TJ, Allan EH, Caple IW et al. Parathyroid hormone-related protein: isolation, molecular cloning and mechanism of action. *Recent Prog Horm Res* (1989) **45**: 467–506.
18. Southby J, Kissin MW, Danks JA et al. Immunohistochemical localization of parathyroid hormone-related protein in human breast cancer. *Cancer Res* (1990) **50**: 7710–16.
19. Moseley JM, Martin TJ. Parathyroid hormone-related protein: physiological actions. In Bilezikian JP, Raisz LG, Rodan GA (eds) *Principles of Bone Biology* (CA, USA: Academic Press) pp 363–76.
20. Grill V, Ho P, Body JJ et al. Parathyroid hormone-related protein: elevated levels both in humoral hypercalcemia of malignancy and in hypercalcemia complicating metastatic breast cancer. *J Clin Endocrinol Metab* (1991) **73**: 1309–15.
21. Kukreja SC, Schavin DH, Wimbiscus S et al. Antibodies to parathyroid hormone-related protein lower serum calcium in athymic mouse models of malignancy associated hypercalcemia due to human tumors. *J Clin Invest* (1988) **82**: 1798–802.
22. Kukreja SC, Rosol TJ, Wimbiscus SA et al. Tumor resection and antibodies to parathyroid hormone-related protein cause similar changes on bone histomorphometry in hypercalcemia of cancer. *Endocrinology* (1990) **127**: 305–10.
23. Ellis AG, Adam WR, Martin TJ. Comparison of the effects of parathyroid hormone (PTH) and recombinant PTH-related protein on bicarbonate excretion by the isolated perfused rat kidney. *J Endocrinol* (1990) **126**: 403–8.
24. Zeimer HJ, Greenaway TM, Slavin J et al. Parathyroid hormone-related protein in sarcoidosis. *Am J Pathol* (1998) **152**: 17–21.
25. Ralston SH, Fogelman I, Gardiner MD, Boyle IT. Relative contribution of humoral and metastatic factors to the pathogenesis of hypercalcaemia in malignancy. *Br Med J* (1984) **288**: 1405–8.
26. Burtis WJ, Wu J, Bunch CM et al. Identification of a novel 17,000-dalton parathyroid hormone-like adenylate cyclase-stimulating protein from a tumor associated with humoral hypercalcemia of malignancy. *J Biol Chem* (1987) **262**: 7151–6.
27. Grill V, Hillary J, Ho PMW et al. Parathyroid hormone-related protein: a possible endocrine function in lactation. *Clin Endocrinol* (1992) **37**: 405–10.
28. Powell GJ, Southby J, Danks JA et al. Localization of parathyroid hormone-related protein in breast cancer metastases: increased incidence in bone compared with other sites. *Cancer Res* (1991) **51**: 3058–61.
29. Guise TA, Yin JJ, Taylor SD et al. Evidence for a causal role of parathyroid hormone-related protein in the pathogenesis of human breast cancer-mediated osteolysis. *J Clin Invest* (1996) **98**: 1544–9.
30. Danks JA, Ebeling PR, Hayman J et al. Parathyroid hormone-related protein: immunohistochemical localization in cancers and in normal skin. *J Bone Miner Res* (1989) **4**: 273–8.
31. Bunn PA, Schechter GP, Jaffe E et al. Clinical course of retrovirus associated adult T-cell lymphoma in the United States. *N Engl J Med* (1983) **309**: 257–64.
32. Burt ME, Brennan MF. Incidence of hypercalcaemia and malignant neoplasm. *Arch Surg* (1980) **115**: 704–7.
33. Firkin F, Seymour J, Watson AM, Grill V, Martin TJ. Parathyroid hormone-related protein in hypercalcemia associated with haematological malignancy. *Br J Haematol* (1996) **94**: 468–92.
34. Kyle RA. Multiple myeloma: review of 869 cases. *Mayo Clin Proc* (1975) **50**: 29–40.
35. Valentin-Opran A, Charhon SA, Meunier PJ, Arlot CME, Arlot ME. Quantitative histology of myeloma-induced bone changes. *Br J Haematol* (1982) **52**: 601–10.

36. Bataille R, Delmas PD, Chappard D, Sany J. Abnormal serum bone gla protein levels in multiple myeloma. Crucial role of bone formation and prognostic implications. *Cancer* (1990) **66**: 167–72.
37. Roodman GD. Osteoclast function in Paget's disease and multiple myeloma. *Bone* (1995) **17**: 57S–61S.
38. Mundy GR, Raisz LG, Cooper RA, Schechter GP, Salmon SE. Evidence for the secretion of an osteoclast stimulating factor in myeloma. *N Engl J Med* (1974) **291**: 1041–6.
39. Garret IR, Durie BGM, Nedwin GE *et al*. Production of lymphotoxin, a bone-resorbing cytokine, by cultured human myeloma cells. *N Engl J Med* (1987) **317**: 526–32.
40. Kawano M, Yamamoto I, Iwato K *et al*. Interleukin-I-beta rather than lymphotoxin as the major bone resorbing activity in human multiple myeloma. *Blood* (1989) **73**: 1646–9.
41. Schneider H-G, Kartsogiannis V, Zhou H, Chou ST, Martin TJ, Grill V. Parathyroid hormone-related protein mRNA and protein expression in multiple myeloma: a case report. *J Bone Miner Res* (1998) **13**: 1640–43.
42. Breslau NA, McGuire JL, Zerwekh JE, Frenkel EP, Pak CYC. Hypercalcaemia associated with increased serum calcitriol levels in three patients with lymphoma. *Ann Intern Med* (1984) **100**: 1–7.
43. Rosenthal N, Insogna KL, Godsall JW, Smaldone L, Waldron JA, Stewart AF. Elevations in circulating 1,25-dihydroxyvitamin D in three patients with lymphoma-associated hypercalcaemia. *J Clin Endocrinol Metab* (1985) **60**: 29–33.
44. Fukumoto S, Matsumoto T, Ikeda K *et al*. Clinical evaluation of calcium metabolism in adult T-cell leukemia/lymphoma. *Arch Intern Med* (1988) **148**: 921–5.
45. Motokura T, Fukumoto S, Takahashi S *et al*. Expression of parathyroid hormone-related protein in a human T cell lymphotrophic virus type 1-infected T cell line. *Biochem Biophys Res Commun* (1988) **154**: 1182–8.
46. Ikeda K, Ohno H, Hane M *et al*. Development of a sensitive two-site assay for parathyroid hormone-related peptide: evidence for elevated levels in plasma from patients with adult T-cell leukaemia/lymphoma and B-cell lymphoma. *J Clin Endocrinol Metab* (1994) **79**: 1322–7.
47. Suki WN, Yium JJ, von Minden M, Saller-Herbert C, Eknovan G, Martinez-Maldonado M. Acute treatment of hypercalcemia with furosemide. *N Engl J Med* (1970) **283**: 836–40.
48. Hosking DJ, Stone MD, Foote JW. Potentiation of calcitonin by corticosteroids during the treatment of hypercalcemia of malignancy. *Eur J Clin Pharmacol* (1990) **38**: 37–41.
49. Fleisch H. *Bisphosphonates in Bone Disease. From the Laboratory to the Patient* (London: Parthenon Publishing Group, 1995).
50. Sahni M, Guenther HL, Fleisch H, Collin P, Martin TJ. Bisphosphonates act on rat bone resorption through the mediation of osteoblasts. *J Clin Invest* (1993) **91**: 2004–11.
51. Brown JH, Kennedy BJ. Mithramycin in the treatment of testicular cancer. *N Engl J Med* (1965) **272**: 111–18.
52. Bonjour JP, Rizzoli R. Antiosteolytic agents in the management of hypercalcemia. *Ann Oncol* (1992) **3**: 589–90.
53. Gurney H, Kefford R, Stuart HR. Renal phosphate threshold and response to pamidronate in humoral hypercalcaemia of malignancy. *Lancet* (1989) **ii**: 241–4.
54. Gurney H, Grill V, Martin TJ. Parathyroid hormone-related protein level predicts response to pamidronate in the treatment of tumor-induced hypercalcemia. *Lancet* (1993) **ii**: 241–4.
55. Hirschel SS, Caverzasio J, Bonjour JP. Inhibition of parathyroid hormone secretion and parathyroid hormone-independent diminution of tubular calcium reabsorption by WR-2721, a unique hypocalcemic agent. *J Clin Invest* (1985) **76**: 1851–6.
56. Goldman ME, McKee RL, Caulfield MP *et al*. A new highly potent parathyroid hormone antagonist: D-Trp12, Tyr34: bPTH-(7-34)NH2. *Endocrinology* (1988) **123**: 2597–9.
57. Murayama E, Miyamoto K, Kubodera N, Mori T, Matsunaga I. Synthetic studies of vitamin D3 analogues. VIII. Synthesis of 22-oxavitamin D3 analogues. *Chem Pharm Bull (Tokyo)* (1986) **34**: 4410–13.
58. Brown AJ, Ritter CR, Finch JL *et al*. The noncalcemic analogue of vitamin D, 22-oxacalcitriol, suppresses parathyroid hormone synthesis and secretion. *J Clin Invest* (1989) **84**: 728–32.
59. Ikeda K, Lu C, Weir EC, Mangin M, Broadus AE. Transcriptional regulation of the parathyroid hormone-related protein gene by glucocorticoids and vitamin D in a human C-cell line. *J Biol Chem* (1989) **264**: 15 743–6.
60. Simonet WS, Lacey DL, Dunstan CR *et al*. Osteoprotogerin: a novel secreted protein involved in the regulation of bone density. *Cell* (1997) **89**: 309–19.

61. Tsuda E, Goto M, Mochizuki S *et al*. Isolation of a novel cytokine from human fibroblasts that specifically inhibits osteoclastogenesis. *Biochem Biophys Res Commun* (1997) **234**: 137–42.
62. Yasuda H, Shima N, Nakagawa N *et al*. Osteoclast differentiation factor is a ligand for osteoprotogerin/osteoclastogenesis inhibitory factor and identical to TRANCE/RANKL. *Proc Natl Acad Sci U S A* (1998) **95**: 3597–602.
63. Lacey DM, Timms E, Tan H-L *et al*. Osteoprotogerin ligand is a cytokine that regulates osteoclast differentiation and activation. *Cell* (1998) **93**: 165–76.
64. Quinn JMW, Elliott J, Gillespie MT, Martin TJ. A combination of osteoclast differentiation factor and macrophage-colony stimulating factor is sufficient for both human and mouse osteoclast formation in vitro. *Endocrinology* (1999) (in press).
65. Wong BR, Rho J, Arron J *et al*. TRANCE is a novel ligand of the tumor necrosis factor receptor family that activates c-Jun N-terminal kinase in T-cells. *J Biol Chem* (1997) **272**: 25 190–4.
66. Horwood NJ, Kartsogiannis V, Lam MHC *et al*. Activated T cells are capable of inducing osteoclast formation: a mechanism for rheumatoid arthritis. *J Bone Miner Res* (1998) **23,5**: S214.
67. Thomas RJ, Guise TA, Yin JJ *et al*. Breast cancer cells stimulate osteoblastic osteoclast differentiation factor (ODF) to support osteoclast formation. *J Bone Miner Res* (1998) **23,5**: S378.

7

Diagnostic nuclear medicine

Gary J R Cook and Ignac Fogelman

Introduction • Radiopharmaceuticals and mechanisms of uptake in the skeleton • Scanning methods • Scintigraphic patterns in the diagnosis of bone metastases • The role of bone scintigraphy in specific tumours • Other radionuclide scanning techniques • Positron emission tomography

INTRODUCTION

Since the first description of bone scintigraphy using strontium-85 (^{85}Sr) by Fleming *et al.* in 1961,[1] there have been many improvements in both radiopharmaceuticals and scanning techniques in the evaluation of metastatic bone disease. Currently, bone scintigraphy with technetium-99m (^{99m}Tc)-labelled diphosphonates remains the most widely used method for diagnosis and surveillance of bone metastases. In recent years there have been major advances in cross-sectional, anatomical imaging techniques such as computed tomography (CT) and magnetic resonance imaging (MRI) but its high sensitivity and ability to image the whole skeleton easily have enabled bone scintigraphy to remain one of the first-line investigations when assessing the skeleton in patients with cancer.

Bone scanning agents, such as methylene diphosphonate (MDP), are labelled with ^{99m}Tc, a radionuclide which is readily available to most departments of nuclear medicine. Other radiopharmaceuticals exist for specific tumours, e.g. iodine-131 (^{131}I) for differentiated thyroid carcinoma metastases and ^{123}I or ^{131}I metaiodobenzylguanidine (MIBG) for neuroendocrine tumours such as neuroblastoma and carcinoid. Some nonspecific, tumour-avid radiopharmaceuticals have also been assessed in the evaluation of bone metastases, including gallium-67 (^{67}Ga), thallium-201 (^{201}Tl), ^{99m}Tc sestamibi, and ^{99m}Tc pentavalent dimercaptosuccinic acid (V DMSA) but are used infrequently in routine clinical management. Positron emission tomography (PET) has previously been regarded as a research tool but now has a number of defined clinical applications, particularly in oncology. Fluorodeoxyglucose-18 (^{18}FDG) is an analogue of glucose and is now commonly used in cancer imaging, both on dedicated PET scanners and more recently on adapted conventional gamma cameras. Fluoride-18 (^{18}F) is also available as a specific PET bone tracer and has been recognized as a potential bone agent for many years.[2]

RADIOPHARMACEUTICALS AND MECHANISMS OF UPTAKE IN THE SKELETON

The uptake of diphosphonate compounds depends on local blood flow but more importantly on local osteoblastic activity. It is thought that diphosphonates are incorporated into the hydroxyapatite crystal by chemisorption on to the surface of bone. ^{99m}Tc-labelled MDP is one of the most commonly used bone tracers and gives near optimal contrast between normal skeletal uptake and lesions, but other diphosphonate-based tracers also exist.[3] The positron emitter, ^{18}F fluoride, accumulates in a similar manner, dependent on blood flow and osteoblastic activity and the fluoride ion is incorporated into the hydroxyapatite crystal to form fluoroapatite.

Once metastases are deposited in the bone marrow, skeletal damage results from increased bone resorption caused by stimulation of osteoclasts by tumour-derived humoral mediators including growth factors and cytokines.[4] Bone destruction by a metastasis is nearly always accompanied by an osteoblastic proliferation and it is the balance between this effect and osteolysis that determines the behaviour of a metastasis. Most cancers are associated with predominantly osteoclastic, lytic lesions but the osteoblastic response means that the vast majority of metastases are associated with increased uptake of bone tracers and a 'hot spot' on a bone scan. Some exceptions exist. For example, myeloma characteristically produces little or no osteoblastic response and may not produce an abnormality on a bone scan. Although radiography is probably a better measure of disease extent in this disease,[5] it is rare that a bone scan is completely normal in widespread myeloma. However, even purely lytic lesions without any significant osteoblastic response may still be detectable as a photopoenic lesion on a bone scan if large enough and are often visible with improvement in spatial resolution on modern gamma cameras. In assessing the skeleton in cancers that characteristically produce purely lytic lesions such as myeloma or renal cell carcinoma, a careful inspection should therefore be made for photopoenic lesions which on first inspection may not be obvious. Photopoenic lesions may also be seen in very aggressive metastases where bone is unable to mount sufficient osteoblastic response, an appearance not uncommonly seen in breast and lung cancer (Fig. 7.1). Although many tumours produce lytic metastases there is usually a rim of increased activity corresponding to bone repair (Fig. 7.2).

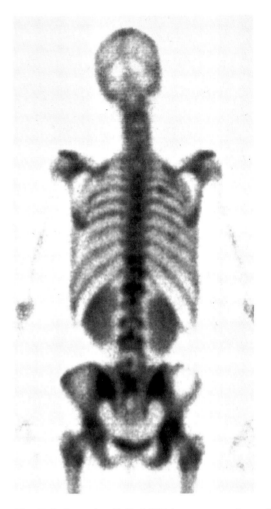

Fig. 7.1 Posterior ^{99m}Tc MDP bone scan of a patient with lung cancer. Note photopoenic lesions in the lumbar spine, particularly at L5 and in the right iliac wing. No accompanying increased uptake is seen.

Tumours are known to exhibit a high glycolytic rate compared to normal tissues[6] and so the glucose analogue ^{18}FDG accumulates selectively in tumour tissue and can be detected with PET or specially adapted gamma cameras. Other mechanisms such as tumour hypoxia may also play a part in uptake of this radiopharmaceutical in some tumours.[7] Because uptake of ^{18}FDG is in tumour cells, this technique images the tumour or metastasis itself rather than a

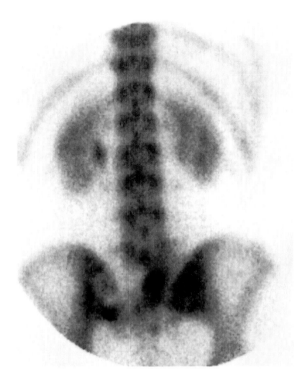

Fig. 7.2 Posterior ^{99m}Tc MDP scan of the lumbar spine of a patient with breast cancer. A large photopoenic lesion is seen at the left sacroiliac joint extending into the sacrum. Areas of increased activity in the periphery correspond with an osteoblastic response.

bone reaction as in bone scintigraphy. Because of this it is possible that this method is more sensitive in the detection of bone metastases, detecting presence of tumour activity before a bone reaction is established.

A number of single photon, tumour-specific tracers exist which have been utilized in both primary and metastatic bone tumours. ^{201}Tl, a radiopharmaceutical which behaves as an analogue of potassium, enters the cell via the sodium/potassium ATPase pump. Uptake reflects the metabolic status of the cell but also relies on local blood flow. ^{99m}Tc sestamibi shows a similar tissue distribution to thallium but accumulates in cells by a different mechanism, the majority being found in mitochondria. The radiopharmaceutical, pentavalent dimercaptosuccinic acid (V DMSA), initially used in detecting medullary thyroid cancer metastases, has been shown to accumulate in bone metastases.[8,9] The mechanism of uptake and the exact role for this radiopharmaceutical are not clear. It may improve the specificity of bone scan findings but is unlikely to have a significant role in routine clinical practice.

Because bone metastases initially seed in bone marrow, there is a stage where the tumour is small enough not to have excited an osteoblastic bone reaction. Bone marrow scintigraphy, where focal marrow defects correspond to marrow replacement by tumour, is therefore a potentially sensitive method for detection. This may account for reports where bone marrow scanning techniques have shown greater sensitivity than conventional bone scans.[10,11] Bone marrow scintigraphy is limited to some extent by obscuration of the spine by uptake of tracer into the liver and spleen and is not able to assess the peripheral skeleton where there is a paucity of red marrow. This technique is unlikely to be used in routine clinical practice for detection of metastases but on occasion a role may exist as an adjunct to ^{99m}Tc MDP scintigraphy where it may increase specificity for individual lesions in which it would otherwise be difficult to differentiate malignant from benign bone lesions.

Nuclear medicine offers a number of tracers which are specific to certain tumours or tumour types. Although uptake of these radiopharmaceuticals is not specific to bone metastases they may often be helpful in the assessment of bone metastases in addition to soft tissue metastases. Examples include ^{131}I iodine for differentiated thyroid cancers, ^{131}I or ^{123}I metaiodobenzylguanidine (MIBG) for neuroblastomas, medullary thyroid cancers, and carcinoid tumours (Fig. 7.3), and ^{111}indium octreotide for a variety of neuroendocrine tumours.

SCANNING METHODS

Historically the majority of bone scans have been performed by acquiring multiple spot

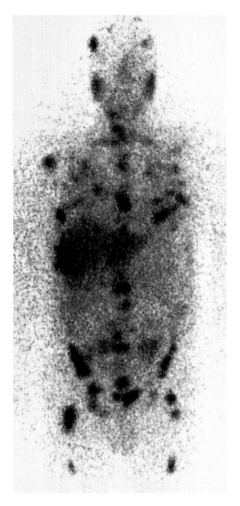

Fig. 7.3 Anterior ^{123}I MIBG scan in a patient with metastatic carcinoid tumour demonstrating multiple skeletal metastases as well as liver lesions.

views or, alternatively, whole-body images. Newer, multiheaded gamma cameras are able to acquire high-resolution, whole-body images of the entire skeleton in a rapid scan time whilst providing both anterior and posterior images simultaneously. If any parts of the skeleton require further images these can be obtained with localized spot views. Nearly all modern gamma cameras have the ability to acquire tomographic images (single photon emission computed tomography, SPECT). Tomography not only allows better anatomical localization of lesions from the inherent three-dimensional data but also increases sensitivity by improving contrast resolution. This is because tomography can separate activity within an organ from superimposed background activity from overlying structures which occurs with planar, non-tomographic imaging. Early reports have suggested that the use of SPECT may not only improve sensitivity in the detection of vertebral metastases but that it may also be possible to improve specificity by examining the pattern and position of abnormalities within the vertebra. For example, lesions involving the vertebral body and also extending into the posterior elements or with involvement of the pedicle alone are more likely to represent metastases than those in the facet joints, anterior vertebral body, or intervertebral disc space (Fig. 7.4).[12–14]

Positron emission tomography relies on the detection of two 511 KeV gamma rays which are emitted at 180° to each other following the annihilation of a positron (a positively charged electron from an unstable nucleus) and a negative electron. The synchronous detection of the gamma rays allows accurate placement of the point of emission and so PET scans show higher spatial resolution than conventional nuclear medicine, single photon imaging. Tomography as a routine and the use of radiolabelled, naturally occurring compounds rather than analogues confer other advantages. PET remains comparatively expensive compared to other nuclear medicine techniques and clinical PET centres are not widespread, but with the growing interest and experience it is sure to play a more significant role in clinical imaging, especially oncology, in the future.

SCINTIGRAPHIC PATTERNS IN THE DIAGNOSIS OF BONE METASTASES

As with any imaging technique it is important that normal variations, artefacts and coexistent benign abnormalities are recognized to aid accurate reporting. A number have been described on bone scans which can mimic metastases.

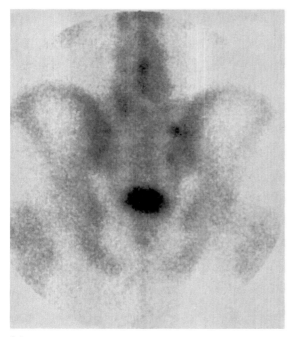

(a)

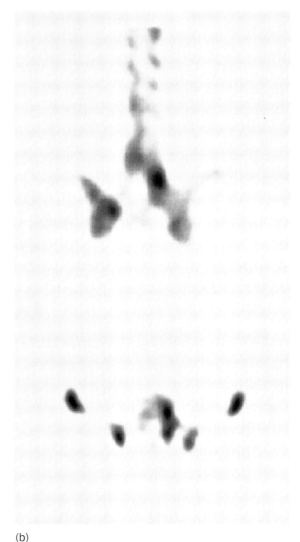

(b)

Fig. 7.4 (a) Posterior 99mTc MDP bone scan of the pelvis in a patient with prostatic cancer. A faint abnormality is seen at the lumbosacral junction on the left with further abnormality in the right sacroiliac joint region. (b) SPECT images (coronal – above, transaxial – below) confirm an abnormality at L5 and show that the abnormality extends from the vertebral body into the posterior elements including the pedicle, greatly increasing the likelihood that this is metastatic rather than degenerative in nature.

A normal variant that is worthy of mention is that of increased uptake at the manubriosternal junction. In patients with breast cancer, more so than other cancers, the sternum is a relatively common site to be affected, probably resulting from local spread from involved internal mammary nodes. If a sternal lesion is situated distant from the manubriosternal junction, is irregular, asymmetrical, or eccentric then malignant involvement should be suspected. In a retrospective series of 1104 breast cancer patients, 3.1% presented with an isolated sternal lesion and 76% of these were found to represent metastatic disease.[15] Other variants that should be recognized as such include focal activity at the confluence of the sutures at the pterion in the skull, the deltoid muscle insertion on the humerus, and symmetrical muscle insertions in the ribs of paraspinal muscles, resulting in a stippled appearance. On occasion the tip of the

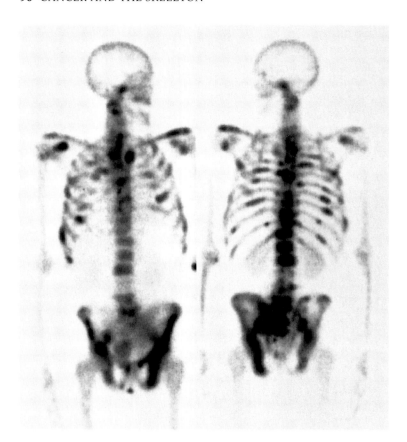

Fig. 7.5 ^{99m}Tc MDP bone scan of a patient with prostatic cancer demonstrating the typical axial distribution of metastases.

scapula overlying a rib may mimic a focal abnormality. This may easily be distinguished by taking a further view with the arms raised thereby moving the tip of the scapula outside the line of the ribs. Abnormalities seen at joints are generally benign. Increased uptake either side of a joint is reassuring although this pattern may be difficult to discern in the spine but SPECT may again be helpful in this situation. Another benign disease which may cause difficulty in interpretation is Paget's disease. In some areas this may be present in up to 5% of the population over 40 years old[16] and is asymptomatic in the majority. The diffuse nature of diphosphonate uptake throughout a bone due to increased osteoblastic activity and vascularity in this disease, together with the appearance of expansion of the affected bone, or the abnormality extending from a joint into the diaphysis of a long bone with a flame-shaped leading edge, will aid correct interpretation. It is usually advisable to confirm the diagnosis with radiographs, however. Even so, radiographic appearances may be difficult to differentiate from confluent osteoblastic metastases such as those commonly seen in prostate cancer.

Bone scintigraphy, using radiopharmaceuticals such as ^{99m}Tc MDP, is undoubtedly a sensitive technique, a false negative rate of only 0.08% being quoted in one of the largest studies of breast cancer including more than 1200 women,[17] but specificity without other correlative imaging or interval follow-up is relatively poor. Specificity may be aided by a knowledge of the common distribution of metastases from most cancers, i.e. the axial skeleton and ribs corresponding to the distribution of red marrow[18] (Fig. 7.5), but peripheral lesions are not that infrequent.[19,20] A small proportion affect the appendicular skeleton (10%), a feature most commonly seen in clinical practice in carcinoma of the lung, prostate, and breast.[21] Opinions differ as to whether the peripheral skeleton should be routinely imaged when assessing cancer patients but few would disagree that this should be the case if the patient has peripheral symptoms. With the reintroduction of whole-body scanning techniques with modern gamma cameras the peripheries are easily included with a greater time efficiency than the multiple overlapping spot view technique. One potential bonus from including the peripheries, especially in patients with lung cancer, is that hypertrophic pulmonary osteoarthropathy (HPOA) may be detected. The typical appearance of this is an increase in uptake extending down the cortical borders at the ends of the long bones resulting in a 'parallel stripe sign'. While clinically HPOA is most evident at the wrists or ankles it is most clearly seen in the lower femora on bone scans.

Rarely, when skeletal metastases are very extensive, a bone scan may appear normal on first inspection because the lesions become confluent. The 'superscan', so-called because of the apparent exceptional quality of the scan, has a number of distinguishing features which should alert the experienced interpreter. In addition to the apparent high quality of the images, the soft tissues, including the kidneys, are inconspicuous or invisible due to the increased ratio between skeletal uptake and soft tissues. On close inspection of a malignant superscan there is often some irregularity of uptake in the ribs or long bones suggesting its metastatic nature and differentiating it from superscans caused by metabolic bone diseases such as hyperparathyroidism (Figs 7.6 and 7.7).

There is usually little doubt as to the nature of irregularly scattered, axial skeletal lesions but solitary lesions may be more problematic. A solitary bone lesion due to a metastasis is not an uncommon finding. In a retrospective study of 301 patients with a variety of cancers, 11% with a solitary, new abnormality had malignancy confirmed.[22] In a further review of 160 consecutive bone scans of patients with breast cancer

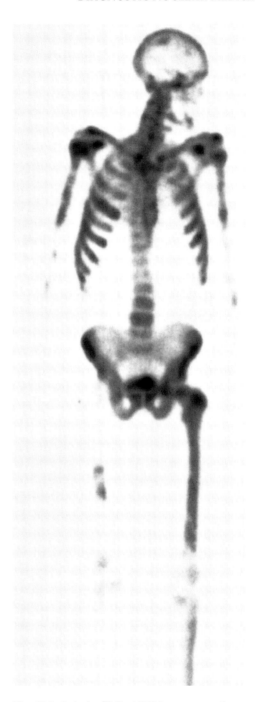

Fig. 7.6 Anterior ^{99m}Tc MDP bone scan of a man with prostatic cancer demonstrating features of a superscan with increased uptake throughout the majority of the skeleton and no visualization of soft tissue structures, including kidneys. Some irregularity seen in the long bones indicates the metastatic nature.

98 CANCER AND THE SKELETON

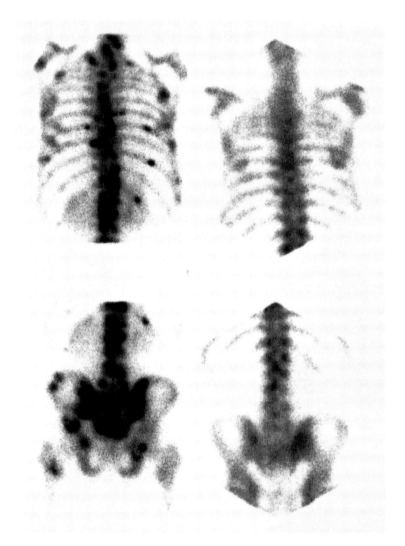

Fig. 7.7 Posterior ^{99m}Tc MDP bone scans. The right-hand scan was performed 6 months after the left. On initial inspection the multiple focal metastases appear to have resolved but on closer inspection the later scan shows evidence of a superscan. Note that soft tissue and renal activity is no longer apparent. These features suggest a progression of disease, the previous focal lesions having coalesced and become uniform.

and new bone metastases, 21% relapsed with a solitary metastasis which was most often located in the spine.[23] A single rib lesion is usually regarded as having a low probability (10%) of being a metastasis in patients with a known primary tumour,[24,25] although a more recent study in a similar mixed population of cancer patients found that more than 40% of these lesions proved to be metastatic in nature.[26] Even focal abnormalities at the anterior ends of ribs, commonly regarded as a benign finding, had a high incidence (36%) of confirmed metastases in this latter series. In patients with breast cancer, a solitary lesion in an upper rib due to osteonecrotic fracture following radiotherapy is not uncommon. Although a focal rib lesion is often the result of trauma, which may not even be recalled by the patient, a lesion that extends along the length of a rib would raise suspicions of malignant involvement. Conversely, a line of foci in adjacent ribs is a situation where one may be certain of a traumatic cause.

The interpretation of lesions in the spine, whether single or multiple, may be especially problematic as there is a high incidence of benign abnormalities in the older population, including osteoarthritis, which may be indistinguishable from metastases without further investigation. The spine is one of the commonest sites for skeletal metastases[18] and in patients with a known primary cancer, solitary vertebral bone scan lesions were reported to be benign in just over half (57%) in one study.[27] The authors then went on to classify distinguishing features on planar scans and found that only complex areas of uptake were a useful feature, with 11 out of 15 showing this pattern being associated with malignant disease. Conversely, all peripheral vertebral body lesions which extended outside the vertebral margin had a benign aetiology. As already mentioned above, it is possible that SPECT might further improve the specificity of the bone scan in the spine.

Vertebral body fractures have a characteristic appearance on bone scintigraphy, showing a linear pattern of increased uptake but it is not possible to differentiate fractures due to benign processes such as osteoporosis from malignant infiltration and subsequent pathological fracture. Multiple, irregularly scattered lesions elsewhere in the skeleton would suggest a malignant aetiology whereas a follow-up scan after an interval of a few months that shows reducing activity would suggest a benign cause. Plain radiographs do not commonly add further information but merely confirm that the pattern seen on a bone scan is due to vertebral collapse. MRI, where altered signal in the bone marrow or evidence of a soft tissue mass confirms malignancy, is the next best noninvasive investigation.

An interval scan may be helpful in the differentiation of bone scan lesions. In a series of patients with a mixture of cancers, 19 out of 21 metastases became more intense whilst benign lesions either remained unchanged (47%) or resolved (41%). Benign rib, pelvic, and peripheral lesions tended to resolve within 12–24 months but benign skull and vertebral lesions persisted.[22] It is clear, however, that even using all the available information from a bone scan there are often cases that remain indeterminate and require further correlative imaging to differentiate benign from malignant lesions. Initially, plain radiographs are most commonly used and it has been shown that if there is a benign radiographic explanation for a bone scan abnormality then there is less than a 1% chance that a coincident metastasis will be missed.[28] Unfortunately the converse is not true. Radiographs are relatively insensitive for detecting metastases, requiring a lesion to be over 1 cm with 50% loss of trabecular bone before it is readily visible.[29] Galasko reported a median lead time of between 12 and 18 months for bone scintigraphy over radiographs[30] although in a study of 6-monthly bone scans in patients with breast cancer, a median lead time of 4 months (range 0–18 months) was found.[31] In view of these observations it can be seen that a negative radiograph does not predict absence of metastatic disease and with current, clinically available technology, cross-sectional, anatomical imaging such as CT or MRI are the next best step in evaluating indeterminate bone scan lesions. MRI is regarded as having greater sensitivity as imaging of the bone marrow is possible, thereby detecting metastases before there has been destruction of bone.[32] The role of ^{18}FDG PET in this situation is still being assessed but would appear a promising method of differentiating benign from malignant disease processes as it has in other clinical situations.[33]

Although not usually of any diagnostic value, extraskeletal accumulation of bone scanning agents is occasionally seen. Uptake may be seen in tumours themselves and is not uncommonly witnessed in malignant breast masses or hepatic metastases, especially from a gastrointestinal primary tumour. Low-grade, diffuse uptake may also be seen in malignant pleural effusions and ascites. Hypercalcaemia due to malignancy may cause diffuse soft tissue uptake in a number of organs. Most commonly the kidneys show enhanced activity but if the hypercalcaemia is severe then lung and rarely stomach activity may occur (Fig. 7.8).

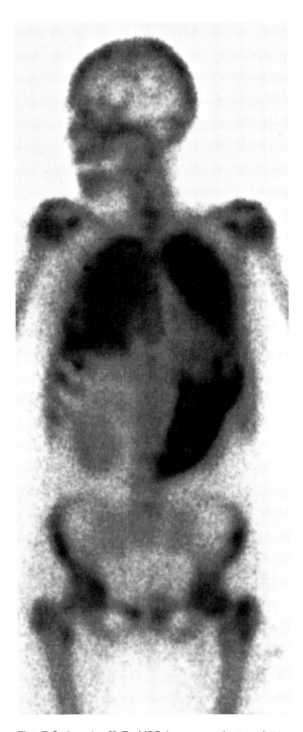

Fig. 7.8 Anterior ^{99m}Tc MDP bone scan in a patient with breast cancer and hypercalcaemia. Extensive soft tissue activity is noted in the stomach and lungs.

THE ROLE OF BONE SCINTIGRAPHY IN SPECIFIC TUMOURS

The clinical use of bone scintigraphy is determined to some extent by the frequency of bone metastases in individual tumours. In current clinical practice bone scintigraphy is most often used in the evaluation and management of breast and prostate cancers, although specific roles exist in other tumours.

Some controversy has existed as to the precise role of bone scanning in patients at different disease stages and its use still varies between institutions. A number of general situations arise where the bone scan is potentially valuable. Included are its use as part of the initial evaluation at presentation as a baseline staging procedure, in the routine follow-up of asymptomatic individuals, to assess response to therapy, and in the investigation of patients with symptoms and/or laboratory investigations which suggest possible bone involvement. Due to the low incidence of bone involvement at presentation in many of the commoner cancers such as bowel, thyroid, melanoma, and head and neck tumours, bone scintigraphy is usually only performed in those with suspicion of bone involvement and in the treatment assessment of those with proven bone metastases.

One complicating factor in the use of bone scintigraphy in the assessment of response to treatment is the flare phenomenon. An increase in lesion activity or in number of lesions within 6 months of systemic therapy does not necessarily indicate disease progression. Indeed these appearances may indicate a better prognosis.[34] Increased osteoblastic activity, as a healing response to successful treatment, is the cause of the flare response and may not only cause lesions to appear more active but may also make lesions appear that were previously invisible. In clinical practice the flare phenomenon is most often encountered in patients with either breast or prostate cancer. In breast cancer the flare phenomenon is maximal at approximately 3 months after treatment and it may not be possible to differentiate response from progression until 6 months. Although often regarded as an infrequent finding it occurs in the majority of patients who are responding and has been reported with both endocrine treatment[34] and chemotherapy.[35]

Breast cancer

Breast cancer is common – the lifetime probability of women in the UK developing this disease being approximately 1 in 12. The skeleton is the most common distant site to which breast cancer spreads. Bone metastases affect 8% of all patients who develop breast cancer, but this rises to nearly 70% in those with advanced disease.[36]

Secondary deposits in bone are the reason for much of the morbidity and disability caused by this disease as the clinical course may be prolonged. The median survival for those whose disease remains confined to the skeleton is 24 months with 20% remaining alive at 5 years.[36] Complications from skeletal metastases include pain, pathological fracture, hypercalcaemia, myelosuppression, spinal cord compression, and nerve root lesions and the costs of treating bone metastases and associated complications make a major demand on health-care resources.[37]

In breast cancer there is usually a predominance of osteoclastic activity causing lytic metastases which are generally associated with greater morbidity, but mixed or purely osteoblastic, sclerotic lesions may occur.

The use of bone scintigraphy in the staging of early breast cancer has previously been and continues, to some extent, to be a controversial area. This particularly applies in stage I and stage II disease. Some of the initial large studies carried out in the 1970s reported skeletal metastases detection rates of between 0 and 18% for stage I[38–42] and 0 and 41% for stage II.[38,40–43] This compares to 0 to 6% and 0.2% to 10%, respectively, in similar studies carried out a decade later.[17,44–46] when equipment and radiopharmaceuticals had improved and had been standardized and when similar criteria for confirming the metastatic nature of lesions were more widely applied. Due to the early reports it was recommended that all patients with breast cancer should have a bone scan performed at presentation. Because of the later results this belief is no longer universally held although some argue that a baseline scan which documents any benign abnormalities is useful for future comparison.

Stage III disease is associated with a detection rate of between 6% and 62% in the studies quoted above and most would agree that bone scintigraphy is justified in this group as a reasonable use of resources. Conversely, the gain in these patients may be less as many with advanced disease would be inoperable, requiring radiotherapy and chemotherapy even without evidence of skeletal metastases. However, the bone scan may be useful in identifying metastases which are at increased risk of pathological fracture or spinal cord compression and aiding in directing palliative radiotherapy.

From one of the largest studies,[17] in which clinical staging, imaging technique, and scan interpretation were well standardized and with at least 1 year of follow-up in all patients ($n = 1267$), the rates for bone scans showing evidence of metastatic disease were 0, 3, 7, and 47%, respectively, for stages I to IV. When staging by primary tumour size alone, it was found that T2 tumours (2–5 cm) were very unlikely to be associated with a positive scan (0.3%) but that T3 (greater than 5 cm) and T4 tumours (any size with infiltration, ulceration, etc.) were associated with positive scans in 8% and 13%, respectively. It was therefore concluded that routine scans are not routinely required in those with tumours of less than 2 cm but only with stage II, III, or IV disease. In addition to aiding immediate management, a positive baseline bone scan also has prognostic significance. Patients with a positive scan have a poorer prognosis[46,47] with the median survival of those with disease confined to the skeleton being approximately 24 months.[36]

The role of the bone scan in the follow-up of asymptomatic and symptomatic patients is perhaps less controversial. Although the pick-up rate of new metastases in those being screened serially varies among reported studies, most authors conclude that follow-up scans in asymptomatic patients are unnecessary and not cost effective. It has been shown that more than 50% of patients may seek medical attention between serial scan follow-up with the majority of relapses being clinically evident.[48] Perhaps more importantly, a large, randomized, multicentre study found that even though more metastases could be detected with 6-monthly bone scans, 5-year survival was not altered.[49] Coleman et al. have tried to rationalize the situation by determining an asymptomatic group who might benefit from serial scans.[31] Using 6-monthly follow-up scans for 2 years in 560 patients, they identified a groups with T4 tumours, more than 4 involved axillary lymph nodes and those with inoperable tumours as having a high enough scan conversion rate (> 6%) to justify serial scanning. It is not known whether earlier detection in this high-risk group affects morbidity or mortality but the psychological value of a negative scan to the patient should not be underestimated.

Few would argue that a bone scan is justified in patients with new symptoms or in whom there are worrying clinical, laboratory, or radiological features as it may subsequently help in decisions on local or systemic palliative therapy as well as providing prognostic information. The bone scan can also play a role in the prediction of complications from metastases. Long bone metastases are worthy of radiological follow-up as these are at increased risk of pathological fracture and may therefore warrant prophylactic orthopaedic intervention, commonly by placing an intramedullary nail. Patients with hypercalcaemia usually have evidence of widespread skeletal involvement although humoral factors may be the cause in up to 15% of cases.[36]

Both systemic (endocrine and chemotherapy) and local (radiotherapy) treatments exist for bone metastases from breast cancer and methods for assessing the response to treatment are an important part of the management of these patients. At present the most standardized way of assessing response is by comparing serial radiographs. The Union Internationale Contre le Cancer (UICC) defined a number of criteria which indicate response to treatment including disappearance of lesions and sclerosis of formerly lytic lesions.[50] Although standardization is improved by using these criteria, the method is otherwise relatively insensitive as it may take between 6 months and a year for radiographic evidence of response to be seen. The assessment of sclerotic disease, although less frequent than in prostatic cancer, is especially problematic. Interestingly it has been noted that the response of skeletal metastases compared to soft tissue disease is often less in the same individual.[36] Rather than there being a different biological response among different types of metastases it is thought that this phenomenon may simply reflect the insensitivity of the UICC radiographic method of response assessment.

In view of these problems other methods have been studied for assessing skeletal response. These include clinical assessment,[51] biochemical markers,[52] tumour markers[53] and bone scintigraphy.[34] Bone scintigraphy shows advantages over other methods in that it is a sensitive technique, assesses the whole skeleton, and localizes sites of disease. An increase in lesion intensity (taking careful account of technical factors in the image display and acquisition) or an increase in the number of lesions is regarded as disease progression. The flare phenomenon, which is described above, means that it may not be possible confidently to differentiate response from progression until 6 months after therapy, however. Conversely, apparent reduction in lesion activity may also not reflect response because very aggressive lytic disease may continue to progress without an osteoblastic response although this observation is rare compared to the flare phenomenon.[54] Although more difficult to explain, occasionally a mixed response may be seen between different lesions within the same individual. Allowing for these confounding factors and by only interpreting scans with a detailed knowledge of previous therapy together with correlative radiography when necessary, the bone scan is nevertheless not only a valuable objective measure of response but also gives prognostic information.[55] To try to improve the assessment of

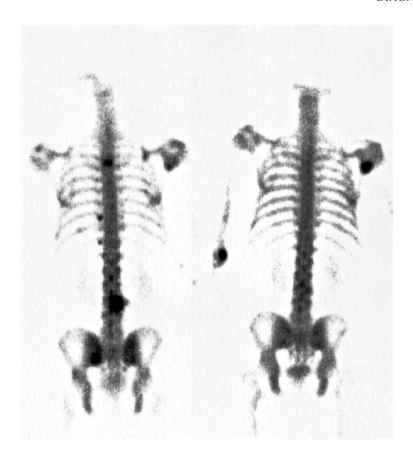

Fig. 7.9 Posterior ⁹⁹ᵐTc MDP bone scans in a patient with breast cancer before (left) and 6 months after (right) chemotherapy. Significant improvement is seen in the vertebral lesions.

disease response with bone scintigraphy some authors have described semi-quantitative means of following bone metastases[56,57] but others have found no advantage over visual interpretation[58] which is the method most commonly used in routine practice (Fig. 7.9).

Prostate cancer

Prostate cancer is one of the commonest cancers in men and 85% of patients dying of this disease have evidence of bone metastases. The majority of skeletal metastases from carcinoma of the prostate are sclerotic and because of this the bone scan is extremely sensitive.

At presentation, the number of patients with bone metastases is high and may be as high as 30–50%[59] but this varies according to the stage of disease. A number of methods of staging the disease exist, including clinical staging,[60] tumour size (T staging),[61] Gleason histologic staging[62] and measurement of the serum prostatic-specific antigen (PSA) levels.[63] The results of a small number of studies using these staging methods are summarized in Table 7.1.

It might be argued that even the lowest stage by clinical and T classification shows a high enough scan positive rate to warrant routine bone scans and therefore a more discerning measurement is required. The measurement of PSA would seem a simple and convenient way of selecting those asymptomatic patients who might benefit from a staging bone scan. A level of between 10 and 20 ng/ml might be considered to give too low a return to be cost effective but most would agree that a level of greater than

Table 7.1 Frequency of bone metastases according to clinical stage, T classification, Gleason histologic grading and PSA measurement

Staging method					
Clinical stage[60]	I	II	III	IV	
	9%	20%	24%	60%	
T classification[61]	T1	T2	T3	T4	
	7.1%	19.3%	39.2%	65%	
Gleason[62]	low (2–5)	high (6–10)			
	0%	47%			
PSA (ng/ml)[63]	< 10	10–20	20–50	50–100	> 100
	0%	1%	7%	38%	71%

20 ng/ml should lead to a bone scan being performed. In symptomatic patients at presentation or during follow-up, whatever the stage, bone scintigraphy should be considered. More controversial is the question of whether serial follow-up scans should be performed routinely in asymptomatic patients. Although a high conversion rate (20%) from scan negative at presentation to scan positive by the second year has been reported,[64] it was also found that many of these patients developed clinical or biochemical evidence of bone involvement, questioning the need for routine serial scintigraphy. It may be possible to select those asymptomatic patients who require a bone scan by following the cheaper and more convenient measurement of PSA.[65]

The bone scan is also valuable as a method of assessing treatment response but, as with breast cancer, the flare phenomenon may occur and so care must be taken in the timing and interpretation of scans. If a flare response is confirmed then a favourable treatment response is predicted.[66] For those in whom bone scan appearances deteriorate after therapy then the prognosis is much worse, the 1-year survival in those with disease progression being 7% compared to 60% in those with no change or improvement.[67]

Miscellaneous cancers

Metastases from renal cell carcinoma are mostly lytic and frequently do not excite much in the way of an osteoblastic reaction. Lesions may therefore be difficult to spot and a careful review of bone scans for cold lesions should be made when assessing the skeleton in this cancer.[68] The presence of skeletal metastases at presentation does not necessarily alter the surgical management of this tumour but is valuable in assessing the extent of disease, predicting complications such as fracture and localizing lesions prior to palliative radiotherapy. Although the incidence of metastases at presentation is relatively high (7.5–32%[69]), the majority of patients have clinical or laboratory evidence of skeletal involvement and there is therefore usually no need to scan all asymptomatic patients routinely at presentation.

The incidence of skeletal involvement at initial presentation of other genitourinary tumours such as bladder, cervical, ovarian, and uterine carcinomas is relatively low and so the role of bone scintigraphy in these cases is limited to the evaluation of symptomatic patients and in assessing response to therapy.

In lung cancer the reported rates of skeletal involvement at presentation varies quite widely (2–19%[69]) but this may in part reflect the different types of lung tumour cases studied in different reports. Small cell lung cancers appear to have a high incidence of bone metastases at presentation (approaching 50%[70,71]) but this type of tumour is only rarely treated surgically having a very poor prognosis even in those without apparent metastases. Non-small cell lung cancers may be curable by surgery if no metastases are present but opinions vary as to whether bone scans should be routinely included in the presurgical investigation of asymptomatic patients. The prognosis of those with bone metastases is very poor with very few surviving more than 12 months.[72] Practice may change with the increased availability of PET as ^{18}FDG scanning can assess local and distant metastatic spread to soft tissues and bone. Although the anatomical detail of mediastinal structures is not present, this technique would appear more sensitive than CT alone. In a recent series, 18% of patients had management changed to a nonsurgical regime because of the detection of previously unsuspected metastases[73] and despite initial caution because of the relatively high cost of individual studies there is increasing evidence that this technique's high sensitivity allows it to be cost effective in preoperative staging.[74]

In lung cancer there is no evidence of increased survival by the detection of presymptomatic bone metastases, and routine follow-up bone scintigraphy is not indicated. Investigation of patients suspected of having bone involvement is helpful in confirmation, localization, and assessing extent and, together with other correlative imaging, helping to exclude benign causes for symptoms. Bone scintigraphy shows specific changes in patients with hypertrophic pulmonary osteoarthropathy which may help to explain the cause of distal limb pain or be noted as an incidental finding in patients with lung cancer.

Neuroblastoma is a rare solid tumour of childhood which deserves separate mention because it frequently metastasizes to the skeleton. Bone scintigraphy has been demonstrated as a sensitive method for assessment of the skeletal involvement but depends on obtaining very good-quality images to avoid false negative interpretations. Photopoenic lesions may occur which can be difficult to resolve in the smaller paediatric skeleton[75] and symmetrical, diffuse uptake of tracer next to the joints, seen as blurring of the borders of epiphyseal activity, requires high-resolution images for detection. Uptake of ^{99m}Tc MDP is often noted in the primary tumour and soft tissue metastases.[76,77] Although ^{123}I MIBG is a specific tracer for staging and follow-up of neuroblastoma, false negatives have been noted in relation to the skeleton and full assessment with both ^{99m}Tc MDP and ^{123}I MIBG is recommended.[78]

OTHER RADIONUCLIDE SCANNING TECHNIQUES

The bone scan is the most commonly utilized method of skeletal evaluation in cancer patients but other radiopharmaceuticals and radionuclide methods have been assessed. Nonspecific tumour agents such as ^{201}Tl have been studied to differentiate benign from malignant lesions which appear as a solitary hot-spot on a bone scan. Van der Wall and colleagues described uptake in seven out of eight malignant tumours compared to only one out of 17 benign lesions.[79] Similarly, the metabolic agent ^{99m}Tc sestamibi shows higher accumulation in malignant bone lesions compared to benign, suggesting the ability to differentiate although 6 out of 42 malignant lesions were not clearly identified.[80] In the same study it was found that a reduction in uptake of ^{99m}Tc sestamibi correlated well with histological response following radiotherapy or chemotherapy.

As previously mentioned, bone scintigraphy may not be optimal for assessing the extent of myeloma involvement of the skeleton. It has been noted however that myeloma lesions accumulate ^{99m}Tc sestamibi and that use of this radiopharmaceutical may be an accurate method of measuring extent of disease.[81] Further, it has been found that those tumours which do not accumulate tracer but which are known to be active may be resistant to chemotherapy as ^{99m}Tc sestamibi is actively

106 CANCER AND THE SKELETON

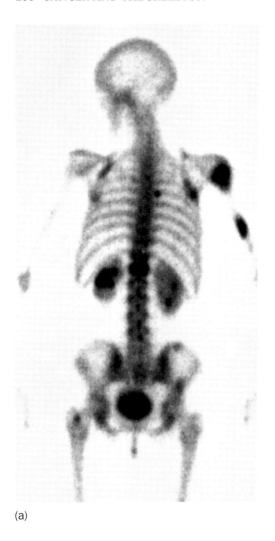

(a)

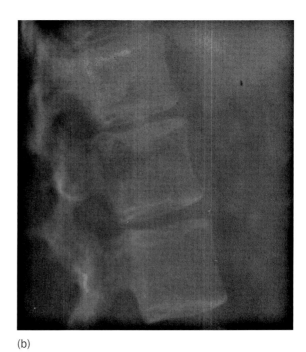

(b)

Fig. 7.10 (a) Posterior ^{99m}Tc MDP bone scan showing a number of metastases throughout the skeleton. (b) Lateral lumbar spine radiograph showing the metastasis in the uppermost vertebra (L1) is sclerotic. (c) Left – ^{18}FDG and right – ^{18}F scan at L1. Note that the L1 sclerotic metastasis (which had not received radiotherapy) shows osteoblastic activity on the ^{99m}Tc MDP and ^{18}F bone scans but little metabolic activity on the ^{18}FDG scan. (The left kidney has dilated upper pole calyces.)

Transaxial   Sagittal   Transaxial   Sagittal

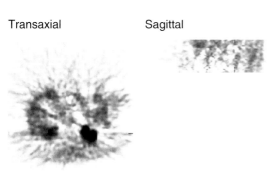
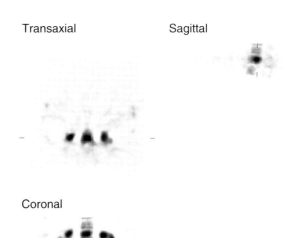

Coronal   Coronal

(c)

eliminated from the cell by P-glycoprotein and it is thought that multidrug resistance may be associated with overexpression of P-glycoprotein, thereby displaying potential as a test for drug resistance.[82]

Other tracers exist which although not specific to bone metastases are specific to individual tumours or groups of tumours and so may be helpful in improving specificity of bone scan lesions. Examples include ^{131}I iodine scintigraphy which is the mainstay of detection of metastases whether in soft tissue or bone in the differentiated thyroid cancers. Because thyroid replacement therapy needs to be stopped some weeks before scanning can take place, the diphosphonate bone scan with radiographic correlation, if necessary, remains the first line in rapid assessment of patients suspected of having bone metastases. If ^{131}I uptake is subsequently confirmed in bone lesions then high doses may be given as therapy.

Similarly, tracers such as ^{111}In octreotide or ^{123}I MIBG show affinity for neuroendocrine tumours and their metastases but their role specifically in the detection of bone metastases has not been studied. It is unlikely that these tracers would be significantly more sensitive than bone scintigraphy but they may have a role in increasing specificity in otherwise indeterminate bone lesions in patients with these tumours.

POSITRON EMISSION TOMOGRAPHY

Fluoride-18 ion was first described as a bone scanning agent many years ago and has been evaluated using PET in skeletal metastases. In addition to high-resolution images this method allows skeletal kinetics to be quantified.[83,84] A recent report of increased sensitivity for detection of bone metastases with ^{18}F PET compared to ^{99m}Tc MDP in a variety of cancers may be partly explained by the better spatial resolution and provision of tomography as a routine with this method.[85]

^{18}FDG PET has been shown to be an accurate method of evaluating patients with breast cancer for metastases[86,87] but the sensitivity for detection of bone metastases has varied, with some authors noting an apparent lower sensitivity for the detection of skeletal disease compared to conventional scintigraphy.[88] We have noted a lower sensitivity and degree of uptake of ^{18}FDG in a subgroup of patients with progressive osteoblastic disease (Fig. 7.10), whilst overall ^{18}FDG detected more bone lesions than ^{99m}Tc MDP bone scans but particularly in those with lytic disease.[89] The overall increase in sensitivity of ^{18}FDG PET may not only be due to the improved resolution and tomographic capabilities of PET but also that bone metastases may be detected in the bone marrow before a significant bone reaction has occurred, this being necessary for successful ^{99m}Tc MDP imaging. The apparent difference in biological behaviour between types of bone metastases is unexplained but, importantly, the greatest sensitivity is in the group with lytic disease, who experience the most skeletal morbidity, have a more aggressive clinical course and a reduced survival and so who may benefit from earlier detection of skeletal involvement.

REFERENCES

1. Fleming WH, McIraith JD, King ER. Photoscanning of bone lesions utilising strontium-85. *Radiology* (1961) **77**: 635–6.
2. Blau M, Ganatra R, Bender MA. ^{18}F—fluoride for bone imaging. *Semin Nucl Med.* (1972) **2**: 31–7.
3. Fogelman I. Diphosphonate bone scanning agents – current concepts. *Eur J Nucl Med* (1982) **77**: 635–6.
4. Mundy GR. Metastatic bone disease. In Fogelman I (ed) *Bone Remodelling and its Disorders* (London: Martin Dunitz, 1995): 104–22.
5. Wolfenden JM, Pitt MJ, Durie BGW et al. Comparison of bone scintigraphy and radiology in myeloma. *Radiology* (1980) **134**: 723–8.
6. Warburg O. On the origin of cancer cells. *Science* (1954) **123**: 306–14.
7. Clavo AC, Brown RS, Wahl RL. Fluorodeoxyglucose uptake in human cancer cell lines is

increased by hypoxia. *J Nucl Med* (1995) **36:** 1625–32.
8. Kashyap R, Babbar A, Sahai I *et al.* Tc-99m (V) DMSA imaging. A new approach to studying metastases from breast carcinoma. *Clin Nucl Med* (1997) **17:** 119–22.
9. Lam AS, Kettle AG, O'Doherty MJ *et al.* Pentavalent 99mTc-DMSA imaging in patients with bone metastases. *Nucl Med Commun* (1997) **18:** 907–14.
10. Dunker CM, Carrio I, Bernal L *et al.* Radioimmune imaging of bone marrow in patients with suspected bone metastases from primary breast cancer. *J Nucl Med* (1990) **31:** 1450–5.
11. Reske SN, Karstens JH, Gloekner W *et al.* Radioimmunoimaging for diagnosis of bone marrow involvement in breast cancer and malignant lymphoma. *Lancet* (1989) **i:** 299–301.
12. Delpassand ES, Garcia JR, Bhadkamkar V *et al.* Value of SPECT imaging of the thoracolumbar spine in cancer patients. *Clin Nucl Med* (1995) **20:** 1047–51.
13. Bushnell DL, Kahn D, Huston B *et al.* Utility of SPECT imaging for determination of vertebral metastases in patients with known primary tumours. *Skeletal Radiol* (1995) **24:** 13–16.
14. Han LJ, Au-Yong TK, Tong WCM *et al.* Comparison of bone SPECT and planar imaging in the detection of vertebral metastases in patients with back pain. *Eur J Nucl Med* (1998) **25:** 635–8.
15. Kwai AH, Stomper PC, Kaplan WD. Clinical significance of isolated scintigraphic sternal lesions in patients with breast cancer. *J Nucl Med* (1988) **29:** 324–8.
16. Barker DJP, Clough PWL, Guyer PB *et al.* Paget's disease of bone in 14 British towns. *Br Med J* (1977) **1:** 1181–3.
17. Coleman RE, Rubens RD, Fogelman I. Reappraisal of the baseline bone scan in breast cancer. *J Nucl Med* (1988) **29:** 1045–9.
18. Galasko CSB. Tumours. In Galasko CSB, Weber DA (eds) *Radionuclide Scintigraphy in Orthopaedics* (New York: Churchill Livingstone, 1984): 65–110.
19. Corcoran RJ, Thrall JH, Kyle RW. Solitary abnormalities in bone scans of patients with extraosseous malignancies. *Radiology* (1976) **121:** 663–7.
20. Rappaport AH, Hoffer PB, Genant HK. Unifocal bone findings in scintigraphy. Clinical significance in patients with known primary cancer. *West J Med* (1978) **129:** 188–92.
21. Tofe AJ, Francis MD, Harvey WJ. Correlation of neoplasms with incidence and localisation of skeletal metastases. An analysis of 1355 diphosphonate bone scans. *J Nucl Med* (1975) **16:** 986–9.
22. Jacobson AF, Cronin EB, Stomper EC *et al.* Bone scans with one or two new abnormalities in cancer patients with no known metastases: frequency and serial scintigraphic behaviour of benign and malignant lesions. *Radiology* (1990) **175:** 229–32.
23. Boxer DI, Todd CE, Coleman RE *et al.* Bone secondaries in breast cancer: the solitary metastasis. *J Nucl Med* (1989) **30:** 1318–20.
24. Tumeh SS, Beadle G, Kaplan WD. Clinical significance of solitary rib lesions in patients with extraskeletal malignancy. *J Nucl Med* (1985) **26:** 1140–3.
25. Jacobson AF, Stomper PC, Jochelson MS *et al.* Association between number and sites of new bone scan abnormalities and presence of skeletal metastases in patients with breast cancer. *J Nucl Med* (1990) **31:** 387–92.
26. Baxter AD, Coakley FV, Finlay DB *et al.* The aetiology of solitary hot spots in the ribs on planar bone scans. *Nucl Med Commun* (1995) **16:** 834–7.
27. Coakley FV, Jones AR, Finlay DB *et al.* The aetiology and distinguishing features of solitary spinal hot spots on planar bone scans. *Clin Radiol* (1995) **50:** 327–30.
28. Jacobson AF, Stomper MD, Cronin EB *et al.* Bone scans with one or two new abnormalities in cancer patients with no known metastases: the reliability of interpretation on initial correlative radiographs. *Radiology* (1990) **174:** 503–7.
29. Edelstyn GA, Gillespie PJ, Grebell FS. The radiological demonstration of osseous metastases: experimental observations. *Clin Radiol* (1967) **18:** 158–62.
30. Galasko CSB. The significance of occult metastases detected by scintigraphy in patients with otherwise early breast cancer. *Br J Surg* (1975) **56:** 757–64.
31. Coleman RE, Fogelman I, Habibollahi F *et al.* Selection of patients with breast cancer for routine follow up bone scans. *Clin Oncol* (1990) **2:** 328–32.
32. Daffner RH, Lupetin AR, Dash N *et al.* MRI in the detection of malignant infiltration of bone marrow. *Am J Radiol* (1986) **146:** 353–8.
33. Gupta NC, Frank AL, Dewan N *et al.* Solitary pulmonary nodules: detection of malignancy

with PET 2–[F-18]-fluoro-2–deoxy-D-glucose. *Radiology* (1992) **184:** 441–4.
34. Coleman RE, Mashiter G, Whitaker KB *et al.* Bone scan flare predicts successful systemic therapy for bone metastases. *J Nucl Med* (1988) **29:** 1354–9.
35. Schneider JA, Divgi CR, Scott AM *et al.* Flare on bone scintigraphy following Taxol chemotherapy for metastatic breast cancer. *J Nucl Med* (1994) **35:** 1748–52.
36. Coleman RE, Rubens RD. The clinical course of bone metastases from breast cancer. *Br J Cancer* (1987) **55:** 61–6.
37. Richards MA, Braysher S, Gregory WM *et al.* Advanced breast cancer: use of resources and cost implications. *Br J Cancer* (1993) **67:** 856–60.
38. Nomura Y, Kondo H, Yamagata J *et al.* Evaluation of liver and bone scanning in patients with early breast cancer based on results obtained from more advanced patients. *Eur J Cancer* (1978) **14:** 1129–36.
39. Davies CJ, Griffiths PA, Preston BJ *et al.* Staging breast cancer. Role of scanning. *Br Med J* (1977) **2:** 603–5.
40. Gerber FH, Goodreau JJ, Kirchner PT, Fonty WJ. Efficacy of preoperative and postoperative bone scanning in the management of breast carcinoma. *N Engl J Med* (1977) **297:** 300–3.
41. Citrin DL, Furnival CM, Bessent RG *et al.* Radioactive technetium phosphate bone scanning in preoperative assessment and follow up study of patients with primary carcinoma of the breast. *Surg Gynecol Obstet* (1976) **143:** 360–4.
42. Campbell DJ, Banks AJ, Davis GD. The value of preliminary bone scanning in staging and assessing the prognosis of breast cancer. *Br J Surg* (1976) **63:** 811–16.
43. Sklaroff RB, Sklaroff DM. Bone metastases from breast cancer at the time of radical mastectomy. *Cancer* (1976) **38:** 107–11.
44. Ciatto S, Pacini P, Bravetti P *et al.* Staging breast cancer – Screening for occult metastases. *Tumori* (1985) **71:** 339–44.
45. Strender LE, Lagergren C, Wallgren A *et al.* Role of bone scans in the initial assessment of operable patients with breast cancer. *Acta Radiol Oncol* (1981) **20:** 187–91.
46. Kunkler IH, Merrick MV, Rodger A. Bone scintigraphy in breast cancer: a nine year follow up. *Clin Radiol* (1985) **36:** 279–82.
47. Furnival CM, Blumgart LH, Citrin DL *et al.* Serial scintiscanning in breast cancer: indications and prognostic value. *Clin Oncol* (1980) **6:** 25–32.
48. Ojeda MB, Alonso MC, Bastus R *et al.* Follow up of breast cancer stages I and II. An analysis of some common methods. *Eur J Cancer* (1987) **23:** 419–23.
49. Rosselli Del Turco M, Palli D, Cariddi A *et al.* Intensive diagnostic follow up after treatment of primary breast cancer. A randomised trial (National Research Council Project on Breast Cancer Follow Up). *JAMA* (1994) **271:** 1593–7.
50. Hayward JL, Carbone PP, Heuson JC *et al.* Assessment of response to therapy in advanced breast cancer. *Eur J Cancer* (1977) **13:** 89–94.
51. Coombes RC, Dady P, Parsons C *et al.* Assessment of response of bone metastases to systemic treatment in patients with breast cancer. *Cancer* (1983) **52:** 610–14.
52. Hortobagyi GN, Libshitz HI, Seabold JE. Osseous metastases of breast cancer. Clinical, biochemical, radiographic and scintigraphic evaluation of response to therapy. *Cancer* (1984) **55:** 577–82.
53. Palazzo S, Liguori V, Molinari B. Is the carcinoembryonic antigen test a valid predictor of response to medical therapy in disseminated breast cancer? *Tumori* (1986) **72:** 515–18.
54. Coleman RE, Rubens RD. Bone metastases and breast cancer. *Cancer Treat Rev* (1985) **12:** 251–70.
55. Bitran JD, Beckerman C, Desser RK. The predictive value of serial bone scans in assessing response to chemotherapy in advanced breast cancer. *Cancer* (1980) **45:** 1562–8.
56. Erdi YE, Humm JL, Imbriaco M *et al.* Quantitative bone metastases analysis based on image segmentation. *J Nucl Med* (1997) **38:** 1401–6.
57. Pitt WR, Sharp PF. Comparison of quantitative and visual detection of new focal bone lesions. *J Nucl Med* (1985) **26:** 230–6.
58. Condon BR, Buchanan R, Garvie N *et al.* Assessment of progression of secondary bone lesions following cancer of the breast or prostate using serial radionuclide imaging. *Br J Radiol* (1981) **54:** 18–23.
59. McKillop JH. Bone scanning in metastatic disease. In Fogelman I (ed) *Bone Scanning in Clinical Practice* (Berlin: Springer-Verlag, 1987): 41–60.
60. Paulson DF and the Uro-oncology Research Group. The impact of current staging procedures in assessing disease extent in prostatic adenocarcinoma. *J Urol* (1979) **121:** 300–2.
61. Biersack HJ, Wegner G, Distelmaier W. Bone metastases of prostate cancer in relation to tumour size and grade of malignancy. *Nuklearmedizin* (1980) **19:** 29–32.

62. Shih WJ, Mitchell B, Wierzbinski B. Prediction of radionuclide bone imaging findings by Gleason histologic grading of prostate carcinoma. *Clin Nucl Med* (1991) **16**: 763–6.
63. Chybowski FM, Keller JJL, Bergstrahl EJ. Predicting radionuclide bone scan findings in patients with newly diagnosed, untreated prostate cancer: prostate specific antigen is superior to all other clinical parameters. *J Urol* (1991) **145**: 313–18.
64. Huben RP, Schellhammer PF. The role of routine follow up bone scan after definitive therapy of localised prostatic cancer. *J Urol* (1982) **128**: 510–12.
65. Terris MK, Klonecke AS, McDougall IR *et al.* Utilisation of bone scans in conjunction with prostate-specific antigen levels in the surveillance for recurrence of adenocarcinoma after radical prostatectomy. *J Nucl Med* (1991) **32**: 1713–17.
66. Sundqvist CMG, Ahlgren L, Lilja B. Repeated quantitative bone scintigraphy in patients with prostatic carcinoma treated with orchidectomy. *Eur J Nucl Med* (1988) **14**: 203–6.
67. Pollen JJ, Gerber K, Ashburn WL. Nuclear bone imaging in metastatic cancer of the prostate. *Cancer* (1981) **47**: 2585–94.
68. Kim EE, Bledin AG, Gutierrez C *et al.* Comparison of radionuclide images and radiographs for skeletal metastases from renal cell carcinoma. *Oncology* (1983) **40**: 284–6.
69. Fogelman I, McKillop JH. The bone scan in metastatic disease. In Rubens RD, Fogelman I (eds) *Bone Metastases: Diagnosis and Treatment* (London: Spinger-Verlag, 1991): 31–5.
70. Bitran JD, Beckerman C, Pinsky S. Sequential scintigraphic staging of small cell carcinoma. *Cancer* (1981) **47**: 1971–5.
71. Levenson RM, Sauerbrum FJL, Ihde DC *et al.* Small cell lung cancer: radionuclide bone scans for assessment of tumour extent and response. *Am J Radiol* (1981) **137**: 31–5.
72. Gravenstein S, Peltz MA, Poreis W. How ominous is an abnormal scan in bronchogenic carcinoma? *JAMA* (1979) **241**: 2523–4.
73. Lewis P, Griffin S, Marsden P *et al.* Whole body 18F-fluorodeoxyglucose positron emission tomography in preoperative evaluation of lung cancer. *Lancet* (1994) **i**: 1265–6.
74. Valk PE, Pounds TR, Tesar RD *et al.* Cost-effectiveness of PET imaging in clinical oncology. *Nucl Med Bio* (1996) **23**: 737–43.
75. Fawcett HD, McDougall IR. Bone scan in extraskeletal neuroblastoma with hot primary and cold skeletal metastases. *Clin Nucl Med* (1980) **5**: 49–50.
76. Howman-Giles R, Gilday DL, Ash JM. Radionuclide skeletal survey in neuroblastoma. *Radiology* (1979) **131**: 497–502.
77. Podrasky AER, Stark DD, Hattner RE *et al.* Radionuclide bone scanning in neuroblastoma: skeletal metastases and primary tumour localisation on 99m-Tc MDP. *Am J Radiol* (1983) **141**: 469–72.
78. Gordon I, Peters AM, Gutman A *et al.* Skeletal assessment in neuroblastoma – the pitfalls of iodine-123-MIBG scans. *J Nucl Med* (1990) **31**: 129–34.
79. Van der Wall H, Murray IP, Huckstep RL *et al.* The role of thallium scintigraphy in excluding malignancy in bone. *Clin Nucl Med* (1993) **18**: 551–7.
80. Caner B, Kitapcl M, Unlu M *et al.* Technetium-99m-MIBI uptake in benign and malignant bone lesions: a comparative study with technetium-99m-MDP. *J Nucl Med* (1992) **33**: 319–24.
81. Pace L, Catalano L, Pinto AM *et al.* Different patterns of technetium-99m sestamibi uptake in multiple myeloma. *Eur J Nucl Med* (1998) **25**: 714–20.
82. Tirovola EB, Biassoni L, Britton KE *et al.* The use of 99mTc-MIBI scanning in multiple myeloma. *Br J Cancer* (1996) **74**: 1815–20.
83. Petren-Mallmin M, Andreasson I, Ljunggren O *et al.* Skeletal metastases from breast cancer: uptake of 18-F fluoride measured with positron emission tomography in correlation with CT. *Skeletal Radiol* (1998) **27**: 72–6.
84. Hawkins RA, Choi Y, Huang SC *et al.* Evaluation of skeletal kinetics of fluorine-18-fluoride ion with PET. *J Nucl Med* (1992) **33**: 633–42.
85. Schirrmeister H, Guhlmann CA, Diederichs H *et al.* Planar bone imaging Vs 18F-PET in patients with cancer of the prostate, thyroid and lung. *J Nucl Med* (1998) **39**: 113P–14P (abst).
86. Tse NY, Hoh CK, Hawkins RA *et al.* The application of positron emission tomographic imaging with fluorodeoxyglucose to the evaluation of breast disease. *Am Surg* (1992) **216**: 27–34.
87. Wahl RL, Cody RL, Hutchins GD *et al.* Primary and metastatic breast carcnoma: initial clinical evaluation with PET with the radiolabeled glucose analogue 2-[F-18]-fluoro-2-deoxy-D-glucose. *Radiology* (1991) **179**: 765–70.

88. Moon DH, Maddahi J, Silverman DH *et al.* Accuracy of whole body fluorine-18-FDG PET for the detection of recurrent or metastatic breast carcinoma. *J Nucl Med* (1998) **39**: 431–5.

89. Cook GJR, Houston S, Rubens RD *et al.* Detection of bone metastases in breast cancer by ^{18}FDG PET: differing metabolic activity in osteoblastic and osteolytic lesions. *J Clin Oncol* (1998) **16**: 3375–9.

8

Radiology and magnetic resonance imaging

David MacVicar

Introduction • Diagnostic approach to bone lesions • Principles of radiological analysis • Primary bone tumours • Metastatic disease in bone • Primary tumours of bone marrow • Image-guided biopsy • Assessment of response to treatment

INTRODUCTION

The skeletal system has been a source of fascination to the radiologist for as long as the speciality has existed. The first radiographic images depicted the bones of Mrs Roentgen's hand in 1895, and for many years X-ray equipment was used primarily for images of the skeleton. Early radiographs could discriminate only four levels of contrast, namely, bone, soft tissue, fat, and air, and it was not until the 1920s that systematic experimentation with contrast agents led to the development of techniques such as angiography and pneumoencephalography. Since the 1970s, computer-based techniques, notably ultrasound (US), computed tomography (CT), and magnetic resonance imaging (MRI), have developed the ability to demonstrate a wide range of contrast within the soft tissues, and spatial resolution has improved to an extent where exquisite anatomical detail is available, with structures of under 2 mm being clearly demonstrable by all three techniques. Nevertheless, the spatial resolution available with high-quality plain film imaging of bone remains unsurpassed. Bony trabeculae and elevated periosteum, structures which are of the order of microns in thickness, may be demonstrated by skeletal radiography.

In oncological practice, lung secondaries are probably less common than primary tumours of the lung, and brain secondaries are certainly more common than brain primaries. Liver secondaries are undoubtedly more common than liver primaries in the UK, although this pattern is reversed in other parts of the world. Bone secondaries are very much more common than bone primaries, but secondary carcinoma of the bone may present with a solitary lesion, and there is a wide differential diagnosis for all such lesions, including a variety of benign conditions. This chapter will begin with a discussion of general principles of radiological diagnosis of bony lesions, followed by a discussion of the salient imaging features of three broad groups, namely, primary bone tumours, secondary deposits, and disorders of the bone marrow.

DIAGNOSTIC APPROACH TO BONE LESIONS

The clinical presentation of patients with bony tumours usually involves pain, sometimes with swelling or pathological fracture. This pain may be attributed to some minor trauma. The examining surgeon, physician, or casualty

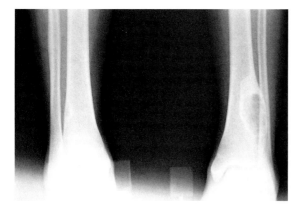

Fig. 8.1 The lateral aspect of the right tibia shows a small oval lesion aligned in the long axis of the bone, with a sclerotic margin. The appearance is typical of a fibrous cortical defect. The left tibia shows a larger lesion with the same characteristics. The increase in size has allowed a 'soap bubble' appearance to develop. By virtue of its size alone, this lesion is designated a nonossifying fibroma. The histology of the lesions is identical. They are benign developmental defects.

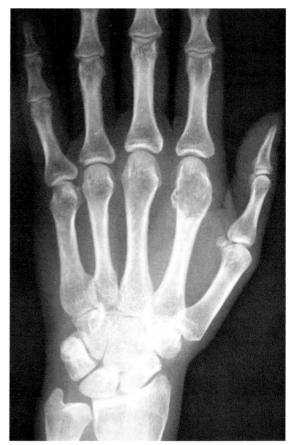

Fig. 8.2 Enchondroma of second metacarpal. The distal end of the bone is expanded. The cortex is thin. There is a narrow zone of transition and flecks of calcification are seen centrally.

officer cannot even suggest the presence of a neoplasm without an imaging procedure of some sort, so the radiologist will be involved in the management of bony tumours from the time of initial diagnosis. Radiology subsequently provides important information for staging tumours once the diagnosis has been confirmed.

It is a truism that the definitive diagnosis of tumour-like conditions of bone is made by the histopathologist, but in bone pathology more than any other the radiologist's role is complementary to that of the pathologist; if radiological input is inadequate, diagnostic errors will ensue. Some lesions can be diagnosed with confidence by the radiologist alone as normal variants or benign conditions. Examples of these are benign cortical defects (nonossifying fibroma), haemangiomas of the vertebral body, fibrous dysplasia, and enchondromas (Figs 8.1 and 8.2). Such lesions have typical appearances and can be left alone or followed with serial imaging.

Neoplasms of bone exhibit a variety of changes including necrosis and dedifferentiation. The pathologist may be presented with a small amount of biopsy material which is not necessarily representative of the majority of the tumour, or may even contain no malignant cells. Radiographic examination provides an invaluable demonstration of the gross anatomy of the entire lesion, particularly if the site of biopsy can be related accurately to the plain radiograph or scan. If the diagnostic features shown on the imaging procedure do not tally with the histological diagnosis, then a repeat biopsy may be necessary. The radiologist will usually be able to decide whether a lesion is growing slowly or rapidly, and the pattern of the image may suggest a certain cell type. However, only the pathologist can make a tissue diagnosis, and will deduce the rate of growth of the lesion from that. Expert skeletal pathologists and radiologists stress the need for regular contact between all members of the diagnostic team to ensure that the final diagnosis is appropriate and acceptable to all parties.

PRINCIPLES OF RADIOLOGICAL ANALYSIS

Before interpreting any radiological procedure, a basic amount of clinical data is essential. This includes the patient's age and sex, presence or absence of pain, duration of symptoms, and history of intervention, including biopsy and treatment. This information can be provided on the radiological request form, but unfortunately is often withheld or inaccurate. The first question to answer is whether a lesion is present at all. A bone may appear entirely normal and, in the presence of painful swelling, ultrasound or even MRI can be very valuable in demonstrating that a 'pseudo-tumour' of the soft tissues may be related to asymmetry of muscle group, accessory muscles, post-traumatic haematoma, or other benign abnormalities.

If a lesion is present, it may be a normal variant or a clinically insignificant abnormality such as a developmental defect. A variety of tumour-like disorders such as fibrous dysplasia and Paget's disease of bone are readily recognizable, and benign or latent lesions (e.g. enchondroma) can be diagnosed with confidence. Some neoplasms have benign characteristics but nevertheless need biopsy (e.g. osteoblastoma), and some lesions can be categorized as likely malignancy, either primary or secondary, which require biopsy for histological diagnosis and typing.

If this analysis suggests a malignant neoplasm, further radiographic assessment concentrates on the rate of growth of the lesion, specific features on the plain film which help in diagnosis, and a consideration of whether other imaging techniques can contribute towards the diagnosis. The plain film remains the most valuable investigation for specific radiological diagnosis. CT may provide clearer evidence of soft tissue calcification or bony destruction where doubt exists on the plain film; MRI is most valuable in demonstrating the extent of tumour within the bone and any associated soft tissue mass. Most of the diagnostic features seen on plain films are well established and documented.[1,2]

From the rate of growth of a lesion, the degree of local aggression can be inferred: the more locally aggressive the lesion appears, the more likely it is to be malignant. There is a certain amount of overlap between benign and malignant neoplasms, as some benign neoplasms may be aggressive radiologically and some malignancies are slow growing. Three patterns of radiographic change are described in ascending order of aggression, namely, *geographic, moth eaten*, and *permeative* patterns of growth.

Geographic lesions show evidence of the slowest growth and can be divided into three subgroups depending on the clarity of their margins and whether peripheral sclerosis due to reactive bone is present. The margin of these lesions may be regular or irregular in shape, but the zone of transition between normal and abnormal bone is no more than 2–3 mm. The three subgroups are:

- type 1A – the slowest growing geographical lesion has clear sclerosis of margins and a very narrow zone of transition, for example, enchondroma (Fig. 8.2) or chondromyxoid fibroma;
- type 1B – a geographical lesion without gross marginal sclerosis, sometimes designated 'punched out'. Examples include subacute infection of bone and some giant cell tumours; and
- type 1C – a geographical lesion with an ill-defined margin, which equates with early infiltrative change at the border. This may be seen with some giant cell tumours and low-grade malignancy such as chondrosarcoma, or even metastases.

Moth-eaten lesions are the most difficult to categorize, which is understandable as they lie between the other two patterns of change. They are less well defined than geographic lesions and have a wider zone of transition.

Permeative lesions are the most rapidly growing infiltrative lesions, giving a coalescent destructive appearance. The exact distinction from surrounding normal bone is difficult to make, and a wide zone of transition is present, often up to several centimetres. Such tumours are epitomized by malignant round cell tumours of bone, and are often shown to be more extensive on MRI than is suggested by plain radiography.

Variations in radiographic technique, for example, if the lesion is towards the end of a bone where the divergent X-ray beam is passing obliquely through the lesion, may make the sharp margin of a geographic lesion less clear; however, the converse is not true, in that a permeative lesion can never look geographic.

Once the rate of growth has been estimated, specific features may assist in diagnosis. The age of the patient is of importance since a solitary metastasis from carcinoma is much more common than a primary tumour of bone in middle-aged and elderly patients. In a child under 5 years, metastases and primary bone tumours are extremely rare, and developmental abnormalities are more common. In the teenage years osteosarcoma and Ewing's, although still rare, enter the differential diagnosis.

Location within the skeleton and bone may be helpful since some neoplasms are found predominantly in one region; for example, osteosarcoma prefers the metaphysis of the bone, and is most frequently found either side of the knee. Some predilections are very striking such as that of the solitary bone cyst, which occurs in the proximal humerus, proximal femur, and calcaneus, rarely straying from these sites, and chordoma occurs in the occipitocervical or sacral region in approximately 90% of cases.

The site of destruction within the bone affects the detectability and interpretation of lesions. A tumour within the medulla must destroy 40–50% of the bone mass before it becomes visible on a radiograph. Most neoplasms begin in the medulla and the initial radiographs may therefore be normal. At this stage, detection of a suspected lesion is more sensitive with scintigraphy or MRI. Once the cortex is involved, the lesion is more clearly visible on the plain film, and as the lesion becomes more peripheral within the cortex a periosteal reaction will ensue. The lifting and separation of the osteoblast-bearing layer of the periosteum result in a linear osteoblastic reaction which is relatively nonspecific and can be seen in the presence of tumour or infection. If the rate of growth of tumour is slow, laminar new bone formation will result in cortical thickening. This may be found in low-grade chondrosarcoma or recurrent osteomyelitis. An aggressive tumour gives less opportunity for the periosteum to form bone, and in some instances the periosteum simply disappears. Although Ewing's sarcoma is aggressive, it has a natural history involving periodic growth. This results in the presence of multilaminar plates of new bone laid down by the periosteum, resulting in the characteristic 'onion skin' appearance (Fig. 8.3).

When a tumour mass becomes extracortical, reactive periosteal triangles may form. A rapidly growing lesion such as an aneurysmal bone cyst will form a clear well corticated triangle close to the site of 'blow-out'. This is essentially a benign feature, and CT will confirm a thin egg shell of periosteal new bone around such lesions. In more permeative lesions, reactive triangles (Codman's triangle) appear to arise beyond the limits of the tumour within bone. This indicates that tumour has permeated the cortex and is growing in the subperiosteal space stimulating reactive elevation at its periphery. Perpendicular fibres of periosteum, intended to hold the periosteum to the bone, may also undergo reactive sclerosis in response to the presence of extracortical tumour. This results in the 'sunburst' calcification or 'hair on end' appearance which is sometimes seen with osteosarcoma and Ewing's tumour. These appearances are of considerable interest, but are unfortunately not specific to a cell type.

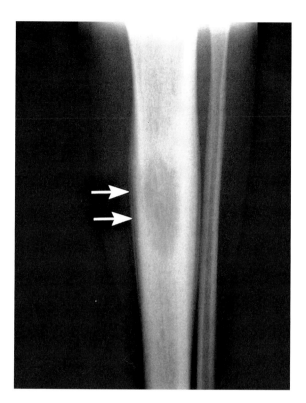

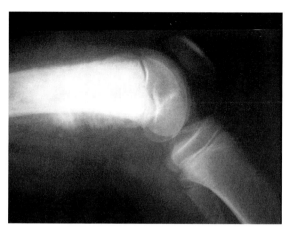

Fig. 8.4 Osteosarcoma. There is a bone-forming tumour of the distal metaphysis of the femur. The lesion extends to the distal epiphysis. It is associated with amorphous, cloud-like calcification in the soft tissues. The appearance of a bone-forming tumour associated with a soft tissue mass is characteristic of classical osteosarcoma.

Fig. 8.3 Ewing's sarcoma. There is a lytic lesion in the diaphysis of the left tibia. It has a wide zone of transition consistent with an aggressive lesion. There is slight thickening of the cortex and laminar periosteal reaction as a result of the periodic growth of the tumour, resulting in an 'onion skin' appearance (arrowed).

However, they are characteristic of aggressive lesions.

Tumour matrix is a useful indicator of tissue type. Certain neoplasms are composed of tissue with a potential for calcification, and these are generally tumours of chondroid or osseous nature. Radiographically, chondromas, chondroblastomas, and chondrosarcomas may all contain areas of calcification which are curvilinear in the most indolent lesions, and punctate or nodular in more rapidly growing tumours. The calcification is less marked towards the growing edge of the lesion. Bone formation is the natural potential of osteomas, osteoblastomas, and osteosarcomas. The most mature trabeculated bone is evident in slow-growing lesions such as osteomas, whereas the most rapidly growing neoplasms such as telangiectatic osteosarcomas form the least bone. The new bone formed in classical osteosarcoma is usually homogeneous and amorphous, and can be seen on both plain film and CT (Fig. 8.4).

Extension of osseous tumours into soft tissues is a feature of aggressive behaviour. Ewing's tumour frequently results in large extraosseous masses, such that a primary soft tissue tumour may be suspected initially (Fig. 8.5). MRI comes into its own in assessing the size of soft tissue components and defining the proximity to neurovascular bundles if surgery is to be contemplated.

PRIMARY BONE TUMOURS

Primary neoplasms of bone are rare, accounting for approximately 0.2% of all malignant

118 CANCER AND THE SKELETON

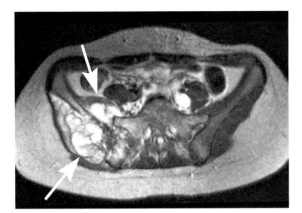

Fig. 8.5 Ewing's sarcoma. A T2-weighted MRI examination shows a high-signal soft tissue mass erupting from a limited abnormality in the posterior aspect of the right iliac bone. The soft tissue tumour (arrowed) is elevating the iliacus muscle and invading posteriorly into the gluteal muscles. The exuberant growth of a soft tissue mass associated with a limited bony abnormality is frequently seen with Ewing's tumour.

Table 8.1   Classification of primary malignant bone tumours

Tumours of osteoid origin
   Conventional intramedullary (high-grade) osteosarcoma
   Parosteal osteosarcoma
   Periosteal osteosarcoma
   Telangiectatic osteosarcoma
   Secondary osteosarcoma, e.g. Paget's sarcoma
   High-grade surface osteosarcoma
   Small cell osteosarcoma
   Low-grade central osteosarcoma

Tumours of chondroid origin
   Chondrosarcoma
   Juxtacortical chondrosarcoma
   Mesenchymal chondrosarcoma
   Clear cell chondrosarcoma

Tumours of fibrous origin
   Malignant fibrous histiocytoma
   Fibrosarcoma

Malignant round cell neoplasms of bone
   Ewing's sarcoma
   Primary malignant lymphoma of bone

Other miscellaneous bone tumours
   Chordoma
   Synovial sarcoma
   Angiosarcoma
   Liposarcoma
   Adamantinoma of long bones
   Malignant giant cell tumours

neoplasms.[3] Malignant change may arise in the various tissues which constitute bone, and the important primary tumours of bone are listed in Table 8.1.

Osteosarcoma

Conventional (high-grade) osteosarcoma
This is the most common primary bone tumour, with a peak age of presentation between 15 and 20 years. The vast majority arise in the metaphysis of long bones, 75% of them around the knee.[4] Pain is the most common presenting feature. The radiographic features of a classical osteosarcoma commence with a destructive medullary lesion showing a permeative pattern with a wide zone of transition. The pathological hallmark of an osteosarcoma is the presence of osteoid, which may mineralize to give a characteristic 'cloud-like' calcification (Fig. 8.4). As the tumour reaches the cortex, it will destroy it, extending into a soft tissue lesion. Reactive new bone at the periosteum may form Codman's triangles or sunburst calcification. The soft tissue mass, like the medullary lesion, is initially uncalcified but may later mineralize. Variations may appear, for example the tumour bone may be extremely sclerotic, and there are a number of recognizable other types of osteosarcoma.

Parosteal and periosteal osteosarcoma

Parosteal osteosarcomas account for approximately 5% of all osteosarcomas[5] and present in adult life as slow-growing low-grade lesions. Most occur in the lower femur, and they develop in the cortex of the bone, often sparing the medulla and growing circumferentially around the bone, presenting as a hard soft tissue mass. They are characterized by dense masses of mature bone wrapping around the shaft. Early in the natural history of the tumour a radiolucent line separates tumour from the normal cortex. It may be difficult to establish by plain radiography that the medulla is not involved, and CT may be helpful. Eventually the tumour will involve the medulla and metastasis to the lungs will be seen. Wide local excision has a high chance of producing long-term survival.[6]

Periosteal osteosarcoma occurs on the surface of the bone, usually in the upper tibial metaphysis. As with parosteal sarcomas, the medulla is not typically involved, but the periosteal osteosarcoma is an aggressive high-grade tumour with chondroblastic elements. Elevation and reaction of the periosteum, often with radiating spicules, are seen, and CT will confirm a hemispherical lesion applied closely to the cortex of the bone.

Telangiectatic osteosarcoma

These aggressive high-grade tumours contain little osteoid, and tumour bone formation is less likely to occur (Fig. 8.6). The radiographic appearance is therefore similar to early classical osteosarcoma, and the natural history of the tumour is similar to other high-grade osteosarcomas.

Paget's sarcoma

Approximately 1% of patients with Paget's disease develop a primary bone sarcoma within the abnormal area.[7,8] The majority occur in the pelvis and femur and present with increasing local pain. Most tumours are osteosarcomas, although some are fibrosarcomas or anaplastic lesions. The differentiation is scarcely relevant as all are highly aggressive. In the age group affected, the differential diagnosis of importance is with metastatic carcinoma occurring in pagetic bone. In all instances the prognosis is poor.

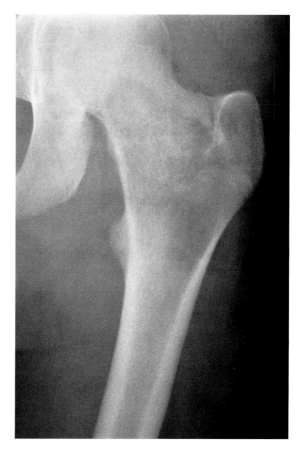

Fig. 8.6 Telangiectatic osteosarcoma. There is a lytic lesion extending from the intertrochanteric region of the left femur into the femoral neck and shaft. There is little evidence of tumour bone formation, and the appearance would be consistent with telangiectatic osteosarcoma or an early high-grade osteosarcoma.

Multifocal osteosarcoma

The demonstration of more than one osteosarcoma of bone at presentation is rare. Although a metastatic explanation for multiple lesions is possible, there is clinical and radiological evidence that a specific entity of multifocal osteosarcoma exists. The radiological appearance is of densely osteoblastic lesions all of much the same size and maturity involving the metaphyses of long bones. Initially, lesions may be relatively benign in appearance, but subsequently show soft tissue extension and typically malignant behaviour. The similar size of the lesions and the absence of pulmonary metastases differentiate the disease from metastatic osteosarcoma. Histologically, each lesion is a typical osteosarcoma. Metastatic spread to the lungs will eventually occur and the disease is difficult to treat and almost inevitably lethal.

Tumours of chondroid origin

Primary chondrosarcoma

This tumour accounts for 10% of malignant bone tumours.[9] Primary chondrosarcomas arise *de novo* where secondary chondrosarcomas may develop within a pre-existing bone lesion, for example enchondroma. The majority of chondrosarcomas are central within the bone, and the most frequent sites are pelvis and upper femur. Patients are usually over 40 years of age and present with pain. Tumour grade varies considerably. Usually the pathologist has little difficulty in identifying the chondroid nature of the tissue, but there is overlap cytologically between entirely benign lesions (enchondromas) and low-grade chondrosarcomas. Similarly, there is overlap of radiographic features between benign and low-grade malignant entities. Slow growth allows reactive growth to sclerosis in adjacent normal bone, and as the medullary tumour enlarges, scalloping of the endosteal surface of the cortex may occur. With more malignant tumours, cortical destruction will identify the malignant nature of the process. A valuable diagnostic aid is the presence of a soft tissue extracortical mass which is frequently out of proportion with the intraosseous lesion. Unfortunately, in the common location of the pelvis, plain radiography fails to demonstrate the soft tissue mass, and cross-sectional imaging with CT or MRI can therefore be helpful. The plain film sometimes shows the characteristic calcification of the tumour matrix, which may be stippled, nodular, or conglomerate.

Other types of chondrosarcoma

Juxtacortical chondrosarcoma, mesenchymal chondrosarcoma, and clear cell chondrosarcoma are all rare variants. Juxtacortical chondrosarcoma is similar to the classical central chondrosarcoma in every way except its initial site. Its segregation as a separate entity is probably illogical. Mesenchymal chondrosarcomas are aggressive whereas clear cell chondrosarcomas are slow-growing lesions which metastasize late. These diagnoses are usually made by the pathologist. The chondrosarcoma is an example of a tumour which may need repeat biopsy, as its clinical, radiological, and pathological interfaces are with benign lesions, some of which may be pre-existent.

Tumours of fibrous origin

Fibrosarcoma

This is the least common of the primary sarcomas of bony connective tissue, with an incidence approximately one tenth of that of osteosarcoma. It is usually a low-grade sarcoma found mostly in long bones and typically gives a moth-eaten pattern of bony destruction commencing in the medulla, although eccentric lesions occur. Fibrosarcoma may also be a soft tissue tumour, and involvement of two adjacent bones such as tibia and fibula suggests a soft tissue neoplasm. Bony fibrosarcoma may expand the bone or cause skip lesions within a single bone. It rarely calcifies, and radiologically is one of the least specific of bone sarcomas.

Malignant fibrous histiocytoma (MFH)

This is a rare tumour, usually of bone but sometimes confined to soft tissues. The differentiation from fibrosarcoma is contentious, causing heated debate among pathologists which radiologists are well advised not to join. Radiologically, it presents as a lytic lesion with a permeative pattern of destruction. It can rarely be diagnosed radiologically with any confidence, but should be considered with a solitary lesion in the patient under 40 years of age.

Malignant round cell tumours of bone

The term 'malignant round cell tumour of bone' has traditionally been used to take in Ewing's sarcoma (and its variants such as Askin's tumour), and primary lymphoma of bone, along with metastatic involvement by neuroblastoma. These lesions overlap with pure marrow neoplasms, such as leukaemia, myeloma, and histiocytosis. The pathologist may have initial difficulty with cytological identification of the cell, and with these lesions, the clinical presentation, radiological appearance, and laboratory tests are very important in guiding the pathologist; special staining techniques have been developed over the past few years which are crucial in diagnosis.

Ewing's sarcoma

Most patients present between the ages of 5 and 15 years, and Ewing's sarcoma is rare over the age of 30 years. The characteristic symptom is persistent pain over several weeks, which may be severe and is associated with constitutional symptoms such as pyrexia. Usually a single bone is involved, although later in the disease Ewing's sarcoma metastasizes readily to other bones. Approximately 75% of Ewing's sarcomas are diaphyseal, and bones commonly involved are marrow-rich bones such as the pelvis and ribs, the femur, tibia, and humerus.

The bony lesion is destructive and infiltrative, and is the epitome of a permeative lesion with a wide zone of transition; extension tends to occur along the length of the marrow so that an extensive segment of the diaphysis is affected compared to other neoplasms which exhibit a more concentric growth pattern. The tumour breaches the cortex and exuberant growth of the soft tissue mass ensues, which may cause a mechanical pressure effect on the outer aspect of the cortex of the bone known as 'saucerization'. The disproportionately large soft tissue mass is an important diagnostic feature which is best demonstrated by CT or MRI.

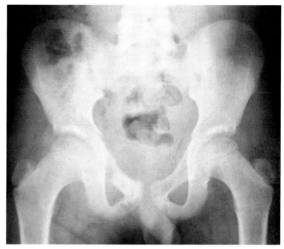
(a)

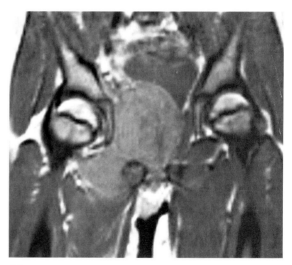
(b)

Fig. 8.7 Ewing's sarcoma. (a) A plain pelvic radiograph shows a sclerotic region in the right superior pubic ramus. The appearance is occasionally seen in Ewing's sarcoma of flat bones. (b) Proton density weighted MR imaging shows a dumbell-shaped tumour returning intermediate signal, rising into the pelvis where it is displacing the urinary bladder superiorly and to the left. The soft tissue tumour also extends into the medial compartment of the upper thigh.

The periodic growth of the tumour sometimes results in the classical onion-skin periosteal reaction. Occasionally a mixed or mainly sclerotic bony appearance is seen, usually in the flat bones (Fig. 8.7). A lytic osteosarcoma may be indistinguishable from Ewing's sarcoma; sunburst calcification is less common in Ewing's sarcoma and tends to give more delicate and sparse perpendicular spicules.

Malignant lymphoma of bone
This entity has also been known as reticulum cell sarcoma of bone and may present as a primary bone tumour. However, it may later transpire that it is the first manifestation of disseminated lymphoma. It is a relatively rare entity with the same distribution as Ewing's sarcoma, namely, to the diaphyses of long bones and marrow-bearing flat bones. The age range is much wider than Ewing's sarcoma, with a mean age at presentation of 45 years. The osseous destruction is usually permeative, although a moth-eaten pattern and varying degrees of reactive sclerosis may be seen. As with Ewing's sarcoma, MRI frequently demonstrates a soft tissue mass, and involvement of the marrow may be much more extensive than suggested by other investigations. Involvement of distant areas of the marrow ('skip lesions') may be identified on MRI.

Chordoma

This tumour originates from ectopic cellular remnants of the notochord. Around 90% of cases affect the sacrum the craniocervical region. It grows slowly and is associated with a large soft tissue mass. Pain is present for a year (on average) before presentation. Other symptoms relate to pressure on local structures, notably the sacral plexus or cranial nerves. Sacral lesions usually show a large area of bone destruction with well defined margins. MRI or CT will show a large soft tissue mass. Amorphous calcification may be detectable by CT, but rarely seen on plain film. Craniocervical chordoma occasionally presents with a mass indenting the nasopharynx and plain radiographic examination may demonstrate destruction of the dorsal aspect of the sella and clivus. The presence of bone destruction and a large soft tissue mass may simulate chronic infection, especially tuberculosis.

Other tumours which may affect bone

Since bone contains other connective tissues, there are a variety of rare lesions which can present as bony tumours. These include angiosarcomas (haemangioendothelioma), intraosseous liposarcoma (very rare, despite the extensive fatty content of bone marrow), and synovial sarcoma. The latter is the commonest of these lesions and is characterized by marked bony destruction, usually on both sides of a joint, associated with a large soft tissue mass. Adamantinoma of long bones is a rare tumour which typically involves the mid-shaft of the tibia. Its pathogenesis is not clear, although it may be of epithelial origin like the histologically similar ameloblastoma of jaw. The shaft of the bone is usually affected by an osteolytic lesion which may be central or eccentric. The margin is moderately well defined and circumferential bone sclerosis is common. It produces satellite lesions and, while metastasis is unusual, it is locally aggressive and early complete resection is advisable.

METASTATIC DISEASE IN BONE

It can scarcely be overemphasized that primary malignant bone tumours are very rare, and bony metastases, particularly from carcinoma, are very common. In the over 40 years' age group, it is not unusual for a metastatic bone lesion to be the first manifestation of disease. In such circumstances, the diagnostic approach to the lesion is similar to investigation of a bone primary; the clinical background and plain film appearance will frequently allow diagnosis and suggest the site of primary disease. Once disseminated cancer is suspected, the most sensitive investigations for defining the extent of bony spread are isotope studies and MRI.

There is good evidence that distant metastasis results from venous tumour emboli.[10] From the primary tumour, venous haematogenous spread should initially be to the lungs. From the lungs, further emboli may 'cascade' to the bones. If skeletal metastases are found in the absence of pulmonary lesions, it is possible that the lung deposits are present but hidden or beyond the resolution of imaging studies used. Transpulmonary passage of malignant cells occasionally occurs, and paradoxical embolism through a patent foramen ovale has been authenticated on rare occasions. Retrograde venous embolism is probably the most important mechanism for involvement of the vertebral column from intra-abdominal tumours. The vertebral venous plexus is valveless, and allows cranial and caudal flow of blood which varies with fluctuating intra-abdominal pressure.

Metastatic cancer to the skeletal marrow occurs in 30–70% of all cancer patients.[3,11] In a series of 1000 consecutive autopsy patients dying from epithelial cancers, the common primary tumours to cause bone metastasis were prostate, breast, lung, kidney, rectum, pancreas, stomach, colon, and ovary. Overall, breast cancer was responsible for approximately 70% of all bony metastases in women and prostate cancer was the cause of 60% of bony metastases in men.[11] Other tumours which have a reputation for metastasizing frequently to bone are uterus, thyroid, and melanoma. While the statistics are interesting, it should be borne in mind that virtually any tumour can metastasize to bone, although this happens sufficiently rarely with some tumours (for example, glioma) that an alternative diagnosis may be sought when apparent bony lesions develop.

Diagnostic features of skeletal metastatic disease

The distribution of skeletal metastases is dictated largely by haematogenous spread. Over 90% of metastatic lesions are found in the distribution of red bone marrow in adults, with only a small percentage outside the red marrow areas.[12] In an autopsy series of 2000 patients dying of cancer with bony metastases, the vertebrae were involved in 69%, pelvis in 41%, proximal femur in 25%, and skull in 14%.[13] Only 9% of autopsy patients with skeletal metastases have solitary bony lesions.[14] The patterns of haematogenous spread can be explained to a large extent on the basis of bony microvascular structure and the microenvironment of the bone marrow, but clearly there is some variation in interaction between tumour cells and host bone. Tumour cells may destroy bone directly by the growth of a mass, or by the production of mediators that stimulate resorption by osteoclasts. Prostaglandins and other tumour-derived growth factors have been implicated.[15,16] As metastatic lesions grow within the marrow, the surrounding bone may undergo osteoclastic (resorptive) and osteoblastic (depositional) activity. The intensity of these activities may differ between tumour types or even at different locations for the same tumour in the same patient, and the balance of these processes determines the radiographic appearance.

Bony involvement by metastatic disease may exhibit an osteolytic, osteoblastic, or mixed pattern (Fig. 8.8). They are most commonly osteolytic and multiple. However, considerable bony loss is required before the marrow abnormality becomes evident radiographically (a 30–50% change in bone density is required before a metastatic lesion becomes visible) and the plain film is therefore an insensitive investigation.[17] While the appearance of a skeletal deposit can often allow a specific diagnosis of an aggressive lesion with a permeative pattern, it is the demonstration of multiplicity which frequently clinches the diagnosis. A sensitive investigation of as many bones as feasible is a direct and noninvasive route of establishing the diagnosis. Isotope studies, which are dealt with in another chapter in this volume, are an established and appropriate first investigation. However, MRI is slightly more sensitive, and is of considerable utility in clinical circumstances where isotope studies are normal, and a strong suspicion of skeletal metastasis persists (Fig. 8.9).[18]

MRI technique need not be complex, but a detailed knowledge of the variable appearance of bone marrow, and the way in which contrast

124 CANCER AND THE SKELETON

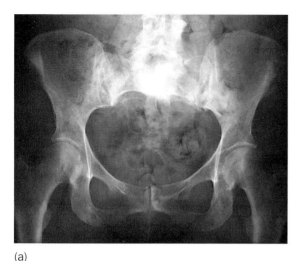

(a)

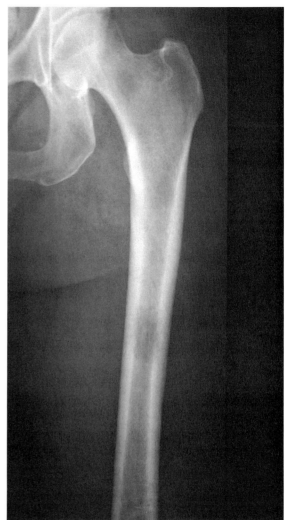

(b)

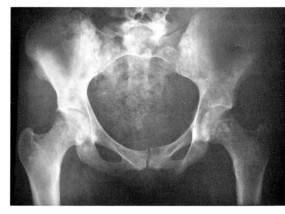

(c)

Fig. 8.8 Bony metastases. (a) Plain radiography of the pelvis shows a large lytic deposit expanding the left iliac bone. There are areas of sclerosis in sacrum and ischial bones (mixed pattern, deposits from carcinoma of breast). (b) There is a lytic lesion in the mid-femoral shaft resulting in some endosteal scalloping (secondary deposit from melanoma). (c) Small sclerotic metastases are scattered throughout the pelvic bones and upper femora (secondary deposits of medulloblastoma).

is generated between tissues within the bone marrow, is of considerable importance. If the marrow cavity is largely filled by yellow marrow, this returns a high signal on simple T1-weighted spin echo sequences, which contrasts markedly with the low signal returned by tumour (Fig. 8.10). This sequence alone may yield convincing evidence of widespread metastatic disease in patients with normal isotope studies. The demonstration of tumour within the marrow does not depend on the presence of increased vacularity or osteoblastic activity, and this accounts for the high sensitivity of this test. Difficulties can arise in those patients whose marrow cavity contains islands of red marrow amongst predominantly yellow marrow. These islands of red marrow can mimic tumour, but an individual patient tends to

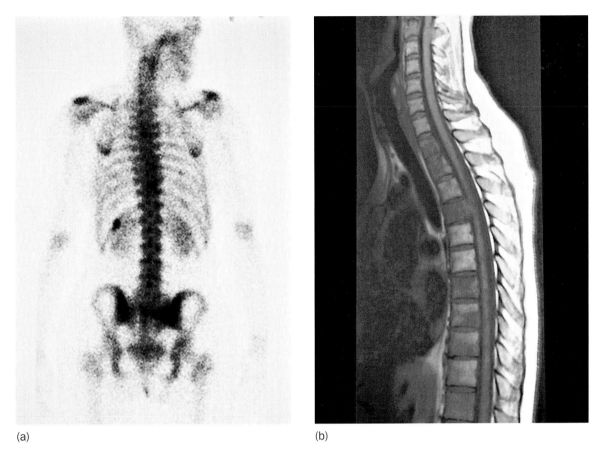

Fig. 8.9 Metastases from carcinoma of breast. (a) The isotope bone scan is within normal limits. (b) MRI study of spine, 2 days after isotope bone scan. T1-weighted spin echo imaging shows abnormal low signal returning from several vertebrae. The appearance is typical of metastatic disease. There is some evidence of soft tissue extension of tumour towards the spinal cord at the T4 level. The tumour within the marrow cavities of the vertebral body has presumably failed to induce an osteoblastic response, resulting in a normal isotope study in this patient.

repeat the same pattern of marrow distribution throughout the vertebral column, and the distribution of marrow in the long bones is generally symmetrical. The radiological literature contains much technical information regarding the efficacy of certain pulse sequences used. The development of MR machines is still in a state of rapid technical flux. Such sequences as the short tau inversion recovery (STIR) sequence are now well established; this technique results in suppression of signal from normal fat, allowing tumour deposits to show as bright high-signal areas. New refinements are tested as the technology becomes available and the complexities of sequence selection are best left to the radiologist who will understand the capabilities and limitations of techniques and the machinery available on site.

Several patterns of marrow involvement have been described on various MRI sequences. It is frequently possible to correlate these patterns with the changes observed on the plain

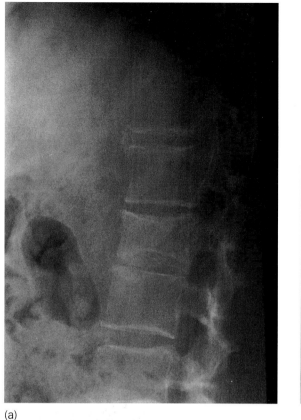 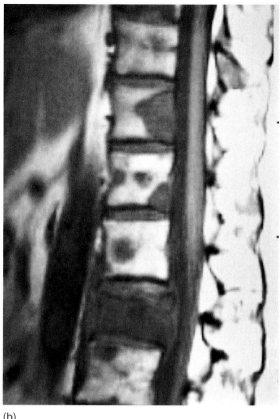

(a) (b)

Fig. 8.10 Metastasis from carcinoma of breast. (a) There is a slight loss of vertebral height in one of the upper lumbar vertebrae, but otherwise no focal abnormality is identified. (b) T1-weighted spin echo imaging of spine in sagittal plane. The compressed vertebra is completely replaced by low-signal tumour. The focal deposits seen in all the other vertebrae show as low signal, contrasting well with the high signal returned by areas of normal fatty marrow.

radiographs. For example, a deposit of prostate carcinoma which returns low signal on a T1-weighted sequence and fails to return the increased signal expected on T2-weighted or STIR images is likely to be sclerotic on plain film radiography (Fig. 8.11). Sometimes the entire marrow cavity is replaced by diffuse homogeneous tumour, which is likely to correlate with a diffusely osteopenic bone. Although many characteristic features exist, the differentiation of metastatic or malignant marrow processes from benign or traumatic conditions is occasionally problematical and, although MRI appears to be a sensitive investigation for marrow disease, its current high cost prevents its use for routine staging. MRI has an extremely important role in the management of patients with bony metastatic disease who present with pain and neurological deficit, particularly where spinal cord compression is being considered. The whole spine should be imaged in sagittal plane, as levels may be multiple, and the possibility of cord compression by soft tissue extension of bony tumour should be borne in mind so that

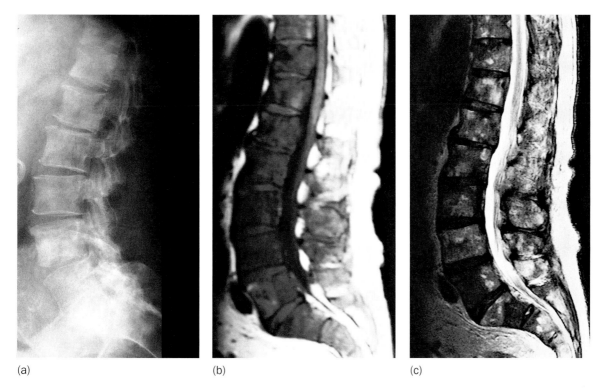

Fig. 8.11 Metastatic disease from carcinoma of prostate. (a) Plain radiograph of the lumbar spine shows sclerotic areas in the vertebral bodies. (b) MRI, T1-weighted spin echo sequence in sagittal plane. Low signal is returned from the marrow cavities. The fatty marrow has been almost entirely replaced by tumour. (c) T2-weighted spin echo sequence in sagittal plane. Tumour tissue usually returns high signal on this sequence. However, areas of low signal on the T2-weighted sequence correspond to areas of sclerosis seen on the plain film. The reduction in signal results from shortening of proton relaxation times as a result of the proximity of dense calcification and sclerosis within the bone.

appropriate images in orthogonal planes may be obtained (Fig. 8.12).

PRIMARY TUMOURS OF BONE MARROW

Haemopoietic elements of the bone marrow may undergo malignant proliferation. Broadly speaking, these may be divided into white cell disorders which include the leukaemias and lymphomas, plasma cell disorders which include plasmacytoma and myeloma, and disorders of the reticulo-endothelial elements which include the histiocytosis spectrum.

White cell disorders

Leukaemia
Acute leukaemia is the commonest malignancy of childhood, with acute lymphoblastic leukaemia (ALL) accounting for the majority of leukaemias in children while acute myelogenous leukaemia (AML) is more common in adults. The disease is often insidious, presenting with nonspecific malaise, but limb pains are common, especially in children. In children, leukaemic infiltration of the long bones may produce a characteristic appearance, although it

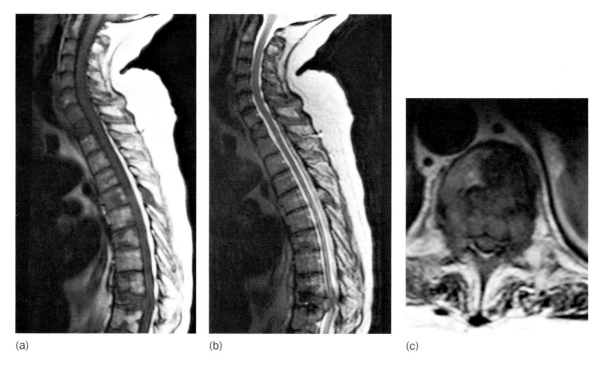

Fig. 8.12 Metastases from carcinoma of breast. (a) MRI examination, T1-weighted spin echo sequence, sagittal plane. Multiple areas of low signal are present in the vertebral bodies indicating the presence of metastatic disease. There is vertebral collapse at T10 with epidural spread of tumour tissue. (b) T2-weighted spin echo sequence, sagittal plane. Using this sequence, CSF shows as high signal, giving a 'myelogram effect'. The spinal cord is mechanically disrupted at the T10 level confirming a diagnosis of cord compression. There is also some degenerative disk disease throughout the spine. (c) T1-weighted spin echo image, axial plane. The axial image shows extensive replacement of the vertebral body by tumour. The pedicles are expanded. Soft tissue extension of tumour is compressing the cord from the anterior aspect. The blood supply of the cord, from the anterior spinal artery, is likely to be disrupted by tumour tissue at this site.

is rarely the means by which the diagnosis is made. Typical features include diffuse osteoporosis, transverse metaphyseal bands of diminished bone density, dense transverse metaphyseal lines caused by growth arrest, subperiosteal new bone formation, discrete osteolytic lesions, and, very occasionally, osteosclerotic lesions.[19] The submetaphyseal lucent bands are seen in approximately 40% of children and probably represent osteoporosis in the rapidly growing region of the long bone. They are most frequently seen in the distal femur, proximal tibia, and vertebral bodies. Focal lytic lesions are more common in AML than ALL. In the skull, they may present with a typical moth-eaten appearance. When MRI was first introduced, there was considerable enthusiasm regarding its potential to evaluate diffuse bone marrow disease. It has transpired that the technique is very sensitive, but the diffuse abnormality has no specific features which allow diagnosis from other causes of diffuse marrow infiltration.

Chronic leukaemias
Chronic lymphatic leukaemia (CLL) and chronic myelocytic leukaemia (CML) are diseases of elderly patients. CLL is characterized by

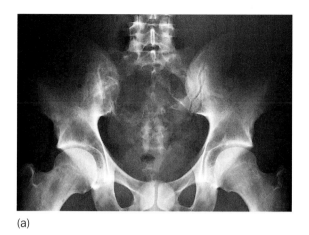 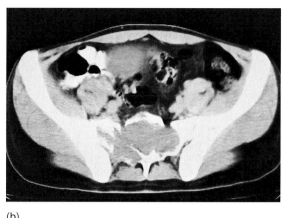

Fig. 8.13 Plasmacytoma. (a) Plain pelvic radiograph shows a destructive lytic lesion replacing the upper sacrum. (b) CT scan shows a large tumour within the sacrum, causing extensive bone destruction without sclerosis.

enlargement of the spleen and lymph nodes. Skeletal involvement does not occur except as a terminal event, particularly if acute blastic transformation has ensued. CML may cause diffuse bone density indistinguishable from myelofibrosis.

Lymphoma
Primary lymphoma of bone is uncommon, but has a similar clinical presentation and radiographic appearance to Ewing's sarcoma. However, both Hodgkin's and non-Hodgkin's lymphoma (NHL) are common diseases of the lymphatic and reticulo-endothelial system, and these tumours are increasing in frequency such that the incidence is predicted to double in southeast England by the year 2010.[20] Involvement of bone indicates extensive or late disease (stage IV).

Hodgkin's disease is fundamentally a disease of the lymph nodes. Unlike carcinoma, very few patients (less than 2%) present with a skeletal lesion at the time of diagnosis. However, in end-stage disease, skeletal involvement is more common, and some autopsy studies report an incidence of bone involvement in up to 75% of patients. Sites of involvement are predominantly in bones containing red marrow, with the majority in the axial skeleton. Lesions may be sclerotic (45%), mixed (41%), or purely lytic (14%) on plain film radiography.[21] A classical lesion is the 'ivory vertebra'. Vertebral bodies are occasionally eroded by paravertebral nodal masses.

NHL involves the bone marrow much more frequently at presentation. Any part of the skeleton may be involved, and lesions are predominantly lytic. Marrow involvement is sufficiently frequent that bone marrow aspiration or trephine is a routine staging procedure at presentation. Radiographic abnormality is frequently absent when the marrow is positive. Children with generalized lymphoma may have osteopenia as a manifestation of widespread skeletal involvement. MRI shows diffusely abnormal signal from the involved bone marrow, but is not used as a routine staging technique. Certain classic lesions are associated with the high-grade B-cell neoplasm Burkitt's lymphoma. This frequently presents as a destructive enlarging lesion centred over the jaw, spreading from the medulla to affect the cortex. Bony destruction and dental displacement give the appearance of 'floating teeth'.

130 CANCER AND THE SKELETON

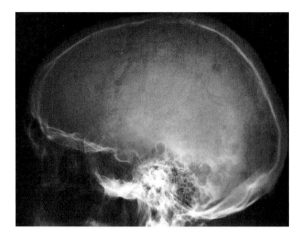

Fig. 8.14 Myeloma. Skull radiograph shows multiple lytic lesions scattered throughout the skull vault.

Lesions in other bones may be similarly lytic with very little periosteal reaction.

Plasma cell disorders

Plasmacytoma is a term which refers to a myeloma lesion, i.e. a proliferation of plasma cells, which is apparently solitary at presentation. It may remain localized at one site for many years, but at any time may make the transition to multiple myeloma. The extremes of the disorder are separated because of their different presentation and management.

Plasmacytoma is a destructive lesion which frequently presents with local pain. Presentation before the age of 40 is unusual. The lesion arises in the medulla, and has a relatively slow growth rate, giving a well defined margin. The lesion is lytic and sclerosis in plasmacytoma is rare (Fig. 8.13). The lesion affects principally the sites containing red marrow. Involvement of the vertebral body is common, sometimes leading to collapse. The differential diagnosis includes metastatic carcinoma.

Multiple myeloma is the commonest primary malignant neoplasm of bone, and widespread involvement of the skeleton is often present at

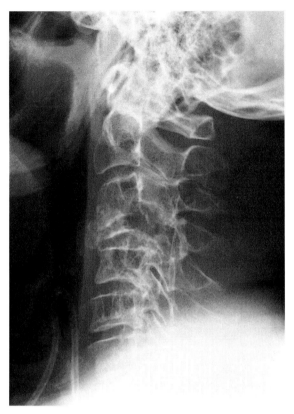

Fig. 8.15 Myeloma. Cervical spine radiograph shows loss of bone density in the vertebral bodies. Vertebral collapse at C4 has resulted in virtual disappearance of the vertebral body. The posterior elements of C4 are preserved. The appearance is typical of myeloma, although not specific.

first attendance. Fever, pain, and backache are common symptoms. In contrast to plasmacytoma, the sedimentation rate is markedly elevated, and paraproteins are detectable in most patients. The classical appearance of myeloma deposits is a well defined 'punched-out' lesion anywhere in the skeleton, often most characteristic in the skull (Fig. 8.14). The only common differential diagnosis of this appearance is multiple secondaries from carcinoma. A distinguishing feature is the lack of reactive sclerosis at the margin of the myeloma lesion; myeloma appears not to engender an osteoblastic bone reaction, which also accounts for the lack of increased

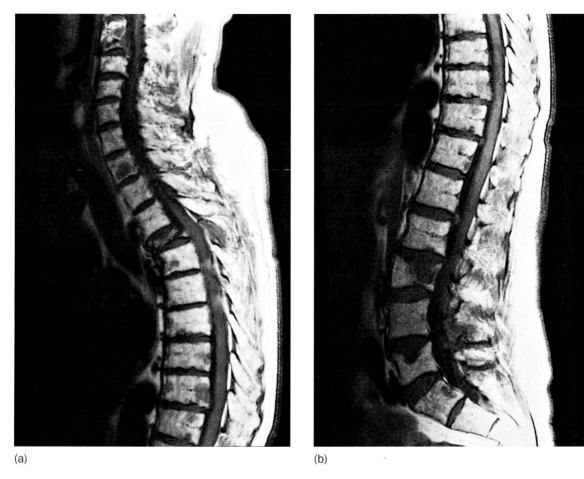

Fig. 8.16 (a) and (b) Myeloma. T1-weighted spin echo images of whole spine show multiple low-signal areas contrasting with normal fatty marrow. There is loss of vertebral height at L3 and T4. The appearance is consistent with a diagnosis of myeloma, but there are no specific features to distinguish this appearance from secondary carcinoma.

activity on isotope studies. Blastic or mixed lesions are extremely rare in the untreated patient, although following radiation this pattern may be modified. Disease may be sufficiently generalized to cause osteopenia throughout the skeleton, which is indistinguishable from senile osteoporosis. This differential diagnosis is difficult, especially in elderly females. Laboratory tests will usually assist in diagnosis. Pathological fractures are common, affecting about half of patients at some time. Many of the fractures are vertebral compressions (Fig. 8.15). Periosteal reaction is uncommon, but fractures of the tubular bones heal readily with normal amounts of callus. Myeloma is frequently associated with a soft tissue mass which may destroy the intervertebral disks, and this helps in differentiation from secondary carcinoma.

The MRI appearance of myeloma is of a diffuse abnormality of signal widespread throughout the marrow cavities.[22] There are no specific MR features which allow differentiation from other diffuse abnormalities of bone marrow (Fig. 8.16). The skeletal survey is still

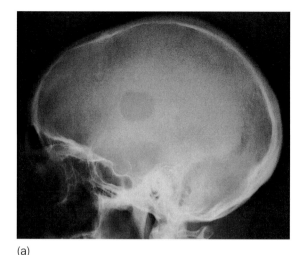

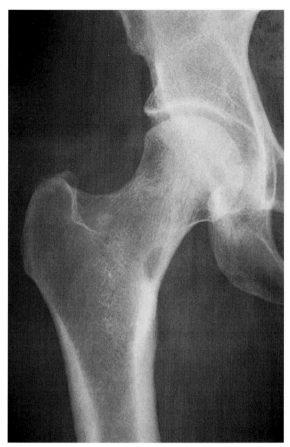

Fig. 8.17 Histiocytosis. (a) Plain skull radiograph shows a cell-circumscribed lytic lesion of the skull vault. (b) Plain radiograph of the upper right femur shows a small lytic lesion at the medial edge of the femoral neck. This is surrounded by reactive sclerosis, consistent with a healing lesion. Classically, the presence of multiple lesions in the skeleton displaying varying degrees of healing response is the hallmark of 'eosinophilic granuloma'.

extensively used in assessment of multiple myeloma. This is a tedious investigation for the patient and the radiographic technician. It is a useful exercise at the time of diagnosis, forming an integral part of the Drury and Salmon staging procedure. However, its value in assessment of response to chemotherapy is debatable, particularly if there are biochemical and haematological parameters which can adequately assess the progress of disease.

Reticulo-endothelial disorders

The histiocytoses are a group of diseases of which the exact pathogenesis is unknown. They are not truly neoplastic, but the bony manifestations are an important differential diagnosis of malignant disease. The histological abnormality is a proliferation of histiocytic elements with a varying number of eosinophil leukocytes, histiocytes, plasma cells, and giant cells. The traditional eponymous labels such as Hand–Schüller–Christian disease have given way to terms such as histiocytosis X and Langerhans' cell histiocytosis. The typical skeletal lesions show geographic destruction of bone, particularly in the skull. Tangental views of these lesions show bevelling of the edges of the defect, indicating that a different degree of destruction affects the inner and outer table of the skull. The classical lesion of the spine is 'vertebra plana', which is a result of wedging of the vertebral

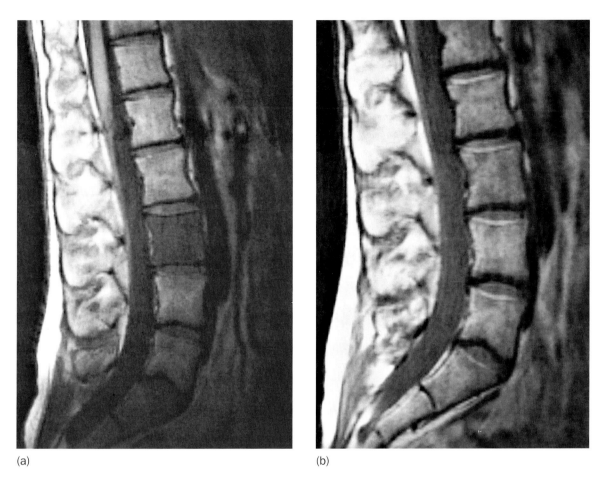

Fig. 8.18 Lymphoma involving bone. (a) MRI examination, T1-weighted spin echo sequence in sagittal plane. There is replacement of the vertebral body of L3 by tumour tissue. The appearance is consistent with marrow replacement by lymphoma. (b) Repeat examination using the same pulse sequences, after 3 months' treatment with cytotoxic chemotherapy. The signal returned from the bone marrow of L3 has returned to normal. This confirms some response to treatment, but does not exclude residual malignancy within the marrow cavity.

body which may become wafer thin. Lesions in flat and long bones commence in the medulla and may result in endosteal erosion of the cortex. These lesions simulate low-grade neoplasms, and biopsy may be necessary to establish the diagnosis. However, if several similar lesions are found in the skeleton, evidence of sclerosis around healing lesions can suggest the diagnosis (Fig. 8.17). Under such circumstances, serial radiography may establish the diagnosis noninvasively. Skull and vertebra are the most commonly affected areas of disease, particularly in children, but no bone is exempt.

IMAGE-GUIDED BIOPSY

There is a growing trend towards 'minimally invasive' techniques. Many radiologists have become adept at needle biopsies of a variety of viscera under ultrasound, CT, and sometimes

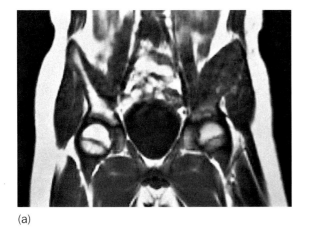
(a)

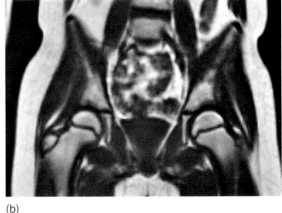
(b)

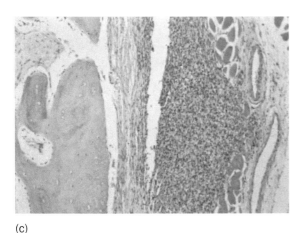
(c)

Fig. 8.19 Ewing's sarcoma. (a) MRI examination, T1-weighted spin echo sequence, coronal plane. There is a tumour mass replacing the marrow cavity of the left iliac bone. This is associated with a low-signal soft tissue mass. (b) MRI repeated with same pulse sequence following chemotherapy. The soft tissue mass has resolved. There are localized areas of low signal within the marrow cavity of the left iliac bone, but the appearance is almost normal. (c) Following resection of the tumour bed, this haemotoxylin and eosin slide shows densely staining small round cells sandwiched between sclerotic reactive bone and muscle fibres. This represents a sheet of active tumour cells at the periphery of the bone. Tumour foci such as this are beyond the resolution of any imaging technique. Even in the presence of apparently complete response to chemotherapy, foci of active tumour cannot be excluded by imaging studies.

MR control. These techniques work best in very cellular neoplasms such as metastases, but it should be remembered that bone is hard and technically difficult to biopsy; fine needle techniques work well on extracortical masses adjacent to bony neoplasms, and tissue may also be obtained through existing cortical defects. Cutting needles give larger samples than aspiration needles. In general, trephine methods give the largest specimens and allow the pathologist to see an interface between tumour and bone.[23,24]

In the diagnosis of primary bone tumours, many still advocate open surgical biopsy. The advantage of this technique is the large amount of tissue which can be provided for histological examination, but it is often accompanied by a relatively long skin incision which may compromise future surgical approaches. The fact that no special skills are necessary to undertake open biopsy is a double-edged sword; if a primary bone neoplasm is suspected, it is probably advisable to refer the patient to a specialist centre for definitive diagnostic procedures, where the appropriate techniques can be selected and suitably skilled personnel are available.

ASSESSMENT OF RESPONSE TO TREATMENT

Most of the tumours described are amenable to a variety of forms of chemotherapy or radiotherapy. Primary bone tumours, particularly osteosarcoma and Ewing's sarcoma, are now treated with chemotherapy prior to consideration for surgery. Dramatic responses to treatment are frequently observed, but evaluating the status of disease at a cellular level remains difficult. Early reports claimed high accuracy in excluding presence of residual or recurrent tumour using signal change properties on MRI.[25] Contrast agent uptake studies following intravenous gadolinium administration also showed some encouraging results.[26,27] It is certainly true that MRI can demonstrate reduction in tumour bulk on treatment. Alteration of signal in bone marrow infiltrating tumours has also been demonstrated in response to treatment (Fig. 8.18). It is more difficult to predict how complete the response is at the cellular level, as no imaging technique can give histological information. It has been demonstrated that in Ewing's sarcoma, MR will demonstrate a favourable response to treatment, but cannot exclude microscopic foci of residual malignant tumour (Fig. 8.19).[28] Although MRI is the most sensitive and sophisticated technique, gross changes such as bony sclerosis may be identified on plain films. While development of such changes (for example, in breast cancer metastases treated with tamoxifen) encourages the physician to believe that some form of healing response has taken place, it is difficult to prove that this is truly the case without histological confirmation.

REFERENCES

1. Lodwick GS, Wilson AJ, Farrell C, Virtama P, Dittrich F. Determining growth rates of focal lesions of bone from radiographs. *Radiology* (1980) **134**: 577–83.
2. Dahlin DC, Unni KK. *Bone Tumours* (4th edn) (Springfield, IL: Charles C. Thomas, 1986).
3. Silverberg E, Lubera J. Cancer statistics. (1987) **27**: 2–20.
4. Dahlin DC, Coventry MB. Osteosarcoma. A study of 600 cases. *J Bone Joint Surg* (1967) **49A:** 101–10.
5. Ahuja SC, Villacin AB, Smith J et al. Juxtacortical (parosteal) osteogenic sarcoma. *J Bone Joint Surg* (1977) **59A:** 532–47.
6. Unni KK, Dahlin DC, Beaubout SW et al. Parosteal osteogenic sarcoma. *Cancer* (1976) **37**: 2466–75.
7. Allwick MR, Siegal GP, Unni KK et al. Sarcomas of bone complicating osteoitis deformans (Paget's disease): 50 years experience. *Am J Surg Pathol* (1981) **5**: 47–59.
8. Greditzer HG, Mcleod RA, Unni KK et al. Bone sarcomas in Paget's disease. *Radiology* (1983) **146**: 333–7.
9. Marcove RC. Chondrosarcoma: diagnosis and treatment. *Orthop Clin North Am* (1977) **8**: 811–20.
10. Galasko CSB. The anatomy and pathways of skeletal metastases. In Weiss L, Gilbert HA (eds) *Bone Metastases* (Boston, MA: GK Hall, 1981): 49–63.
11. Abrams HL, Spiro R, Goldstein N. Metastases in carcinoma. Analysis of 1000 autopsy cases. *Cancer* (1950) **2**: 74–85.
12. Tofe AJ, Francis MD, Harvey WJ. Correlation of neoplasms with incidence and localisation of skeletal metastases: an analysis of 1355 diphosphonate bone scans. *J Nucl Med* (1975) **16**: 986–9.
13. Clain A. Secondary malignant disease of bone. *Br J Cancer* (1965) **19**: 15–29.
14. Johnston AD. Pathology of metastatic tumours in bone. *Clin Orthop* (1970) **73**: 8–32.
15. Galasko CSB. Mechanisms of lytic and blastic metastatic disease of bone. *Clin Orthop* (1982) **169**: 20–7.
16. Manishen WJ, Sivanathan K, Orr FW. Resorbing bone stimulates tumour cell growth: a role for the host microenvironment in bone metastasis. *Am J Pathol* (1986) **123**: 39–45.
17. Edelstyn GA, Gillespie PJ, Grebbell FS. The radiological demonstration of osseous metastases: experimental observations. *Clin Radiol* (1967) **18**: 158–62.

18. Jones AL, Williams MP, Powles TJ et al. Magnetic resonance imaging in the detection of skeletal metastases in patients with breast cancer. *Br J Cancer* (1990) **62:** 296–8.
19. Thomas LG, Forkner CE Jr, Frei E III et al. The skeletal lesions of acute leukaemia. *Cancer* (1961) **14:** 608.
20. Cancer in South East England. *Thames Cancer Registry* (Sutton, Surrey, 1996).
21. Fisher AMH, Kendal B, van Leuven BD. Hodgkin's disease: a radiological survey. *Clin Radiol* (1962) **13:** 115–27.
22. Libshitz HI, Malthouse SR, Cunningham D, MacVicar D, Husband JE. Multiple myeloma: appearance at MR imaging. *Radiology* (1992) **182:** 833–7.
23. Kreicbergs A, Bauer HCF, Brosio O et al. Cytological diagnosis of bone tumours. *J Bone Joint Surg (Br)* (1966) **78B:** 258–63.
24. Stoker DJ, Cobb JB, Pringle JAS. Needle biopsy of musculoskeletal lesions: a review of 208 procedures. *J Bone Joint Surg (Br)* (1991) **73:** 498–500.
25. Vanel D, Lacombe MJ, Couanet D et al. Musculoskeletal tumours: follow up with MR imaging after treatment with surgery and radiation therapy. *Radiology* (1987) **164:** 243–5.
26. Erlemann R, Reiser MS, Peters PE et al. Musculoskeletal neoplasms: static and dynamic Gd-DTPA-enhanced MR imaging. *Radiology* (1989) **171:** 767–73.
27. Vanderwoude A, Bloem JL, Holscher HC et al. Monitoring the effects of chemotherapy in Ewing's sarcoma of bone with MR imaging. *Skeletal Radiol* (1994) **23:** 493–500.
28. MacVicar AD, Olliff J, Pringle J et al. Ewing sarcoma: MRI of chemotherapy induced changes with histological correlation. *Radiology* (1992) **184:** 859–64.

9

Biochemical markers of malignant bone disease

Robert E Coleman

Introduction • Biochemical markers for diagnosis of bone metastases • Evaluation of the patient • Monitoring bisphosphonate treatment of metastatic bone disease • Conclusions

INTRODUCTION

Metastatic bone destruction results from the invasion of malignant cells from the bone marrow cavity.[1] These cells secrete a variety of paracrine factors which stimulate bone cell function. The stimulation of osteoclast function is of particular importance, resulting in osteolysis and typically associated with disruption of the normal coupling between osteoblast and osteoclast function.[2] These effects on bone cell function may in turn influence serum and urinary levels of biochemical markers of bone metabolism. In recent years, the number of available markers has increased rapidly (Table 9.1), and their clinical relevance is under investigation in several tumour types.

Markers of bone formation

Type I collagen is the major protein of bone and accounts for about 90% of the organic matrix. It is a complex molecule consisting of a heterotrimer of two pro-α1 and one pro-α2 peptide chains. The molecule is tightly coiled due to the presence of regular glycine residues which do not possess a bulky side chain and allow the helical structure to form.

Table 9.1 Biochemical markers of bone resorption and formation

Resorption	Formation
Urine	*Serum*
Calcium	Alkaline phosphatase
Hydroxyproline	Osteocalcin
Pyridinoline	PICP
Deoxypyridinoline	PIIINP
Ntx	
Crosslaps	
Free Dpd	
Free Pyr	
Galactosyl hydroxylysine	
Serum	
Calcium	
ICTP	
Galactosyl hydroxylysine	

Dpd = deoxypyridinoline; Pyr = pyridinoline; Ntx = N-telopeptide of Type I collagen; ICTP = Type I collagen C-telopeptide; PICP = serum procollagen I extension peptide; PIIINP = serum procollagen Type III propeptide.

The steps involved in collagen synthesis are multiple and complicated and include a number of post-translational modifications. Essentially a large precursor protein, Type I procollagen, is synthesized by osteoblasts, the three chains are assembled, intra- and intermolecular cross-links bind the peptide chains together making the molecule insoluble, and the collagen fibrils are formed by precise spatial alignment of the collagen chains prior to mineralization of the resulting matrix. The available biochemical markers of bone formation reflect different aspects of this process.

Type I procollagen (PICP) is believed to be a marker of early bone formation, appearing principally during the phase of osteoblast proliferation. Assay of the carboxy terminal propeptide is now possible by radioimmune assay.[3,4] Osteoblasts are naturally rich in alkaline phosphatase, and release of the enzyme into the circulation occurs predominantly during the matrix maturation phase of bone formation, and provides a slightly different indication of osteoblast activity.

Total alkaline phosphatase is routinely measured in clinical practice, but to exclude the contribution from the liver and other organs, bone isoenzyme estimation (ALP-BI) is required. Raised levels reflect increased new bone formation and in oncology the highest values are found with osteoblastic metastases or in response to healing.[5] Osteocalcin (BGP) is a marker of the late phase of bone formation, appearing during mineralization.[4] It is also synthesized in osteoblasts, and contains three residues of the vitamin K-dependent amino acid γ-carboxy-glutamic acid. Osteocalcin binds strongly to hydroxyapatite, but a small fraction of the newly synthesized protein appears in the circulation from which it is rapidly cleared by the kidney. Measurement of serum levels is possible by a variety of radioimmune assays.

Markers of bone resorption

Resorption of bone releases calcium, hydroxyproline, and collagen fragments into the circulation. These are cleared by the kidney and excreted largely unchanged into the urine. Urinary calcium excretion is a frequently measured indicator of alterations in calcium homeostasis. The molar ratio of calcium to creatinine in an early-morning urine sample collected after an overnight fast is a convenient reproducible method of quantifying calcium excretion. The problem with urinary calcium is that it is not a specific resorption inhibitor, but reflects the net effects of bone formation and resorption. It is also influenced by diet, the circulating levels of both parathyroid hormone (PTH) and parathyroid-related peptide (PTHrP), and the concommitant administration of drugs such as bisphosphonates which influence bone resorption independently of any tumour-related effects.[6,7] Urinary hydroxyproline excretion is a conventional parameter for measuring bone resorption in benign bone disease where it indicates bone matrix destruction with quite high specificity. However, it has been generally unreliable in the monitoring of metastatic bone disease due to the contributions from dietary intake and the soft tissue destruction which may result from the metastatic process.[6,8,9]

Serum calcium measurements are routinely performed during clinical management, but changes within the normal range give little guide to disease activity. Hypercalcaemia typically indicates uncontrolled progressive malignancy, although rarely hypercalcaemia can be a manifestation of the tumour flare, occurring within a week or so of starting tamoxifen, and may herald a subsequent response to treatment.[10] Hypocalcaemia is seen when osteoblastic metastases predominate. Hypocalcaemia is more typically associated with prostate cancer but does sometimes occur in advanced breast cancer.

It is hoped that the recently introduced measurements of the intermolecular cross-linking compounds of collagen will overcome the poor specificity of the old markers. Pyridinoline (Pyr) and deoxypyridinoline (Dpd), also called hydroxy-lysylpyridinoline and lysyl-pyridinoline, respectively, are two cross-linking amino acids which hold together the extracellular telopeptide region at the ends of adjacent collagen chains. Pyr is found in bone, cartilage, and, to a lesser extent, other connective tissues, while Dpd is almost exclusive to bone.[6] They can be measured accurately in urine by reverse-phase high-peformance liquid chromatography (HPLC) and have been reported as specific measures of the rate of bone resorption.[11]

Although levels of both Pyr and Dpd have provided useful information in benign and malignant skeletal conditions, the HPLC assays are too complex and time-consuming to be suitable for routine laboratory practice. Crosslinks exist in both free (40%) and peptide-bound forms (60%), and, recently, new enzyme-linked immunoassays (ELISA) have been developed to measure the protein-bound cross-links at either the N-terminal (Ntx),[12] or the C-terminal[13] portion (Crosslaps) of Type I collagen, as well as the free portions of both pyridinoline (F-Pyr) and deoxypyridinoline (F-Dpd),[14] thereby providing a range of relatively simple assays for specific assessment of the rate of bone resorption. A recent study in hypercalcaemia of malignancy has shown that the simpler ELISA assays correlate closely with the HPLC-based Dpd and Pyr measurements and accurately reflected the clear clinical differences observed between treatment for hypercalcaemia of malignancy with either pamidronate or clodronate.[15]

There is also great interest in developing a reliable serum assay for cross-links. At present the only commercially available serum assay is the C-telopeptide cross-links (ICTP) developed by Risteli et al.[16] This assay, unlike the Crosslaps assay for urine, recognizes elements from the helical part of both the α1 and α2 chains. Despite some interesting and encouraging preliminary data of ICTP measurements in oncology,[17,18] its clinical value remains uncertain. ICTP levels have been reported to change very little during the management of Paget's disease of bone or osteoporosis, clinical situations where resorption rates are known to be profoundly affected by treatment, and increase during treatment with anabolic steroids which are believed to decrease bone resorption and stimulate collagen synthesis.[6,19] ICTP appears therefore to be more a marker of collagen turnover than a specific indicator of bone resorption.

Technical aspects

Considerable progress has been achieved in developing reliable assays for markers of bone metabolism. However, their interpretation requires an understanding of not only the analytical performance characteristics of the method but also the biological variability of the markers and the influence of preanalytical conditions. Confounding factors include a circadian rhythm to bone metabolism, variations in the age and sex of the subjects studied, the menstrual cycle, changes in liver function and renal clearance, and the possible influences of thermal stability, storage conditions, and repeat freeze–thaw cycles on assay performance.

The bone markers show a significant diurnal variation, with the highest values noted in the early morning and the lowest levels occurring during the afternoon and at night. The time of sampling is therefore crucial to provide clinically relevant information. In addition, considerable day-to-day variability may be seen due to a true variation in the level of the markers,[20] and not analytical imprecision; this intraindividual variability is greater for urine markers than for serum markers.

Specimen collection and storage conditions are other confounding factors. Alkaline phosphatase and osteocalcin may be affected by divalent cations, such that collection tubes containing ethylenediamine tetra-acetic acid (EDTA) or citrate are inappropriate. After collection, alkaline phosphatase and Type I collagen propeptides are fairly stable and can be stored at 4 °C and for longer periods at –20 °C. However, osteocalcin is much more labile and should be frozen within 1–2 hours of collection and for long-term storage should be maintained at –70 °C. Assays which measure both the intact and N-mid-fragment are preferred because of their greater accuracy.[21] The urinary pyridinolines are fairly stable at room temperature, although somewhat light sensitive, and long-term storage at –20 °C is probably adequate.

Table 9.2 Bone resorption and tumour markers in newly diagnosed bone metastases. Mean values (95% confidence intervals) shown.

Marker	Units	Controls	Patients	% patients with increased value
Ntx	(nmol BCE/mmol)	55 (25–120)	84 (66–107)	41
Hydroxyproline	(mmol/mmol)	24 (11–48)	30 (26–35)	24
Urinary calcium	(mmol/mmol)	0.33 (0.13–0.053)	0.27 (0.21–0.034)	28
CA15-3	U/ml	35[a]	48 (32–71)	69
CASA	U/ml	6[a]	6.7 (4.4–10.1)	50

[a] = upper limit of reference range; CASA = cancer-associated serum antigen.
Source: Adapted from Hannon et al.[20]

Cross-linked telopeptides probably have similar stability. For all markers, repeated freeze–thaw cycles may influence their concentrations and should be avoided.

BIOCHEMICAL MARKERS FOR DIAGNOSIS OF BONE METASTASES

None of the bone markers has been shown to be useful in screening asymptomatic patients for metastases. In general, fairly extensive skeletal damage is required before a significant change in marker levels can be expected. In a recent study of patients with new bone metastases from breast cancer diagnosed within the previous 6 weeks, only 41% had raised levels of the resorption marker Ntx, while in this study urinary calcium and hydroxyproline were increased in only 28% and 24%, respectively[22] (Table 9.2). As the disease process progresses the number of patients with raised levels increases[6] and this probably explains the variable data published to date on bone markers and diagnosis. However, a few general observations can be made.

Bone formation markers

Osteocalcin levels have been shown to be significantly increased in metastatic bone disease from breast and prostate cancers when compared to normal subjects,[23] but this is not the case in multiple myeloma where bone formation is typically impaired.[24] Osteocalcin levels are significantly higher in patients with radiologically blastic as opposed to lytic metastases, and there appears to be some correlation of osteocalcin levels with tumour bulk in prostate cancer.[25] Similar trends are reported with ALP-BI with highest levels in patients with multiple blastic metastases.[5] The correlation between ALP-BI and osteocalcin is variable, reflecting their relationship to different phases of the bone formation process.[4] PICP levels typically correlate well with ALP-BI, especially for patients with blastic metastases.[5] Increased levels are seen in over half of patients with prostatic metastases[26] and around 25% with breast cancer[5] but PICP is usually normal in multiple myeloma.[27]

Bone resorption markers

Urinary calcium excretion is not significantly increased in the majority of patients with metastatic bone disease,[6] reflecting the additional effects of cancer on bone formation and of PTHrP on the renal handling of calcium. Hydroxyproline excretion, which indicates matrix destruction more specifically, is typically

Table 9.3 Biochemical evidence of increased bone resorption irrespective of tumour type. Ratio of mean values in cancer patients with bone metastases to mean values in age and sex-matched controls. All markers measured in urine and corrected for creatinine.

	Breast (n = 29)	Prostate (n = 10)	Others* (n = 7)
Ntx	2.55	7.61	3.19
Crosslaps	1.84	4.93	2.86
Free Dpd	2.22	3.19	2.47
Hydroxyproline	1.66	2.92	2.27
Urinary calcium	0.78	1.77	2.46

Note: Others included 2 sarcoma, 2 myeloma, 1 lung, 1 melanoma, and 1 unknown primary.

increased in breast cancer[8,9] and myeloma, but high, intermediate, and low levels have been reported in prostate cancer.[26]

It is clear that the collagen cross-links are much more reliable in confirming metastatic bone disease. In a review of six studies, elevated levels of Pyr and Dpd were reported in 58–88% and 60–80%, respectively.[6] Increased bone resorption marker levels are also seen in prostate cancer. Despite its sclerotic radiographic appearance there is biochemical[5,28–30] and histological[31,32] evidence of increased bone resorption. Indeed in a series of patients included in a clinical trial of pamidronate for metastatic bone pain,[33] the levels of bone resorption markers appeared to be even higher, in comparison to age and sex-matched controls, in prostate cancer patients than in those with breast cancer or other predominantly lytic forms of metastatic bone disease (Table 9.3).

In breast cancer, levels of Pyr and Dpd have also been slightly elevated in breast cancer patients without evidence of skeletal metastases, perhaps indicating subclinical involvement or, more likely, the effects of PTHrP and other bone-mobilizing tumour products on the skeleton.[34]

Tumour markers

In breast cancer, unlike the germ cell malignancies, there is not a highly specific tumour marker for either diagnosis or monitoring of disease. However, most breast tumours do express cell surface mucins which can be detected by radioimmunoassay. The most widely studied are carcinoembryonic antigen (CEA) which is elevated in 50–80% of patients with metastatic breast cancer and carcinoma antigen (CA) 15-3 which is elevated in 60–90% of cases with advanced disease.[35] There are some data to suggest that tumour markers may identify metastatic disease before symptoms are reported.[36,37] Large multicentre studies are planned to see if tumour markers are a cost-effective component of breast cancer follow-up and whether, as preliminary data would seem to suggest,[37] the treatment of rising tumour markers in an otherwise well patient improves survival.

Prostate specific antigen (PSA) is a marker of prostatic pathology and may be elevated in any prostate disease: benign prostatic hypertrophy (BPH), prostatitis, and cancer. The highest tissue production occurs in prostate cancer and PSA has proved useful in the early diagnosis, staging, and follow-up of patients.[38] The level of PSA is dependent on the volume of cancer, the volume of BPH in the prostate, and the differentiation of the tumour with less production of PSA from poorly differentiated tumours.

EVALUATION OF THE PATIENT

A variety of treatments, including radiotherapy, endocrine treatment, chemotherapy, and bisphosphonates, are used for the treatment of metastatic bone disease and evaluation of their effects is important for both routine clinical practice and research. The current imaging methods used to assess response to these treatments are qualitative and routinely include plain radiographs, radionuclide bone scans, and, in particular situations, computerized tomography (CT) and magnetic resonance imaging (MRI).

The response assessment of bone metastases to therapy is notoriously difficult, as the events in the healing process are slow to evolve and quite subtle, and more difficult than evaluation of disease in viscera and soft tissues where tumour measurements can usually be taken. A complete review of the bone radiographs since the start of a treatment is necessary to evaluate response, a time-consuming and tedious process with marked inter- and intraobserver error. Sclerosis of lytic lesions generally only begins to appear 3–6 months after the start of therapy.[39]

Bone has separate criteria for evaluation of response to treatment, based on bone repair and destruction rather than changes in tumour volume.[40] This results in reports of lower response frequencies to systemic treatments in the skeleton compared with other sites of disease. Complete response in nonosseous sites affected by breast cancer occurs in 10–20% of patients but a complete response (CR) in bone with return of normal trabecular pattern, or resolution of sclerotic metastases, is very rare. This is almost certainly a reflection of the insensitivity of the assessment methods rather than representing some biological phenomenon of site-specific resistance. Consequently, patients with metastatic disease confined to the bone are frequently excluded from many therapeutic trials and patients with widespread metastatic disease (including bone) rely on the changes observed in soft tissue or visceral disease to judge response to treatment.

Although it is recognized that the changes seen on serial radiographs remain the 'gold standard' for evaluating response to therapy, new methods of assessing response are needed, both to improve patient management and to evaluate specific treatments. A number of alternatives or adjuncts to assessment based on plain radiographs have been suggested. None is ideal, each having advantages and disadvantages, but the recent developments in biochemical evaluation of bone metabolism offer the possibility of real progress in this area.

Biochemical assessment of response

When treatment is prescribed for a patient with bone metastases the effects of that treatment on the tumour cell population will influence bone cell activity. These changes probably occur within the first few weeks of starting effective therapy, and therefore biochemical markers which reflect the respective rates of bone formation and resorption could provide an early assessment of response to treatment.

In the mid-1980s there were several studies which investigated the use of biochemical assessment of response to systemic therapy.[8,9,41,42] These generally showed that radiological response is correlated with a reduction in bone resorption. But, perhaps because at the time urinary calcium and hydroxyproline were the only available resorption markers, the reliability of biochemical monitoring was not established.

Breast cancer
Urinary calcium excretion was initially reported as a marker of response in advanced breast cancer more than 10 years ago;[43] follow-up studies have confirmed that a rapid fall in urinary calcium excretion is typical of response. In one prospective study of 70 unselected patients with advanced breast cancer receiving systemic treatment,[9] 15/16 radiographically confirmed objective responders (94%) had a > 10% reduction in calcium excretion compared with 10/21 (48%) with progressive disease ($p < 0.01$). Markers of osteoblast activity were also evaluated in this study. After 1 month 15/16 responding patients (94%) showed a > 10% rise

in both ALP-BI and osteocalcin compared with 7/22 (31%) with radiological evidence of progression ($p < 0.001$). The serum concentration of ALP-BI and osteocalcin subsequently fell steadily after 1–2 and 3–4, months respectively. Variable changes in bone formation have been reported by others, depending on the timing of sample collection and the confounding changes induced by the healing flare.[41]

With the development of the cross-link assays, there has been renewed interest in biochemical monitoring.[44] A preliminary report of deoxypyridinoline (Dpd) and pyridinoline (Pyr) measurements in breast cancer patients receiving endocrine treatment has shown that pretreatment levels of Dpd and Pyr were two to threefold higher in patients who progressed on treatment compared to stable or responding patients; during treatment cross-link excretion increased in patients with progressive disease (PD) but remained stable or fell in the responders.[45] In another study, Blomqvist and colleagues monitored the serum C-telopeptide of Type I collagen (ICTP). Increased levels of ICTP generally indicated progressive disease, although a few patients with increasing ICTP subsequently showed a response or disease stabilization.[46]

A more detailed study has recently been published.[22] Bone resorption and tumour markers were assessed as possible alternatives to serial plain radiographs in an EORTC study of 37 patients with newly diagnosed radiographically assessable bone metastases from breast cancer. The markers of bone metabolism measured included urinary calcium (uCa), hydroxyproline (Hyp), the N-telopeptide cross-links of Type I collagen (NTx), and total alkaline phosphatase. The tumour markers measured were CA15-3 and cancer-associated serum antigen (CASA). The choice of specific anti-cancer treatment was left at the discretion of the patient's treating physician and included radiotherapy, chemotherapy, and endocrine therapy. Bone metastases were identified by radionuclide bone scan and confirmed by plain radiographs or CT scanning. Radiographs of involved sites, and a fasting morning serum sample and a second voided urine sample, were obtained regularly, and at each time there was either a change in systemic therapy or a skeletal complication.

For assessment of response and identification of progression, Ntx was the most useful bone marker. There was a significant difference in mean NTx levels between PD patients versus no change (NC) or partial response (PR) patients at 1 ($p = < 0.05$) and 4 months ($p = < 0.01$). There was also a significant difference in the CA15-3 levels between PD patients versus NC or PR patients at 4 months ($p = < 0.05$), but not at 1 month, and no significant difference at either time point with CASA ($p = 0.09$). Ntx was the only bone resorption marker able to discriminate reliably after 1 and 4 months of treatment between patients progressing early after commencing treatment (time to progression [TP] ≤ 7 months) from those with a longer period of disease control (TP of > 7 months).

An algorithm based on the least significant change in an individual parameter to predict response was constructed to try to incorporate a panel of biochemical markers with symptomatic response. The best combination to predict response was found to be the combination of a rise in Ntx and alkaline phosphatase with a fall in clinical (pain score) response (Table 9.4). The predictive values of an increase in markers to predict for progression were also calculated. The diagnostic efficiency (DE) for prediction of PD following a > 50% increase in Ntx or CA15-3 was 78% and 62%, respectively (Table 9.5).

The clinical relevance of these results lies in the context of the treatment of bone metastases being palliative rather than curative, where the aim of treatment in metastatic bone disease is to keep patients symptom-free and active for as long as possible, with the fewest adverse effects from treatment. Early information indicative of either response or progressive disease would be particularly helpful in determining whether or not treatment should be continued.

Prostate cancer

Biochemical monitoring of bone metabolism in prostatic cancer is perhaps less relevant as serial measurements of PSA are relatively easily inter-

Table 9.4 Predictive values of changes in markers at 1 month for response to treatment as determined at 4 months. Values given as %.

Marker(s)	PV+	PV–	DE
Ntx (≥ 30% fall)	95	41	69
CA15-3 (≥ 10% fall)	82	41	61
tAP (≥ 10% fall)	94	47	69
Pain score (≥ 20% fall)	94	47	69
Ntx + CA15-3	95	35	44
Ntx + pain score	95	53	56
tAP + pain score	89	53	53
Ntx + tAP	95	58	64
Ntx + tAP + pain score	95	70	72
Ntx + CA15-3 + pain score	95	53	58
Ntx + tAP + CA15-3	100	53	56
Ntx + tAP + CA15-3 + pain score	100	58	61

PV+ = positive predictive value; PV– = negative predictive value; DE = diagnostic efficiency.

Table 9.5 Predictive value for PD of a 50% increase in markers or pain whenever it occurs. Values given as %.

	PV+	PV–	DE
Ntx	81	76	78
Hyp	57	62	59
uCa	62	25	46
tAP	94	33	59
CA15-3	75	52	62
CASA	50	52	51
Pain score	100	6	42

PV+ = positive predictive value; PV– = negative predictive value; DE = diagnostic efficiency.

preted and, as indicated below, correlate well with disease activity. However, in prostate cancer, effective endocrine treatment typically also leads to control of bone resorption, with a fall in Dpd levels to within the normal range whereas, in patients with PD, persistently increased levels of Dpd are found.[47] In a study run by the Finnish Prostate Cancer Group, PICP levels were measured. Pretreatment levels were elevated, reflecting increased osteoblast activity,[26] and then fell during treatment. However, the significance of this change was difficult to interpret. Initially the fall may have been due to a reduction in both tumour burden and removal of tumour stimulation of osteoblast function but, as patients started to progress again, the levels continued to fall; this was attributed by the investigators to enhanced catabolism and tumour-induced cachexia associated with the late stages of the disease.

Multiple myeloma
In myeloma, one study has suggested that serial measurements of the serum resorption marker ICTP could discriminate between PD and disease response or stabilization.[27] In this study, PICP was also measured. Multiple myeloma is a condition characterized by a depressed bone formation and, not suprisingly, levels of PICP were low to normal before treatment, reflecting the inhibition of osteoblast function, and re-

mained so despite a reduction in tumour mass.

Tumour markers

In metastatic breast cancer, serial measurements of CA15-3 and CEA appear to correlate closely with response in measurable disease.[48] As a result their use is being increasingly advocated, particularly in patients with sclerotic or mixed lytic and sclerotic disease which is so difficult to assess radiologically.[49] There are also a number of other mucin markers which are potentially of value, and it is probably realistic to expect that a panel of tumour markers will be identified which collectively can provide reliable information on tumour response.

PSA is under androgen regulation and, as a result, levels usually decline after androgen deprivation. This decrease may not accurately reflect the response of the tumour to treatment, but is the most reliable marker available for following patients after definitive therapy, and has superceded the use of acid phosphatase.[50] Additionally, elevations of PSA usually antedate other clinical evidence of progression by at least 6 months.[51]

MONITORING BISPHOSPHONATE TREATMENT OF METASTATIC BONE DISEASE

Bisphosphonates are an important new treatment modality in the management of metastatic bone disease. Through their potent inhibitory effects on bone resorption they have become the treatment of choice for hypercalcaemia of malignancy,[52] and are able to reduce the number and rate of skeletal complications in multiple myeloma[53] and advanced breast cancer,[54] delay the onset of progressive disease in bone following palliative chemotherapy for both breast cancer and myeloma,[55,56] and relieve metastatic bone pain caused by a variety of solid tumours with a consequent improvement in quality of life.[57]

The effects of bisphosphonates on bone pain are now well recognized. Quite consistently the phase II studies have reported relief of bone pain in around one half of patients.[57] However, the reason(s) for a lack of symptomatic response in the other 50% of patients treated are unclear. Bone pain is a complex process and mechanical factors such as spinal instability or nerve entrapment may contribute. Nevertheless much of the morbidity associated with bone metastases is secondary to focal tumour-induced osteolysis.

Changes in cross-link excretion have been evaluated in patients receiving bisphosphonate treatment for hypercalcaemia of malignancy. Before treatment, Dpd and Pyr excretion is four times the upper limit of normal and the levels of the peptide-bound cross-links (Ntx and Crosslaps) increased up to seven times normal.[15] After treatment, with full doses of either pamidronate,[15,58] clodronate,[15] or ibandronate,[59] levels of Pyr and Dpd fall by 30–60%, and reduction in Ntx and Crosslaps of 80–90% occurs.[15,58]

Cross-link excretion has also been used to monitor response to bisphosphonates in normocalcaemic subjects, with significant falls of 40–50% in Dpd and 25–35% in Pyr following either intravenous[60] or oral[44] pamidronate for metastatic breast cancer and oral residronate for multiple myeloma.[24]

Two studies have been performed in Sheffield which recruited 86 normocalcaemic patients with heavily pretreated painful progressing bone metastases (52 breast, 17 prostate, 17 others) to investigate a possible link between inhibition of bone resorption and symptomatic response.[7,33] In the first study, total pyridinoline (Pyr) and deoxypyridinoline (Dpd) were measured, while in the second study the easier and more sensitive ELISA assays for Ntx, Crosslaps, and free deoxypyridinoline (F-Dpd) were measured.

Patients received pamidronate 120 mg as a 2-hour outpatient infusion. The first study ($n = 34$) was an open uncontrolled phase-II evaluation of the clinical and biochemical effects of a single infusion.[7] In the second study,[33] 52 patients were randomized to receive either pamidronate or a placebo infusion of saline alone. Four weeks later, or earlier in the event of worsening symptoms ($n = 13$), all patients received an infusion of pamidronate 120 mg. In both studies, patients experiencing subjective benefit received

Table 9.6 Influence of biochemical response on probability of clinical response to intravenous pamidronate

		Clinical response
Ntx response	Yes	12/19 (63%)
	No	0/11 (0%)
	Always normal	7/13 (53%)
Crosslaps response	Yes	13/24 (54%)
	No	0/7 (0%)
	Always normal	6/12 (50%)
Free Dpd response	Yes	8/15 (53%)
	No	3/15 (20%)
	Always normal	8/13 (61%)

Yes = raised pretreatment level returned to the normal range; no = raised pretreatment level failed to return to the normal range.

further infusions when their symptoms worsened again. No concomitant systemic anticancer treatment or radiotherapy during the course of the study were allowed. Prior to commencing therapy and then weekly for 12 weeks, patients were asked to complete a pain intensity (P) and analgesic consumption (A) questionnaire and their WHO performance status (P) was recorded. These three parameters were combined to produce an overall pain score (PPA) as described previously.[9] Clinical response to treatment was defined as ≥ 20% decrease in PPA recorded on at least two consecutive measurements. Patients with a decrease in PPA of < 20% were considered nonclinical responders.

In the first study, the first evidence in oncology to suggest a link between metastatic bone pain and bone resorption was seen.[7] Patients achieving a ≥ 50% reduction in Dpd were more likely to respond than those with a < 50% fall in this specific marker of bone resorption ($p = < 0.05$). In addition, as patients returned requesting further treatment because of an increase in bone pain, the levels of Dpd were noted also to be rising at this time. A similar link between pain and resorption rate has also been reported in a study of intravenous alendronate for bone pain from prostate cancer.[61]

In the more recent study, the relationships between bone pain and bone resorption rates were evaluated more thoroughly. First, the pretreatment values of Ntx (N-terminal protein-bound cross-linking fragment of Type I collagen) predicted for clinical response to treatment. Patients with an initial NTx value more than twice the upper limit of normal rarely (13%) showed a response to therapy, while clinical response was frequent (63%) in those patients with pretreatment levels of NTx below this cut-off level.

Additionally, patients in whom the rate of bone resorption, as measured by NTx, Crosslaps, or F-Dpd, did not return to normal after pamidronate had a very poor clinical response (0–20% depending on the marker),

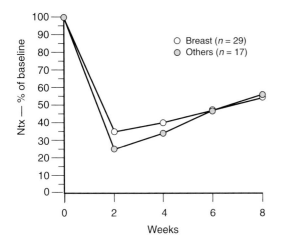

Fig. 9.1 Changes in the bone resorption marker Ntx following treatment with a single infusion of pamidronate 120 mg in patients with bone metastases and breast cancer ($n = 29$) or other tumour types ($n = 17$; 10 prostate, 2 sarcoma, 2 lung, 1 melanoma, 1 renal, 1 unknown primary), indicating very similar responses irrespective of tumour type or radiographic appearance of the bone metastases. Median % of baseline values shown.

while in those patients in whom a biochemical response was achieved or with marker levels always in the normal range, the frequency of response was much higher (53–63%, again depending on the marker – $p < 0.01$) (Table 9.6). Interestingly the changes in collagen cross-link excretion were very similar, irrespective of tumour type, with patients with prostate cancer responding similarly to those patients with breast cancer (Fig. 9.1).

These results suggest that patients with bone metastases and a very high rate of bone resorption will probably respond poorly to bisphosphonates, and that the aim of bisphosphonate treatment should be to restore the rate of bone resorption to normal. This is similar to the aims of bisphosphonate treatments for osteoporosis and Paget's disease of bone. If these results continue to be confirmed by others, patients most likely to benefit from bisphosphonate treatment could in the future be selected on the basis of biochemical measures of bone resorption, and treatment only continued in those patients where the rate of bone resorption can be successfully controlled. For patients with more aggressive disease, more potent bisphosphonates, a higher dose or dose intensity, may be required.

Lipton and colleagues have also reported on the use of collagen cross-link measurements following systemic therapy associated with bisphosphonates. In this trial, 51 patients (49 breast cancer, 2 myeloma) with bone metastases were treated with either pamidronate 90 mg intravenously monthly or placebo in addition to standard systemic therapy. During the 6 months of the trial, NTx was the marker that showed the most significant decrease ($p = 0.0006$), while there was a smaller difference with deoxypyridinoline ($p = 0.03$) and no detectable difference with pyridinoline.[62]

CONCLUSIONS

There are now reliable, specific measures of bone resorption and formation which are relatively simple to measure. The use of modern biochemical markers of bone metabolism, tumour markers, subjective response, and quality-of-life assessment need continued refinement. However, in the future biochemical monitoring is likely to provide more clinically and biologically relevant information than has been available hitherto which can be used to supplement or possibly even replace the use of serial plain radiographs for monitoring the response of bone metastases to treatment.

REFERENCES

1. Mundy GR. Mechanisms of bone metastasis. *Cancer* (1997) **80 (Suppl 8)**: 1546–56.
2. Kanis JA, McCloskey EV. Bone turnover and biochemical markers in malignancy. *Cancer* (1997) **80 (Suppl 8)**: 1538–45.
3. Melkko J, Niemi S, Ristelli J, Risteli L. Radioimmunoassay for human procollagen. *Clin Chem* (1990) **36**: 1328–32.
4. Koizumi M, Maeda H, Yoshimura K, Yamauchi T, Kawai T, Ogata E. Dissociation of bone formation markers in bone metastasis of prostate cancer. *Br J Cancer* (1997) **75**: 1601–4.
5. Berruti A, Panero A, Angelli A *et al*. Different mechanisms underlying bone collagen resorption in patients with bone metastases from prostate and breast cancer. *Br J Cancer* (1996) **73**: 1581–7.
6. Vinholes J, Coleman R, Eastell R. Effects of bone metastases on bone metabolism: implications for diagnosis, imaging and assessment of response to cancer treatment. *Cancer Treat Rev* (1996) **22**: 289–331.
7. Vinholes JJ, Guo C-Y, Purohit OP, Eastell R, Coleman RE. Metabolic effects of pamidronate in patients with metastatic bone disease. *Br J Cancer* (1996) **73**: 1089–95.
8. Coombes RC, Dady P, Parsons C, McCready VR, Gazet J-C, Powles TJ. Assessment of response of bone metastases to systemic treatment in patients with breast cancer. *Cancer* (1983) **52**: 610–14.
9. Coleman RE, Whitaker KD, Moss DW, Mashiter G, Fogelman I, Rubens RD. Biochemical monitoring predicts response in bone to systemic treatment. *Br J Cancer* (1988) **58**: 205–10.
10. Villalon AH, Tattersall MH, Fox RM, Woods RL. Hypercalcaemia after tamoxifen for breast cancer: a sign of tumour response. *Br Med J* (1979) **20**: 1329–30.
11. Siebel MJ, Robins SP, Bilezikian JP. Urinary pyridinium crosslinks of collagen. Specific marker of bone resorption in metabolic bone disease. *Trends Endocrinol Metab* (1992) **3**: 263–70.
12. Hanson D, Weis MAE, Bollen AM *et al*. A specific immunoassay for monitoring human bone resorption: quantification of type 1 collagen cross-linked N-telopeptides in urine. *J Bone Miner Res* (1992) **7**: 1251–8.
13. Bonde M, Qvist P, Christiansen C *et al*. Applications of an enzyme immunoassay for a new marker of bone resorption (Crosslaps): follow-up on hormone replacement therapy and osteoporosis risk assessment. *J Clin Endocrinol Metab* (1995) **80**: 864–8.
14. Robins SP, Woitge H, Lindsay R *et al*. Direct, enzyme-linked immunoassay for urinary deoxypyridinoline as a specific marker for measuring bone resorption. *J Bone Miner Res* (1994) **9**: 1643–9.
15. Vinholes JJ, Purohit OP, Abbey ME, Eastell R, Coleman RE. Evaluation of new bone resorption markers in a randomized comparison of pamidronate or clodronate for hypercalcaemia of malignancy. *J Clin Oncol* (1997) **15**: 131–8.
16. Risteli J, Elomaa I, Risteli L. Radioimmunoassay for the pyridinoline cross-linked carboxyterminal telopeptide of type 1 collagen: a new marker of bone resorption. *Clin Chem* (1993) **39**: 635–40.
17. Koizumi M, Aiba K, Ogata E. Bone metabolic markers in bone metastases. *J Canc Res Clin Oncol* (1995) **121**: 542–48.
18. Rudnicki M, Jensen LT, Iverson P. Collagen derived serum markers in carcinoma of the prostate. *Scand J Urol Nephrol* (1995) **29**: 317–21.
19. Hassager C, Jensen LT, Podenphant J, Thomsen K, Christiansen C. The carboxy-terminal pyridinoline cross-linked telopeptide of type I collagen in serum as a marker of bone resorption: the effect of nandrolone decanoate and hormone replacement therapy. *Calcif Tissue Int* (1994) **54**: 30–3.
20. Hannon R, Blumsohn A, Naylor K, Eastell R. Response of biochemical markers of bone turnover to hormone replacement therapy: impact of biological variability. *J Bone Miner Res* (1998) **13**: 1124–33.
21. Garnero P, Grimaux M, Demiaux B, Preaudat C, Sequin P, Delmas PD. Measurement of serum osteocalcin with a human-specific two-site immunoradiometric assay. *J Bone Miner Res* (1992) **7**: 1389–98.
22. Vinholes J, Lacombe D, Coleman R *et al*. Assessment of bone response to systemic therapy in an EORTC trial of oral pamidronate. *Br J Cancer* (1999) (in press).
23. Coleman RE, Mashiter G, Fogelman I, Rubens RD. Osteocalcin: a marker of metastatic bone disease. *Eur J Cancer* (1988) **24**: 1211–17.
24. Roux C, Ravaud P, Cohen-Solal M *et al*. Biologic, histologic and densitometric effects of oral residronate in patients with multiple myeloma. *Bone* (1994) **15**: 41–9.

25. Kymala T, Ristell J, Elomaa I. Type 1 collagen degradation product (ICTP) gives information about the nature of bone metastases and has prognostic value in prostate cancer. *Br J Cancer* (1995) **71:** 1061–4.
26. Kylmala T, Tammela T, Risteli L, Risteli J, Taube T, Elomaa I. Evaluation of the effect of oral clodronate on skeletal metastases with type I collagen metabolites. A controlled trial of the Finnish Prostate Cancer Group. *Eur J Cancer* (1993) **29A:** 821–5.
27. Elomaa I, Virkkunen P, Risteli L, Risteli J. Serum concentration of the cross-linked carboxyterminal telopeptide of type I collagen (ICTP) is a useful prognostic indicator in multiple myeloma. *Br J Cancer* (1992) **66:** 337–41.
28. Myamato KK, McSherry SA, Robins SP, Besterman J, Mohler JL. Collagen crosslink metabolites in urine as markers of bone metastases in prostate cancer. *J Urol* (1994) **151:** 909–13.
29. Sano M, Kushida K, Takahashi M *et al*. Urinary pyridinoline and deoxypyridinoline in prostate carcinoma patients with bone metastases. *Br J cancer* (1994) **70:** 701–3.
30. Takeuchi S-I, Arai K, Siatoh H, Yoshida K-I, Miura M. Urinary pyridinoline and deoxypyridinoline as potential markers of bone metastases in patients with prostate cancer. *J Urol* (1996) **156:** 1691–5.
31. Clarke NW, McClure J, George NJR. Disodium pamidronate identifies differential osteoclastic bone resorption in metastatic prostate cancer. *Br J Urol* (1992) **69:** 64–70.
32. Taube T, Tammela TLJ, Elomaa I *et al*. The effect of clodronate on bone in metastatic prostate cancer. Histomorphometric report of a double-blind randomised placebo controlled study. *Eur J Cancer* (1994) **30:** 751–8.
33. Vinholes JJ, Purohit OP, Abbey ME, Eastell R, Coleman RE. Relationships between biochemical and symptomatic response in a double-blind trial of pamidronate for metastatic bone disease. *Ann Oncol* (1997) **8:** 1243–50.
34. Demers LM, Costa L, Lipton A. Biochemical markers of bone turnover in patients with metastatic bone disease. *Clin Chem* (1995) **41:** 1489–94.
35. Martoni A, Zamagni C, Bellanova B *et al*. CEA, MCA, CA15.3 and CA549 and their combinations in expressing and monitoring metastatic breast cancer: a prospective comparative study. *Eur J Cancer* (1995) **31:** 1615–21.
36. Jager W, Kramer S, Lang N. Disseminated breast cancer: does early treatment prolong survival without symptoms? *Breast* (1995) **4:** 62–3.
37. Nicolini A, Anselmi L, Michelasi C, Carpi A. Prolonged survival by early salvage treatment of breast cancer patients: a retrospective study. *Br J Cancer* (1997) **76:** 1106–1110.
38. Stamey TA, Yang N, Hay AR, McNeal JE, Freisha FS, Redwine E. PSA as a serum marker of the prostate. *N Engl J Med* (1987) **317:** 909–16.
39. Coleman RE. Evaluation of bone disease in breast cancer. *Breast* (1994) **3:** 73–8.
40. Hayward JL, Carbone PP, Heuson JC, Kumaoka S, Segaloff A, Rubens RD. Assessment of response to therapy in advanced breast cancer. *Cancer* (1977) **3:** 1389–94.
41. Hortobagyi GN, Libshitz HI, Seabold JS. Osseous metastases of breast cancer. Clinical, biochemical, radiographic and scintigraphic evaluation of response to therapy. *Cancer* (1984) **53:** 577–82.
42. Blomqvist C, Elomaa I, Virkkunen P *et al*. The response evaluation of bone metastases in mammary carcinoma. The value of radiology, scintigraphy, and biochemical markers of bone metabolism. *Cancer* (1987) **60:** 2907–12.
43. Campbell FC, Blamey RW, Woolfson AMJ, Elston CW, Hosking DT. Calcium excretion CaE in metastatic breast cancer. *Br J Surg* (1983) **70:** 202–4.
44. Coleman RE, Houston S, James I *et al*. Preliminary results of the use of urinary excretion of pyridinium crosslinks for monitoring metastatic bone disease. *Br J Cancer* (1992) **65:** 766–8.
45. Downey S, Eastell R, Howell A *et al*. Pyridinoline excretion can monitor bone metastases in breast cancer. *Breast Cancer Res Treat* (1994) **32 (Suppl 1):** 83.
46. Blomqvist C, Sarna S, Elomaa I *et al*. Markers of type I collagen degradation and synthesis in the monitoring of treatment response in bone metastases from breast carcinoma. *Br J Cancer* (1996) **73:** 1074–9.
47. Ikeda I, Miura T, Kondo I. Pyridinium cross-links as markers of bone metastases in patients with prostate cancer. *Br J Urol* (1996) **77:** 102–6.
48. Robertson JFR, Pearson D, Price MR, Selby C, Blamey R, Howell A. Objective assessment of therapeutic response in breast cancer using tumour markers. *Br J Cancer* (1991) **64:** 757–63.
49. British Association of Surgical Oncology. BASO guidelines for the management of metastatic bone disease. *Eur J Surg Oncol* (1999) **25:** 3–23.

50. Reni M, Bolognesi A. Prognostic value of prostate specific antigen before, during and after radiotherapy. *Cancer Treat Rev* (1998) **24:** 91–9.
51. Killian CS, Emrich LJ, Vargas FP *et al*. Relative reliability of five serially measured markers for prognosis of progression in prostate cancer. *J Natl Cancer* (1986) **76:** 179–84.
52. Coleman RE. Pamidronate disodium in the treatment and management of hypercalcaemia. *Rev Contemp Pharmacother* (1998) **9:** 147–648.
53. Berenson JR, Lichtenstein A, Porter L *et al*. Efficacy of pamidronate in reducing skeletal events in patients with advanced multiple myeloma. *N Engl J Med* (1996) **334:** 488–93.
54. Hortobagyi GN, Theriault RL, Porter L *et al*. Efficacy of pamidronate in reducing skeletal complications in patients with breast cancer and lytic bone metastases. *N Engl J Med* (1996) **335:** 1785–91.
55. Conte PF, Mauriac L, Calabresi F *et al*. Delay in progression of bone metastases treated with intravenous pamidronate: results from a multicentre randomised controlled trial. *J Clin Oncol* (1996) **14:** 2552–9.
56. Lahtinen R, Laakso M, Palva I, Virkkunen P, Elomaa I for the Finnish Leukaemia Group. Randomised, placebo-controlled multicentre trial of clodronate in multiple myeloma. *Lancet* (1992) **340:** 1049–52.
57. Purohit OP, Anthony C, Radstone CR, Owen J, Coleman RE. High-dose intravenous pamidronate for metastatic bone pain. *Br J Cancer* (1994) **70:** 554–8.
58. Body JJ, Delmas PD. Urinary pyridinium crosslinks as markers of bone resorption in tumour associated hypercalcaemia. *J Clin Endocrinol Metab* (1992) **74:** 471–5.
59. Pecherstorfer M, Herrmann Z, Body JJ *et al*. Randomized phase II trial comparing different doses of the bisphosphonate ibandronate in the treatment of hypercalcemia of malignancy. *J Clin Oncol* (1996) **14:** 268–76.
60. Body JJ, Dumon JC, Delmas PD. Comparative evaluation of markers of bone resorption after a single dose of pamidronate in patients with breast cancer induced osteolysis. *Bone Miner* (1994) **25 (Suppl 1):** S77.
61. Adami S. Bisphosphonates in prostate cancer. *Cancer* (1997) **80 (Suppl):** 1674–9.
62. Lipton A, Hortobagyi G, Reitsma D *et al*. Markers of bone resorption in patients treated with pamidronate. *Bone* (1995) **17:** 615.

10

Bone metastases – general approaches to systemic treatment

Robert D Rubens

Introduction • Specific systemic anti-tumour treatment • Assessment of response to treatment • Conclusion

INTRODUCTION

Most patients with bone metastases have malignant disease which cannot be eradicated by current anti-cancer treatments and for them a therapeutic approach with curative intent is normally unrealistic. Exceptions to this general rule are rare, one example being skeletal involvement in lymphoma. Treatment of metastatic bone disease is therefore usually aimed at palliating symptoms and the reversal or prevention of specific complications. A variety of methods of treatment are available. They include external beam radiotherapy (Chapter 11), radioisotopes (Chapter 12), bisphosphonates (Chapter 16), orthopaedic surgical procedures (Chapter 17), and the management of hypercalcaemia (Chapter 6). Optimal management therefore requires a multidisciplinary team comprising oncologists, orthopaedic surgeons, nuclear medicine physicians, and palliative care specialists. This chapter is concerned with the use of systemic anti-tumour treatments, principally endocrine treatment, for breast and prostate cancer, and cytotoxic chemotherapy for breast and, occasionally, other cancers.

SPECIFIC SYSTEMIC ANTI-TUMOUR TREATMENT

Breast cancer

Although metastatic disease in some patients with breast cancer may apparently be confined to the skeleton, extraosseous disease is also commonly present. Frequently involved sites include soft tissues (breast, skin, and lymph nodes), intrathoracic structures (lung metastases, pleural effusions, and mediastinal involvement), intra-abdominal organs (liver, ascites, and pelvic and retroperitoneal masses), and the brain. When visceral lesions are present, symptoms from them usually dominate the disease and, particularly when the liver is involved, determine that prognosis is poor. In such circumstances, the presence of metastatic bone disease may be of relatively minor importance. In the more common slowly progressive form of metastatic breast cancer without rapidly advancing visceral lesions, skeletal disease, when present, is likely to be the dominant clinical problem. As this metastatic pattern is compatible with prolonged survival, treatment may be needed over a long period of time, often years. Endocrine treatments are generally considered first for the control of metastatic disease but, when rapidly progressing visceral disease is imminently life-threatening, it is usual to initiate systemic treatment with cytotoxic chemotherapy.

The optimal selection of specific systemic treatment for advanced breast cancer is based on a consideration of the extent, pattern, and aggressiveness of the disease, indices of likely hormone sensitivity, such as steroid receptor status, and menopausal status.[1] For patients with rapidly progressing visceral lesions, such as lymphangitis carcinomatosa causing severe breathlessness, or hepatic metastases with deranged liver biochemistry, death is likely to ensue rapidly unless disease progression can be reversed. This type of disease is rarely responsible to hormonal treatment, and chemotherapy is needed if there is to be a chance of disease remission. For patients with less aggressive disease, including the majority with bone metastases, it is helpful to consider the oestrogen and progesterone receptor status of the tumour. Patients with low tumour levels of these receptors are unlikely to respond to hormone treatment and chemotherapy is likely to be more effective. If patients have steroid receptor-positive tumours endocrine therapy is appropriate and menstrual status can assist in the selection of treatment. Chemotherapy can be used when the disease becomes resistant to hormonal approaches. This sequential use of systemic treatments is illustrated in Fig. 10.1.

Endocrine treatment
The rationale for endocrine therapy is to reduce oestrogenic stimulation to tumour growth. This may be achieved by removal of the sources of either oestrogens (ovarian ablation, adrenalectomy) or gonadotrophins (hypophysectomy), inhibiting gonadotrophins (luteinizing hormone-releasing hormone [LH-RH] agonists, e.g. goserelin), blocking the oestrogen receptor (tamoxifen), antagonizing oestrogens (androgens or progestogens), or inhibiting oestrogen synthesis (aromatase inhibitors). The established first-line endocrine treatment for premenopausal patients with receptor-positive tumours

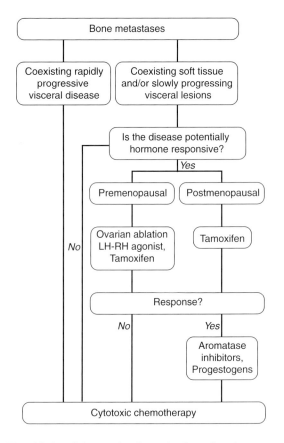

Fig. 10.1 Schema for the selection of anti-tumour treatment in patients with bone metastases from breast cancer

is ovarian ablation, although either LH-RH agonists or tamoxifen are reasonable alternatives. Postmenopausal patients with receptor-positive tumours are treated with tamoxifen.

Metastatic disease which has responded to tamoxifen ultimately, sometimes after several years, becomes resistant to treatment and disease progresses. Possible mechanisms underlying resistance include modification of the structure of the oestrogen receptor so that its binding to tamoxifen forms a complex which is a transcription factor for growth. Another potential mechanism to render tamoxifen ineffective is its metabolism to predominantly oestrogenic metabolites. Hence, although the disease may no longer respond to tamoxifen, this does not necessarily imply that a tumour is no longer amenable to treatment by hormonal approaches.

When disease progresses after a response to primary endocrine treatment, other types may be considered before chemotherapy is needed. Of particular current importance are agents which interfere with oestrogen synthesis.[2] Aminoglutethimide was the first such agent to be used clinically and was originally introduced to inhibit the desmolase enzyme which catalyses the conversion of cholesterol to pregnenolone in the adrenal cortex, so interfering with the production of all adrenocortical hormones. It was subsequently discovered that the principal action of the drug is to inhibit the conversion of C19 androgens to C18 oestrogens by aromatase and this was a more specific effect achieved at drug concentrations which do not inhibit desmolase significantly. This reaction is responsible for the synthesis of oestrogens in peripheral tissues, including breast cancers.

This fundamental understanding of the biochemistry involved has led to the development of more specific aromatase inhibitors which are of two types. Type I inhibitors are steroidal molecules such as formestane (4-hydroxyandrostenedione) and exemestane which bind irreversibly to the catalytic site. The Type II inhibitors are nonsteroidal molecules which bind to cytochrome P-450, the coenzyme for steroidal hydroxylation, and so are less selective than Type I agents. The Type II inhibitors recently introduced for clinical use are letrozole and anastrozole.

Progestational agents, such as medrogesterone acetate, norethisterone acetate, and megestrol acetate, are additional useful agents for second-line endocrine therapy of breast cancer. They act at both the level of the tumour cell and by inhibiting gonadotrophins.

The endocrine treatments in current use are easily administered and lack serious side-effects. There is no clear evidence for the supremacy of one approach over another and the sequential use of treatments as indicated above is usual for routine practice. There is no evidence to support the combined use of hormone treatments other than the addition of prednisolone to either ovarian ablation or tamoxifen.[3] With the variety of endocrine agents now available, there is no longer a place for the use of either high-dose oestrogens or androgens in the treatment of this disease. Oestrogens may cause serious cardiovascular and gastrointestinal toxicity, while the virilizing effects of androgens can be extremely distressing to female patients. The major surgical endocrine ablation procedures of hypophysectomy and bilateral adrenalectomy are now obsolete.

Cytotoxic chemotherapy

The principal cytotoxic agents used for the treatment of metastatic breast cancer are the anthracyclines (doxorubicin and epirubicin), cyclophosphamide, methotrexate, 5-fluorouracil, mitomycin C, and mitozantrone. They are frequently used in combination, common examples being CMF (cyclophosphamide, methotrexate, and 5-fluorouracil), MMM (mitomycin C, methotrexate, and mitozantrone), and FAC (5-fluorouracil, doxorubicin, and cyclophosphamide). No clearly superior combination has emerged, and it is uncertain whether any is significantly more effective than either doxorubicin or epirubicin used alone in optimal dosage. Few new drugs for the treatment of patients with breast cancer have become established in recent years, although the taxoids (paclitaxel and docetaxel) are effective in anthracycline-resistant disease and are being increasingly used.

Dose–response relationships have been demonstrated for cytotoxic drugs and dose intensification has been facilitated by use of haemopoietic growth factors and autologous bone marrow stem cell support. However, there are no convincing data indicating that this approach either enhances palliation of advanced breast cancer or improves the survival of affected patients. There are no good predictors of response to chemotherapy, although crude measures of tumour bulk and performance status give some indication; a large tumour burden and poor performance status correlate with low response rates.

Although the response rate of metastatic breast cancer to first-line chemotherapy in patients selected for clinical trials is in the range 50–70%, in unselected patients receiving such treatment in routine practice the objective response rate is closer to 30%.[4] This discrepancy is a consequence of the highly restrictive entry criteria in trial protocols. Patients in clinical trials are, therefore, not necessarily representative of the whole population with advanced breast cancer. Patients excluded from clinical trials may include the elderly, in addition to those with poor performance status, non-evaluable disease, haematological and biochemical parameters deviating from defined ranges, concomitant illnesses, or previous treatments. It is readily seen that many patients with metastatic bone disease may be excluded from clinical trials because they exhibit one or more of these features.

When selecting cytotoxic chemotherapy, side-effects that most need to be avoided should be considered. For example, the presence of bone marrow involvement or previous extensive skeletal radiotherapy may preclude drugs that are particularly toxic to the bone marrow such as mitomycin C. Considerable progress has been made in reducing the toxic effects of chemotherapy, particularly use of the highly effective anti-emetic 5-hydroxytryptamine ($5HT_3$) inhibitors (ondansetron and granisetron).

Chemotherapy can be particularly hazardous in patients with extensive bone disease as a result of replacement of functioning bone marrow by tumour. Additionally, prior radiotherapy may further compromise bone marrow function. Hence, chemotherapy in patients with metastatic bone disease needs to be used with caution. Although it is possible that the use of haemopoietic growth factors could allow patients with extensive bone metastases to receive intensive chemotherapy regimens, the clinical benefit of this approach for palliative treatment has not yet been demonstrated.

Prostate cancer

Bone is the principal site of metastatic disease in prostate cancer. For many patients it is the only symptomatic problem. Deprivation of the androgenic stimulation to tumour growth is the basis for the endocrine therapy of this disease, about 80% of patients with metastatic prostate cancer showing some response to hormone treatment. The most widely used approach is bilateral orchidectomy. Stilboestrol, once a frequently adopted treatment, is no longer used because of its adverse cardiovascular effects. More recently introduced endocrine treatments include LH-RH agonists and the anti-androgens.

The LH-RH agonists (for example leuprolide, buserelin, goserelin) contain amino acid substitutions which render them resistant to degradation by pituitary peptidases in contrast to the natural decapeptide hormone. The agonists saturate LH-RH pituitary receptors rendering them insensitive to further stimulation. These compounds therefore lead to an initial increase in circulating luteinizing hormone, follicle-stimulating hormone, and testosterone levels which is then followed by a permanent reduction in blood gonadotrophins and androgens. As a result of this mechanism of action, some patients experience a temporary worsening of bone pain. This can be counteracted by the combined administration of an anti-androgen, in addition to analgesics. Cyproterone acetate acts as an anti-androgen by competing with dihydrotestosterone for its receptor. Other, more specific anti-androgens have been developed and are undergoing clinical trial. These pharmacological agents are not any more effective than surgical orchidectomy, but for many patients are more acceptable. Complete androgen blockade in which either orchidectomy or an LH-RH agonist is combined with an anti-androgen has been claimed to provide improved results in the endocrine treatment of prostatic cancer, but this approach remains controversial.[5]

Patients with advanced prostate cancer are usually elderly and often of poor performance status. Consequently, and in the presence of widespread bone involvement, their tolerance to toxic chemotherapy regimens is low and this has significantly limited the use of this type of treatment. There is no evidence that cytotoxic drugs prolong survival in advanced prostate cancer, but a randomized trial of mitozantrone combined with prednisolone has suggested that improved palliation of symptoms and quality of life can be achieved than with prednisolone alone.[6] The use of chemotherapy however is still largely restricted to clinical trials that carefully evaluate pain control, mobility, and quality of life in addition to tumour response.

Other tumours

Skeletal involvement in disseminated cancers which are curable by systemic treatment is relatively rare. It is occasionally seen in patients with germ cell tumours and, although an adverse prognostic feature, cure with chemotherapy is usually achieved. Similarly, bone involvement in lymphoma is uncommon and, although it is associated with a poorer prognosis, curative treatment is still possible.

Chemotherapy is not routinely adopted for the management of bone metastases from the relatively chemoresistant carcinomas of the lung, kidney, thyroid, or elsewhere. Skeletal lesions from these tumours are more appropriately treated by local palliative radiotherapy.

ASSESSMENT OF RESPONSE TO TREATMENT

Assessing response to treatment in bone is considerably more difficult than evaluating disease elsewhere.[7] In soft tissues and viscera, direct estimations of tumour volume can usually be made. By contrast, measurement of disease in bone relies on indirect indices of either bone recalcification in response to treatment or progression of lytic destruction using imaging techniques. As a consequence, lower response frequencies to systemic treatment are usually reported for bone than for disease elsewhere. Complete clinical response of non-osseous metastases from breast cancer is reported in up to 20% of patients on systemic treatment, but complete response in bone with either a return of normal trabecular pattern or resolution of sclerotic metastases is rare. Although this phenomenon might reflect site-specific biological differences in response to treatment, this seems unlikely; the discrepancy is almost certainly a consequence of the insensitivity of assessment methods for disease in the skeleton. It is therefore common for patients with metastatic disease confined to bone frequently to be excluded from clinical trials, while in those with co-existing non-osseous disease, assessment of response to treatment relies on the effect of treatment on soft tissue or visceral lesions.

Radiological assessment of response of skeletal metastases to treatment is based on the observation of recalcification at sites of lytic disease. It is generally accepted that sclerosis of lytic metastases with no radiological evidence of new lesions constitutes tumour regression (a partial response). A confounding factor is the appearance of sclerosis in an area which was previously normal on the radiograph. While this may represent progression of a hitherto unsuspected metastasis, it could also indicate a response within a lesion which, although present when treatment was started, was not sufficiently destructive to be visible radiologically. Interpretation of radiographs is further complicated by variations in film exposure and the effects of overlying intestinal gas. The evaluation of response in osteosclerotic lesions is even more difficult, most patients with sclerotic metastases being categorized as having unassessable disease. Decisions on the effectiveness of treatment have to rely on either symptomatic response and/or changes in existing extraskeletal disease. Although the plain radiograph is an inadequate technique, it continues to be the main assessment criterion for response in clinical trials. Computerized tomography and magnetic resonance imaging provide images of higher quality and with greater sensitivity (Chapter 8). However, they are expensive high-technological tests and less readily applicable in routine practice, although they may give valuable and practical clinical information in specific instances.

The use of isotopic bone scanning (Chapter 7) for assessment or response to therapy is contentious. To interpret a reduction in the intensity and number of lesions on a bone scan as a response to treatment, or an increase in intensity and number as progressive disease may be incorrect. Because an isotope scan images function, rather than structure, increased uptake of radioisotope may be due to enhanced osteoblastic function in response to either bone healing or disease progression. Following successful therapy for metastatic disease, new bone formation causes an increase in tracer uptake and scans performed during the early months of treatment often show heightened intensity and an apparent increase in number of lesions.[8] After about 6 months of treatment, the bone scan appearances may be seen to improve as the increased production of immature new bone wanes and isotope uptake gradually falls. This apparent deterioration followed by subsequent improvement in the bone scan appearances following successful therapy has been termed the flare response and is now a well recognized phenomenon in breast and prostate cancer. Bone scanning in advanced disease should, therefore, be interpreted with caution when performed during treatment and is of most value in screening for bone metastases at relapse, both to identify sites for radiological assessment and to bring to attention sites of disease at high risk of pathological fracture for which prophylactic surgery may be indicated.

Tumour markers have so far had little application to the problem of bone metastases. For breast cancer, unlike germ cell tumours, there is no highly specific biological marker either for diagnosis or monitoring the disease. Some breast cancers produce antigens detectable by radioimmunoassay including carcinoembryonic antigen and CA15-3. Serial measurements are reported to correlate with response in measurable disease, but this has so far not provided useful additional information to aid clinical management nor are these markers specific for breast cancer.

Prostate specific antigen (PSA) is a marker of prostatic pathology and circulating levels may be elevated in any prostatic disease including benign hypertrophy, prostatitis, and cancer. The highest tissue production occurs in prostate cancer. Measurement may enable early diagnosis, assist in staging, and be used in follow-up.

PSA levels usually decline after androgen deprivation for advanced disease and provide a guide to response; a rise in PSA levels often precedes other clinical evidence of progression by several months.

In metastatic bone disease, stimulation of osteoclastic bone resorption by tumour-derived cytokines and disruption of the normal coupling between osteoblast and osteoclast function lead to changes in a variety of bone-specific biochemical parameters, particularly the components of Type 1 collagen (Chapter 9). With successful anti-tumour treatment, a reduction in bone resorption markers can be observed within a few weeks of its commencement providing a much earlier indication of response to treatment than is possible with radiographic techniques. The importance of these biochemical tests relates to the palliative objective of treating bone metastases. Early reliable information on either response or disease progression is likely to be helpful in deciding whether or not treatment, particularly if toxic, should be pursued.

Relief of symptoms is the principal aim of palliative therapy and is the most important index of response to treatment from a patient's point of view. However, the assessment of pain is difficult to quantify and is often omitted from clinical trials. Subjective response to treatment for bone disease needs information on pain intensity, analgesic consumption, and mobility to be recorded. A useful questionnaire which incorporates these factors is illustrated in Table 10.1.

CONCLUSION

For most patients the systemic treatment for metastatic bone disease is palliative, rather than curative. The selection of treatment depends upon the tumour type. Endocrine treatment is important for the two principal causes of bone metastases, breast and prostatic cancer, its rationale being to reduce respectively the oestrogenic or androgenic stimulus to tumour growth. Chemotherapy can also provide valuable palliation in breast cancer for hormone-resistant

Table 10.1 Scoring system for the symptomatic assessment of patients with pain from bone metastases

Parameter	Description	Score
Pain	None	0
	Mild	1
	Moderate	2
	Severe	3
	Very severe	4
	Intolerable	5
Analgesic use	None	0
	Simple analgesic or NSAID[a]	1
	Simple analgesic + NSAID[a]	2
	Moderate analgesic (e.g. dihydrocodeine)	3
	Opiates ($\leq$ 40 mg morphine daily)	4
	Opiates ($>$ 40 mg morphine daily)	5
Mobility	Normal	0
	Vigorous exercise/activity impaired	1
	Climbing stairs/walking/bending impaired	2
	Difficulty with dressing/washing	3
	Difficulty with all activities	4
	Totally dependent and bed-bound	5
Performance status	Normal	0
	Light work possible	1
	Up and about $>$ 50% of the day	2
	Confined to bed $>$ 50% of the day	3
	Completely bed-bound	4
Symptom score expressed as percentage of maximum total		19 (100%)

[a]Nonsteroidal anti-inflammatory drug.
Source: Rubens and Fogelman.[9]

disease, but its use in prostatic cancer is controversial. Rarely, the skeleton may be involved by lymphoma or germ cell tumours and for these diseases a curative approach with chemotherapy is realistic. For other carcinomas, particularly those of the kidney, thyroid, and lung, leading to bone metastases, there is little place for systemic anti-tumour treatment, other palliative approaches being more appropriate. The assessment of metastatic bone disease can be difficult and has relied largely on information from imaging techniques. Biochemical monitoring is showing considerable promise and is likely to become important in the future.

REFERENCES

1. Rubens RD. Routine management of disseminated disease (including anti-osteoclastic therapy). In Bonadonna G, Hortobagyi GN, Gianni AM (eds) *Textbook of Breast Cancer: A Clinical Guide to Therapy* (London: Martin Dunitz, 1997): 169–80.
2. Miller WR. Aromatase inhibitors and breast cancer. *Cancer Treat Rev* (1997) **23**: 171–87.
3. Rubens RD, Tinson CL, Coleman RE et al. Prednisolone improves the response to primary endocrine treatment for advanced breast cancer. *Br J Cancer* (1988) **58**: 626–30.
4. Gregory WM, Smith P, Richards MA, Twelves CJ, Knight RK, Rubens RD. Chemotherapy of advanced breast cancer: outcome and prognostic factors. *Br J Cancer* (1993) **68**: 988–95.
5. Dowling AJ, Tannock IF. Systemic treatment for prostate cancer. *Cancer Treat Rev* (1999) **24**: 283–301.
6. Tannock IF, Osaba D, Stockler MR et al. Chemotherapy with mitozantrone plus prednisone or prednisone alone for symptomatic hormone resistant prostate cancer: a Canadian randomised trial with palliative end-points. *J Clin Oncol* (1996) **14**: 1756–64.
7. Hayward JL, Rubens RD, Carbone PP, Heuson J-C, Kumaoka S, Segaloff A. Assessment of response to therapy in advanced breast cancer. *Br J Cancer* (1977) **35**: 292–8.
8. Coleman RE, Mashiter G, Whitaker KB, Moss DW, Rubens RD, Fogelman I. Bone scan flare predicts successful therapy for bone metastases. *J Nucl Med* (1988) **29**: 1354–9.
9. Rubens RD, Fogelman I (eds). *Bone Metastases: Diagnosis and Treatment* (: Springer-Verlag, 1991): 114.

11

Bone metastases – radiotherapy

Philip J Hoskin

Introduction • Radiotherapy for localized bone pain • Radiotherapy for scattered bone pain • Radiotherapy for complications of bone metastasis • Radiotherapy for neurological complications of bone metastasis • Conclusion

INTRODUCTION

Radiotherapy has a major role in the management of bone metastases. The delivery of ionizing radiation to a bone containing metastatic tumour can be achieved using either radiation from an external X-ray or gamma-ray beam or injected radioisotopes which localize to bone. This latter aspect will be discussed in the next chapter. Radiation beams are classified according to their energy and this is shown in Table 11.1 together with the relevance of each beam type to the treatment of bone metastases. In practice in a modern radiotherapy department most bone metastases will be treated by high-energy X-ray beams from a linear accelerator with an energy of 4–6 million volts.

The process of delivering radiotherapy to an area including a bone metastasis involves a number of steps as follows:

- *Positioning* of the patient in a comfortable yet stable position so that the site can be reliably immobilized and the position reproduced if a course of several treatments is to be delivered. Particular attention to this aspect of treatment is important where the patient may have significant pain, and appropriate analgesia prior to treatment is also a vital consideration.

Table 11.1 Radiation beams in the treatment of bone metastases

Type	Energy	Use for bone metastases
Superficial X-rays	50–150 kV	none
Orthovoltage X-rays	250–500 kV	superficial bones, e.g. ribs, scapula, sacrum
Cobalt gamma rays	2.5 MV	spine, skull, pelvis, long bones
Megavoltage X-rays	4–6 MV	spine, skull, pelvis, long bones
Electron beams	4–20 MeV	superficial bones, e.g. ribs, scapula, sacrum

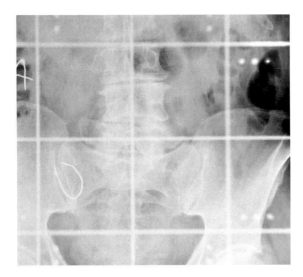

Fig. 11.1 X-ray showing field definition using simulator crosswires to treat spinal and sacral bone metastases

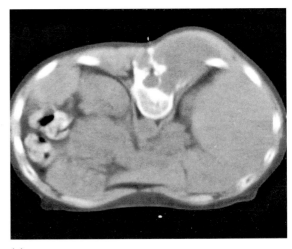

(a)

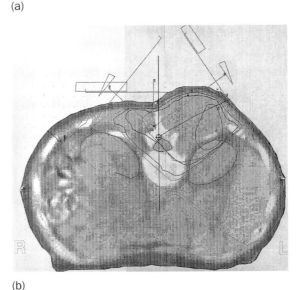

(b)

Fig. 11.2 CT scan to show spinal metastasis with large paraspinal mass (a) and subsequent radiotherapy plan to show treatment of tumour area using two oblique X-ray beams with an even dose distribution (b)

- *Localization* of the bone metastasis to be treated is required and usually achieved by the use of diagnostic X-ray beams using a treatment simulator. X-ray films taken on a treatment simulator showing localization of a beam to treat bone metastases in the spine and pelvis are shown in Fig. 11.1. For superficial bones, however, such as the spine and ribs, simple palpation of tender bones may be sufficient where previous radiology has been used to demonstrate the presence of bone metastasis.
- *Beam arrangement* can then be defined according to the site to be treated. For superficial bones such as the ribs and spine a single direct field will be adequate; for deeper bones such as the long bones and pelvis then opposed beams from front and back will give the best even distribution of radiation dose across the bone. More complex planning using more than two beams is rarely required for bone metastases receiving palliative doses of radiation. Occasionally, however, a localized bone metastasis may be in a site which has already received high-dose irradiation to surrounding tissues or be extending into surrounding soft tissues, when more accurate planning to avoid critical normal structures and the delivery of an even dose of radiation may be required. An example is

shown in Fig. 11.2. In general, however, for palliative treatment a simple pragmatic technique using one or two beams will be chosen.
- *Radiation delivery* follows completion of the above steps using a linear accelerator or if appropriate an orthovoltage X-ray machine. The patient may be prescribed a single dose of radiation or a course of treatment delivering smaller doses on a daily basis over 5–10 treatments encompassing 1–2 weeks. The relative merits of such approaches will be discussed below.

The first description of radiation therapy for bone metastases is found soon after the original discovery of X-rays by Roentgen in 1896 by Freund in 1907, who treated painful metastases in the pelvis from carcinoma of the breast with Roentgen therapy.[1] One of the largest early series was reported from the Mayo Clinic in which 32 patients were treated for the relief of pain from bone metastasis due to breast cancer, of which 30 patients acquired relief of pain.[1] It is also interesting to note that this is probably the only published data which record placebo radiotherapy treatment 'largely for its psychic effect' given to eight patients, though the results of treatment in this group are not commented upon further. This series looked for an association between X-ray energy and dose, and heralding more recent controversy found no constant association between dose of Roentgen rays and degree of pain relief and indeed noted that 'paradoxically, great relief resulted occasionally from low doses of Roentgen rays'.

Subsequently most major radiotherapy centres have published results of their treatment for metastatic bone pain and all uniformly demonstrate the efficacy of this treatment in achieving pain relief. Many of these series can be criticized in their methods of pain measurement, often representing only a retrospective review of clinical case records, but there is striking consistency across the different publications.[2,3]

Currently external beam radiotherapy is widely regarded as the treatment of choice for localized bone pain and is also indicated for some of the more common complications of metastatic bone disease including pathological fracture and neurological complications such as spinal cord compression, peripheral nerve compression, and cranial nerve involvement. It also has a role in the treatment of more scattered symptoms from multiple sites of bone pain. In the future this may be a less common indication as the newer radioisotopes and bisphosphonate drugs will provide alternative treatment options.

RADIOTHERAPY FOR LOCALIZED BONE PAIN

Despite the fact that the vast majority of bone metastases arise from blood-borne dissemination with multiple sites of skeletal involvement, commonly patients present with pain localized to a particular anatomical region. In this setting treatment with local external beam radiotherapy to the painful sites is highly successful. Radiological confirmation should always be obtained and accurate anatomical definition of the site of origin of the pain is essential to enable precise radiation delivery. Using this information an external beam treatment can be planned and delivered to the appropriate site.

The major area of controversy in this treatment relates to the required dose for best effect. Patients presenting with metastatic bone pain are by definition incurable and the principles of palliation demand that treatment should be kept as simple as possible and require as little disturbance to the patient's lifestyle as possible, both in terms of commitment to hospital visits and induced side-effects from the treatment. Clearly the lowest dose and least number of treatments (fractions) compatible with efficacy should be recommended in this setting. There is a large and ever-increasing body of literature which now supports the fact that single doses of radiation delivering 6–10 Gy are highly effective with a response rate in terms of pain relief seen in 70–80% of patients.[4] In general, randomized controlled trials with prospective pain assessments using validated pain scores have failed to show any significant advantage for more

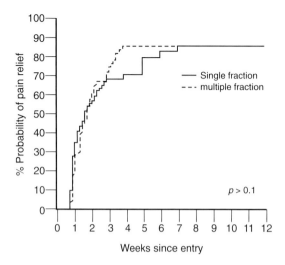

Fig. 11.3 Onset of pain relief after external beam radiotherapy for localized bone pain in a trial comparing a single dose of radiation with 10 doses. (Reproduced from ref. 6, with permission.)

prolonged higher-dose radiation schedules. Only one study[5] performed over 15 years ago randomizing over 1000 patients into five different fraction schedules has reported results supporting more protracted treatment and these results have now been counterbalanced by several more recent prospective randomized trials supporting the use of single doses.[6–10]

The rate of onset of pain relief after external beam radiotherapy is not immediate and as shown in Fig. 11.3 a continued likelihood of response occurs for up to 4 weeks after initial treatment with very few patients experiencing analgesia within the first 24–48 hours but 50% having some pain relief within 2 weeks.

A recent review of published prospective randomized trials conforming to rigorous pain assessment methodology has largely confirmed the view that there is no advantage for high-dose radiotherapy in this setting.[11] Its results, reported in terms of the number needed to treat (NNT) to achieve the therapeutic endpoint of pain relief, estimated that for every four patients treated with external beam radiotherapy one could be expected to achieve complete pain relief.

One trial has sought to define the minimum effective dose of radiotherapy to achieve pain relief and found that a single dose of 4 Gy was statistically less effective than a single dose of 8 Gy although even in the lower dose arm approximately two thirds of patients had some pain relief from treatment.[7]

The duration of pain relief after treatment is variable. Most prospective studies have only looked with systematic pain assessments out to 3 months and it would seem that around 50% of patients maintain their response for this duration. This needs to be put into the context of a population of patients with a median survival of only 6–8 months. A recently published randomized trial[9] comparing a single dose of 10 Gy with 10 treatments delivering a total of 30 Gy found no difference in outcome with a mean duration of benefit of 22.5 weeks in the single treatment and 24.9 weeks in the fractionated group. Preliminary analysis of a recently completed trial again comparing a single dose, on this occasion 8 Gy with 20 Gy in 5 fractions, has performed systematic evaluations out to 1 year from treatment and again shows no effect between the high and low-dose treatment.[12]

Whilst the majority of patients in the published data have primary tumours of breast, prostate, or lung most series also include a number of other histologies. In general breast and prostate patients have a longer survival and may also have hormonal manipulation, but it has yet to be demonstrated that there is any consistent influence of primary histology upon the likelihood of pain relief after local radiotherapy for bone pain. This is important and contrasts with perceptions for radical treatment when certain histological types, for example melanoma, prostate, and kidney, are considered relatively radioresistant with supporting evidence from radiobiological experiments. In the palliative setting patients should not be denied active treatment for metastatic bone pain on the basis of primary histology. Similarly there is no evidence to suggest that osteosclerotic metastasis is more or less radiosensitive than osteolytic metastasis although in the latter case clearly the risk of pathological fracture is an important consideration in management. The absence of a differential effect in different histological or morphological types of bone metastasis, together with failure to demonstrate a dose–response relationship, has been used as a strong argument to support the notion that tumour cell kill may not be important in achieving pain relief after local radiotherapy to a bone. Further observation which supports this is the often rapid relief seen after irradiation to a bone, many patients having pain relief within 24 hours of hemibody radiotherapy, for example. Alternative mechanisms that have been proposed include an effect upon the osteoclasts analogous to the impact of bisphosphonates, an effect upon intraosseous pressure, or a direct effect upon pain transmitters such as prostaglandins, kinins, and substance P. It must however be remembered that none of this excludes an effect upon tumour cells and that small doses of only 2 Gy in experimental systems result in a high level of cell loss and indeed doses less than 1 Gy can result in chemical disruption within the cell. It may well be therefore that a balance between tumouricidal effects and modifications of normal tissue responses to the tumour work together in achieving and maintaining pain relief in a bone after irradiation.

RADIOTHERAPY FOR SCATTERED BONE PAIN

Since multiple sites of bone metastasis are the rule then many patients will ultimately present with pain in anatomically diffuse sites often flitting from one site to another during the day. This presents a much more difficult therapeutic dilemma since it is not possible to identify precisely localized anatomical sites for treatment. In this setting systemic radioisotopes or bisphosphonate therapy alongside specific hormonal or chemotherapy have a major role but localized external beam therapy should also be considered. The technique of wide-field irradiation or hemibody radiotherapy is well established. Conventionally this involves delivering radiation through an external beam treatment to the upper or lower half-body, typically above or below the umbilicus, but pragmatically a patient may well receive treatment to a similar volume encompassing sites of painful bone metastasis in the mid-body, for example pelvis, lumbar, and thoracic spine. Because these techniques require much larger X-ray fields to be used the treatment machine, usually a linear accelerator, may need to be used under nonstandard conditions with, in particular, an increased distance from the beam source to the patient which, with beam divergence, allows for a larger field to be covered. Other than this however the treatment remains relatively simple and for the patient will require no more than a single visit to the treatment machine for the exposure to be delivered. Indeed in contrast to localized treatment there is far less controversy regarding dose and duration of treatment. Whilst there are advocates for longer courses of hemibody radiotherapy in an attempt to deliver somewhat higher doses, there is general consensus that a single dose of 6 Gy to a volume which includes the lungs, i.e. an upper half-body, or 8 Gy to a lower half-body in which there is no lung tissue included are standard doses. There are no randomized trials comparing different dose levels for this type of treatment but both retrospective and prospective studies confirm a response rate of around 80% independent of dose.[2,3,13]

The characteristics of response when larger volumes of the body are treated may differ with a more rapid response than after local radiotherapy, many patients reporting pain improvement within 24 hours and for many patients pain relief being maintained until death. This latter parameter however may reflect the fact that this treatment is often delivered to patients with very advanced disease whose mean survival may be only 3–4 months. One study has compared the response rate in myeloma and prostate cancer patients[14] indicative of two extremes of theoretical radiosensitivity and as in the case of localized treatment found no difference in the likelihood of response in terms of pain relief between these two patient groups.

Perhaps inevitably the major drawback of wide-field irradiation is the fact that there is greater associated toxicity due to the larger volume of tissue included. This is most commonly manifest as gastrointestinal upset as a result of irradiating stomach or bowel and bone marrow depression. Falls in blood count are commonly seen within 2–4 weeks of external beam hemibody radiotherapy but return to normal levels within 6–8 weeks and rarely reach clinical significance, although one study[15] comparing hemibody radiotherapy with radioisotope therapy reported a significant requirement for blood transfusion in patients with carcinoma of the prostate amongst whom 48% required a transfusion within 3 months of hemibody radiotherapy, which compared to only 25% of patients receiving radioisotope therapy with strontium. Clinically hazardous falls in other parameters, however, including neutropenia and thrombocytopenia are not usually seen after this form of treatment. The one potentially fatal complication of wide-field radiotherapy is that of radiation pneumonitis seen in fewer than 1% of patients and catastrophic if it does occur. Its development appears to be idiosyncratic in patients having whole lung volumes included.

Prophylactic wide-field radiotherapy

Wide-field radiotherapy has been investigated as a prophylactic treatment. A randomized trial of the Radiation Therapy Oncology Group (RTOG) took patients receiving local treatment for a painful bone metastasis and randomized them to receive hemibody radiotherapy or not.[16] There was no effect on survival but some reduction in subsequent bone morbidity and requirements for further radiotherapy to sites of bone pain. However, the principal influence of the added wide-field irradiation was to delay events rather than prevent further disease; thus while the median time to new disease within the targeted hemibody region was 12.6 months when hemibody treatment was given, compared to 6.3 months where only local treatment was given, the 1-year survival was only 33% and 30%, respectively. In general therefore this approach has not been widely adopted in routine clinical practice although it has long been recognized that sites receiving radiotherapy which incidentally include bones may, when the patient develops disseminated bone metastasis, demonstrate sparing of bones within the previously irradiated field, the commonest example of this being the dorsal spine in patients with breast cancer.

RADIOTHERAPY FOR COMPLICATIONS OF BONE METASTASIS

Pathological fracture

The mainstay of treatment for pathological fracture is that of surgical fixation. There is however also an important role for radiotherapy in those patients for whom surgery is not possible and in the postoperative setting. These indications are outlined in Table 11.2. The use of radiotherapy in the patient with actual or impending pathological fracture can be considered as follows.

Pain relief may be required in a patient who has pathological fracture but who has other advanced disease with a limited life expectancy

Table 11.2 Indications for radiotherapy in pathological fracture

Inoperable sites of fracture
    ribs
    vertebrae (unless unstable)
    pelvis
    scapula
    clavicle

Long bones
    postoperative
    immobile terminal patient
    ? prophylaxis for high-risk lesions (see text)

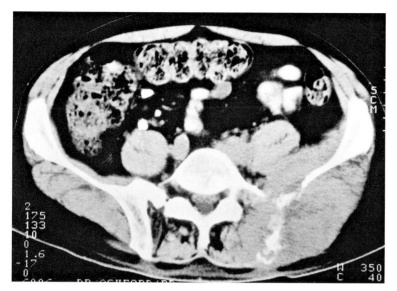

(a)

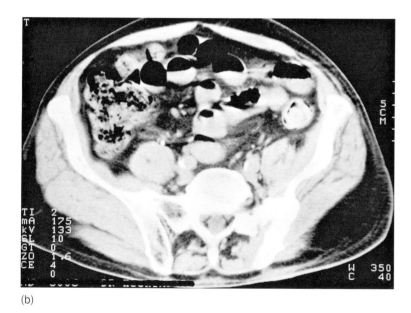

(b)

Fig. 11.4 Large lytic lesion in ilium prior to radiotherapy (a) and 3 months after completion of treatment delivering 30 Gy (b)

which precludes general anaesthesia and surgery. In this setting, particularly where mobility is not a major concern, local radiotherapy is given in doses for pain relief rather than any specific anti-tumour effect. As discussed above, in general this can be achieved by delivering a single dose of 6–10 Gy to the painful fractured bone.

Established pathological fracture in an inoperable bone, for example a rib or pelvic bone, will be best managed by local radiotherapy which will enable fracture healing to proceed. Whilst single doses may be effective in this setting it is more conventional to deliver a fractionated course of treatment over 1–2 weeks delivering 20–30 Gy as a total dose. Fracture healing will then proceed in a similar manner to that following traumatic fracture with ultimate remineralization and remodelling if the underlying malignancy is under control and the patient has a sufficiently long prognosis. X-ray surveillance of such patients shows bone healing 2–3 months after radiotherapy as demonstrated in Fig. 11.4. Pain relief will occur much sooner.

Postoperative radiotherapy is recommended following internal fixation where there remains viable tumour within the bone.[17] This may be omitted in patients who have a relatively short prognosis but for those who are likely to live for more than a few months then there is a possibility of tumour regrowth around the prosthesis with further pain or even bone destruction and fracture in the adjacent area. Local radiotherapy to cover the operative field including the entire prosthesis is recommended, again typically delivering doses of 20–30 Gy in 1–2 weeks.

A more controversial role of radiotherapy proposed by some is for *prophylaxis* of fracture when long bone metastases are identified. On radiological criteria, high-risk lesions for fracture can be identified, notably those with greater than 50% cortical destruction, lesions greater than 2.5 cm diameter with associated pain, or diffuse lytic infiltration of a long bone. These are considered indications for surgical fixation.[18] The role of prophylactic radiotherapy in high-risk lesions has been evaluated in one study[19] in which 85 patients with high-risk lesions received local radiotherapy and from completion of treatment no subsequent episodes of fracture were seen suggesting that this may be an appropriate treatment for those patients who are at risk from an anaesthetic procedure.

RADIOTHERAPY FOR NEUROLOGICAL COMPLICATIONS OF BONE METASTASIS

Spinal canal compression

Vertebral metastases are common and may, either by vertebral collapse or soft tissue extension, impinge on the spinal canal. This can have catastrophic neurological effects with either cord damage or cauda equina compression. The clinical result will be paraplegia or if the cervical spine is involved quadraplegia. Even in advanced cancer with a very limited life expectancy these events have a major impact upon quality of life and all attempts to avoid them should be made. The most important issue in the management of spinal canal compression is early diagnosis, the outcome from treatment invariably relating directly to the performance status of the patient at the time of diagnosis and initiation of treatment. Some 25% of cases of spinal canal compression result directly from spinal bone metastasis, the remainder being associated with extradural metastatic deposits of tumour.[20] Today the diagnosis is made on magnetic resonance imaging.

Radiotherapy has a major role in the management of spinal cord compression. Only in cases where there is demonstrated spinal instability are there significant advantages for surgery when clearly spinal stabilization should be considered with postoperative radiotherapy, as shown in Fig. 11.5. In other cases of spinal canal compression primary radiotherapy is an appropriate treatment with no published evidence to suggest that it is inferior to operative decompression.[21] Where there is no definite histological diagnosis of malignancy then this should be confirmed prior to radiotherapy by needle biopsy. It is important to identify those patients who may be better treated with primary chemotherapy, for example those with lymphoma. Those with primary malignancies from solid tumours should then receive external beam radiotherapy to cover the area of canal compression and typical doses are 20–30 Gy in 1–2 weeks although there is some evidence that single doses of 10–12 Gy are effective also.

The outlook for patients presenting with spinal canal compression is poor. Overall survival is rarely more than a few months although one recent series of patients with prostate cancer[22] and spinal cord compression reports that although the median survival was only 115 days, 25% of patients survived for 2 years, demonstrating that a subgroup of patients presenting with previously undiagnosed disease

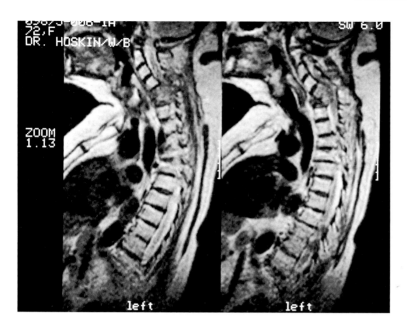

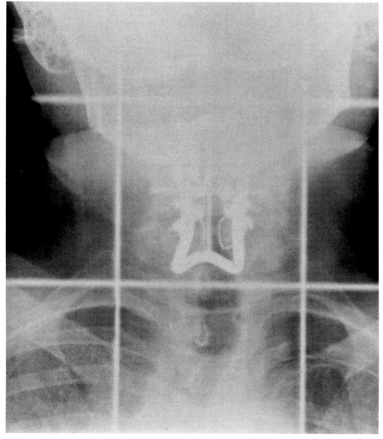

Fig. 11.5 MR scan of cervical spine showing gross vertebral destruction and spinal instability (a) and subsequent radiotherapy planning film following surgical fixation (b)

responsive to hormone treatment may survive for some time after treatment. In this series[22] other predictors of a favourable outcome were single sites of compression compared to multiple levels of involvement and a haemoglobin greater than 12 g/dl. Compression due to bone disease is associated with a worse outcome than where the compression is due to simply soft tissue epidural metastasis.

Patients who are treated primarily with surgery, whether anterior spinal surgery with stabilization or posterior decompression, should receive postoperative radiotherapy. Similar doses to those delivered during primary treatment will be used. A large retrospective review[21] has shown that patients receiving radiotherapy have far better pain control than those having laminectomy alone and another series has suggested that the addition of radiotherapy to laminectomy is superior to laminectomy alone.[23] However, both series are open to criticism, being retrospective analyses with considerable heterogeneity within the treatment subgroups.

Peripheral nerves

In addition to posterior intrusion into the spinal canal, spinal metastases can invade laterally into the root canal resulting in neuropathic pain and other peripheral nerve symptoms. The management of such complications is often difficult, neuropathic pain being notoriously resistant to pharmacological intervention which may include the use of analgesics, anti-convulsants or antidepressants, and nonpharmacological methods such as transcutaneous electrical nerve stimulation (TENS). Many of these patients are referred for and receive local radiotherapy although there are few published data on the results of treatment. Undoubtedly some patients benefit from pain relief and similar doses to those used for other bone metastasis sites are given, either single doses of 8–10 Gy or fractionated courses of 20–30 Gy for 1–2 weeks. Currently a systematic evaluation of radiotherapy for neuropathic bone pain is underway in a prospective randomized trial which may give better information on the precise role of radiotherapy in this setting.

Cranial nerves

The spectrum of bone metastases may include skull infiltration and in particular infiltration of the skull base with compression of cranial nerves as they pass through the tight foramina and canals within the skull. Most commonly it is the 5th, 6th, and 7th cranial nerves which are affected but any may be involved. Again this represents a major morbidity and reduction in quality of life in the final months of life. Two retrospective analyses[24,25] suggest that there is a good response in terms of cranial nerve function to local radiotherapy to the skull base delivering doses of 30 Gy in 10 daily fractions and this should be considered for all patients having symptomatic skull base metastasis.

CONCLUSION

External beam radiotherapy has a long tradition and is well established in the management of bone metastases. Its principal roles are in the relief of localized bone pain and the management of spinal canal compression. It is also of value in selected cases with pathological fracture or impending pathological fracture where surgical fixation is not indicated or clinically desirable and in the less common complications of peripheral and cranial nerve compression. Evidence is strengthening for the role of single-dose treatments for pain and short fractionated treatments for neurological complications using simple beam arrangements. Treatment should be preceded by careful evaluation and accurate localization of the treatment field to ensure maximal benefit with fewest side-effects. Wide-field hemibody radiotherapy still has an important role in the management of more widespread bone pain although greater toxicity is to be expected and alternative treatments where available, such as radioisotope therapy or bisphosphonate therapy, may be preferable.

REFERENCES

1. Leddy ET. Roentgen treatment of metastasis to the vertebrae and bones of the pelvis from carcinoma of the breast. *Am J Roentgen Rad Ther* (1930) **24:** 657–72.
2. Hoskin PJ. Scientific and clinical aspects of radiotherapy in the relief of bone pain. *Cancer Surv* (1988) **7:** 69–86.
3. Hoskin PJ. Palliation of bone metastases. *Eur J Cancer* (1991) **27:** 950–1.
4. Hoskin PJ. Radiotherapy In Body JJ (ed) *Cancer Metastases to Bone* (New York: Marcel Decker, 1998) (in press).
5. Blitzer PH. Reanalysis of the RTOG study of the palliation of symptomatic osseous metastasis. *Cancer* (1985) **55:** 1468–72.
6. Price P, Hoskin PJ, Easton D et al. Prospective randomised trial of single and multifraction radiotherapy schedules in the treatment of painful bony metastases. *Radiother Oncol* (1986) **6:** 247–55.
7. Hoskin PJ, Price P, Easton D et al. A prospective randomised trial of 4Gy or 8Gy single doses in the treatment of metastatic bone pain. *Radiother Oncol* (1992) **23:** 74–8.
8. Cole DJ. A randomized trial of a single treatment versus conventional fractionation in the palliative radiotherapy of painful bone metastases. *Clin Oncol* (1989) **1:** 59–62.
9. Gaze MN, Kelly CG, Kerr GR et al. Pain relief and quality of life following radiotherapy for bone metastases: a randomised trial of two fractionation schedules. *Radiother Oncol* (1997) **45:** 109–16.
10. Nielsen OS, Bentzen SM, Sandberg E, Gadeberg CC, Timothy A. Randomized trial of single dose versus fractionated palliative radiotherapy of bone metastases. *Radiother Oncol* (1998) **47:** 233–40.
11. McQuay HJ, Carroll D, Moore RA. Radiotherapy for painful bone metastases: a systematic review. *Clin Oncol* (1997) **9:** 150–4.
12. Yarnold JR. Bone pain trial: a prospective randomised trial comparing a single dose of 8 Gy and a multifraction radiotherapy schedule in the treatment of metastatic bone pain. *Br J Cancer* (1998) **78 (Suppl 2):** 6.
13. Salazar OM, Rubin P, Hendricksen F et al. Single-dose half body irradiation for palliation of multiple bone metastases from solid tumours. *Cancer* (1986) **58:** 29–36.
14. Hoskin PJ, Ford HT, Harmer CL. Hemibody irradiation (HBI) for metastatic bone pain in two histological distinct groups of patients. *Clin Radiol* (1989) **1:** 67–9.
15. Dearnaley DP, Bayley RJ, A'Hern RP et al. Palliation of bone metastases in prostate cancer. Hemibody irradiation or strontium-89. *Clin Oncol* (1992) **4:** 101–7.
16. Poulter CA, Cosmatos D, Rubin P et al. A report of RTOG 8206: a Phase III study of whether the addition of single dose hemibody irradiation to standard fractionated local field irradiation is more effective than local field irradiation alone in the treatment of symptomatic osseous metastases. *Int J Radiat Oncol Biol Phys* (1992) **23:** 207–14.
17. Hardman PDJ, Robb JE, Kerr GR, Rodger A, MacFarlane A. The value of internal fixation and radiotherapy in the management of upper and lower limb bone metastases. *Clin Oncol* (1992) **4:** 244–8.
18. Hipp JA, Springfield DS, Hayes WC. Predicting pathologic fracture risk in the management of metastatic bone defects. *Clin Orthop* (1995) **312:** 120–35.
19. Cheng DS, Seitz, Eyre HJ. Nonoperative management of femoral, humeral and acetabular metastases in patients with breast carcinoma. *Cancer* (1980) **45:** 1533–7.
20. Pigott KH, Baddeley H, Maher EJ. Pattern of disease in spinal cord compression on MRI scan and implications for treatment. *Clin Oncol* (1994) **6:** 7–10.
21. Findlay CFG. Adverse effects of the management of spinal cord compression. *J Neurol Neurosurg Psychiatry* (1984) **47:** 139–44.
22. Huddart RA, Balakrishnan R, Law M et al. Spinal cord compression in prostate cancer: treatment outcome and prognostic factors. *Radiother Oncol* (1997) **44:** 229–36.
23. Young RF, Post E, King GA. Treatment of spinal epidural metastases. Randomised prospective comparison of laminectomy and radiotherapy. *J Neurosurg* (1980) **53:** 741–8.
24. Vikram B, Chu F. Radiation therapy for metastases to the base of the skull. *Radiology* (1979) **130:** 465–8.
25. Hall SM, Buzdar AV, Blumenschein GR. Cranial nerve palsies in metastatic breast cancer due to osseous metastasis without intracranial involvement. *Cancer* (1983) **52:** 180–4.

12

Clinical use of radioisotopes for bone metastases

Stephen J Houston

Introduction • Site-directed radiotherapy • Problems with studies of radioisotopes in treatment of skeletal metastases • Specific radioisotopes • Side-effects • Cost benefits of radioisotopes • Future directions • Conclusion

INTRODUCTION

Bone metastases account for much cancer-related morbidity and pose a major problem for clinicians involved in treating malignant disease. They are the most common cause of cancer pain.[1] Affected patients may develop pathological fractures, spinal cord compression from epidural extension of the tumour, hypercalcaemia, or bone marrow failure. The costs of treating bone metastases and associated complications make a major demand on health-care resources.[2]

The clinical importance of bone metastases becomes obvious when one considers that at any one time there are 15 000–20 000 women in the UK alive with bone metastases from breast cancer, while 85% of men with advanced prostate cancer and 65% of patients with lung cancer will develop skeletal metastases.[3]

Most morbidity from bone metastases is seen in breast and prostate cancer because of the long clinical course of these diseases. At Guy's Hospital, London, a study of patients with bone metastases from breast cancer patients found a median survival of 24 months for those whose disease was confined to the skeleton, while 20% remained alive at 5 years.[4] Prostate cancer which involves the skeleton is associated with a median survival of 17 months.[5] However, in carcinoma of the lung, bone metastases carries a poor prognosis with median survival of only 3.5 months after diagnosis,[6] and so morbidity is rarely a long-term health-care problem.

Treatment of bone metastases is primarily palliative. The aims of treatment are to relieve pain, prevent development of pathologic fractures, improve mobility and function, and, if possible, prolong survival. A knowledge of current specific anti-cancer and symptomatic pharmacological therapies along with an understanding of specific clinical syndromes and associated morbidities is essential. A multidisciplinary approach is usually required to get the best results, involving medical oncologists, radiotherapists, surgeons, nurses, specialists in pain control, and teams who can support the patient in the community in collaboration with the primary health-care team who can act as a liaison between the patient and the hospital.

Aside from appropriate systemic anti-cancer therapy, several treatment options are available to palliate symptomatic disease, each with specific advantages and drawbacks. These

Table 12.1 Radionuclides suitable for palliative therapy

Radionuclide	Half-life (days)	E_{MAX} (MEV)	Max gamma energy (KEV)	Ligand
Iodine-131	8.1	0.60	364	—
Phosphorus-32	24.5	0.25	—	phosphate orthophosphate
Tin-117m	13.6	0.16	158.6	DTPA
Yttrium-90	2.7	2.27	—	
Samarium-153	1.9	0.81	103	EDTMP
Strontium-69	52.0	1.49	—	chloride
Rhenium-186	3.7	1.07	137	HEDP

DTPA = diethylenetriaminepenta acetic acid; HEDP = hydroxyethylenediphosphonic acid; EDTMP = ethylenediaminetetramethylenephosphonic acid.

options include the use of bone-seeking radioisotopes. This chapter describes the experience with, and future potential of, radionuclide therapy.

SITE-DIRECTED RADIOTHERAPY

Treatment using tracer molecules to target radiation to tumour is well established. Phosphorus-32 (^{32}P) was used more than 40 years ago to treat bone metastases in breast cancer[7] while radioiodine (^{131}I) has an accepted place in the management of follicular thyroid carcinoma.[8]

Targeted radiotherapy offers several potential advantages over external beam radiotherapy. As treatment is site selective with minimal damage to surrounding healthy cells, toxicity should be minimal, while theoretically there is no limit to the absorbed dose that can be delivered to tumour nor to the number of individual treatments that can be administered. The treatment has minimal penetration to the central nervous system which could be a disadvantage in patients with vertebral metastases and coexisting epidural spinal cord compression. Meticulous attention needs to be paid to excluding incipient spinal cord compression in patients being considered for radionuclide treatment. Another attractive feature of radioisotope treatment is the possibility of outpatient treatment. This could be particularly cost effective although presently the price of radiopharmaceuticals is very high.

These agents are best reserved for patients with multifocal pain where the effectiveness of external beam radiotherapy is limited. It is important to remember that response to targeted radiotherapy is dependent upon the osteoblastic activity induced in the adjacent bone to disease which is why the pain of multiple myeloma does not respond to targeted radiotherapy and the bisphosphonates may offer a better treatment option in this condition.

There are several radioisotopes with differing properties now under investigation (Table 12.1) which have been used as therapy for painful bone metastases. They are all beta emitting and so their ionizing radiation has a short range thereby avoiding damage to nontarget tissue. The beta particles of the different radionuclides have different maximum energy and ranges of penetration while some have an additional gamma emission that may be used for imaging. Most work has been undertaken in prostate and breast cancer metastatic to bone using phosphorus-32, strontium-89, samarium-153, and rhenium-186. Certain characteristics are shared. First they are incorporated into bone by virtue of their elemental nature or through the chemical properties of an attached ligand. Next, the therapeutic radiation emitted is that of low-energy electrons (beta emissions) as opposed to gamma radiation which is normally used in nuclear medicine imaging. Finally, they are preferentially incorporated into bony lesions undergoing repair compared to normal bone.

It is not fully understood how these agents work to relieve pain because often pain relief can be observed within 48–72 hours of administration. This is too short a time to achieve any tumour shrinkage and suggests other mechanisms such as reductions in cytokines or alteration in the function of osteoclasts and osteoblasts.

Considerable clinical experience in the use of these agents to treat painful bone metastases has accumulated, particularly in patients with hormone refractory prostate cancer and to a lesser extent in those patients with breast cancer metastatic to bone. There is a lack of suitable systemic options available when prostate cancer is truly hormone refractory and the predominant disease site is skeletal, with visceral metastases only appearing late in the course of the disease, which makes radionuclide therapy for this group of patients an attractive proposition, particularly when there is pain at multiple sites of disease.

PROBLEMS WITH STUDIES OF RADIOISOTOPES IN TREATMENT OF SKELETAL METASTASES

Most of the studies involving the use of radioisotopes to treat bone metastases have shown the usefulness of these agents to control pain. However, there are several weaknesses both in terms of trial design and analysis of results, making comparison between agents and with other treatment options difficult.

Most of the studies only have small numbers of patients with different criteria used for judging symptomatic relief. Some studies note the proportion of patients obtaining 'some' pain relief without quantifying the degree of pain relief while others use complex unvalidated scoring systems that look at analgesic intake, mobility, general condition, and pain analysis. This lack of consistency between different studies makes it difficult truly to compare different rates of response between reports and different radioisotopes.

Further problems of interpretation are encountered because of the large number of patients ineligible for response assessment. Many of these patients died early, were lost to follow-up, or had concomitant therapy within the assessment period.

SPECIFIC RADIOISOTOPES

Phosphorus-32

Phosphorus-32 (^{32}P) was the first radionuclide to be used for the systemic treatment of pain arising from bone metastases.[7] Phosphorus localize in bone marrow, trabecular, and cortical bone, influenced by the chemical form used.[9] Following intravenous administration in humans, 5–10% of ^{32}P orthophosphate is excreted in the urine in the first 24 hours and 20–30% within a week,[10] but less than 2% appears in the faeces.[11] The metastases to normal bone uptake ratio is only in the order of 2:1, which prompted studies to try to increase bone uptake.[9]

Hertz[12] demonstrated that androgen pretreatment with testosterone had the effect of stimulating bone turnover in the vicinity of metastatic deposits which in turn stimulated an increase in phosphate uptake in new bone. Androgen priming has obvious disadvantages in the context of potentially hormone-sensitive tumours. Soft tissue tumour growth may be stimulated and spinal cord compression is a recognized complication.[13]

Pretreatment with parathyroid hormone (PTH) has also been shown to increase uptake of ^{32}P by mobilizing calcium and then making use of the rebound phase of increased osteoblastic activity following PTH withdrawal.[14] By using these methods phosphorus uptake was

Table 12.2 Palliative responses in patients with metastatic bone pain

Radionuclide	Response rate (%)	Average onset	Average duration	Haematologic toxicity
^{89}Sr	50–90	2–4 weeks	3–6 months	moderate and reversible
^{186}Re-HEDP	50–80	< 2 weeks	4–8 weeks	mild and reversible
^{153}Sm-EDTMP	50–80	< 2 weeks	4–16 weeks	mild and reversible

increased in normal bone by a factor of 2–3 and in tumour by a factor of 15–20.

Significant data have now accumulated using ^{32}P with collated results demonstrating a response in terms of subjective reduction of pain in 60–70% of those treated.[15]

The major clinical problem found with ^{32}P, resulting in the reduction of its clinical use, was the associated high incidence of myelosuppression, particularly in patients who had previously been treated with cytotoxic chemotherapy or who already had a high degree of myelosuppression secondary to their metastatic burden.[16]

Since then investigators have identified physical characteristics important for clinically useful radiopharmaceuticals (physical half-life, emission energy, and affinity for bone tissue[17]). Ideally, the half-life should be long enough to deliver therapeutic doses of radiation with a reasonable dosing schedule, but short enough to limit myelotoxicity. To minimize toxicity further, the β particle energy should be less than 1.5 MeV. The range of a β particle of 1.5 MeV energy is about 3 mm in bone. The range of 3 mm will limit excessive irradiation of nearby bone marrow. The radionuclide should localize to bone with minimal marrow uptake. At present there is no completely satisfactory radiopharmaceutical but strontium-89, samarium-153, and rhenium-186 appear to have the most favourable characteristics and have been the most studied (Table 12.2).

Strontium-89

Strontium-89 (^{89}Sr) is approved for treatment of metastatic bone pain in the USA, Canada, and Europe. Clinical experience dates from 1942 when Pecher[18] treated one patient with prostate cancer to bone with ^{89}Sr but his death in the war meant interest waned until the 1970s when Schmidt and Firusian[19] reported on the successful use of ^{89}Sr in four patients with prostate cancer and painful bone metastases. Since that time ^{89}Sr has been extensively investigated and has been shown to be both effective and tolerable for the treatment of the bone pain of skeletal metastases (Table 12.3).

^{89}Sr is a pure β emitter with a long physical half-life of 50.5 days. It is chemically similar to calcium and when taken up into bone it is incorporated into the mineral structure. The β particle has a maximum energy of 1.46 MeV giving a range of 3–8 mm in bone. Following intravenous injection approximately 50% of the ^{89}Sr localizes in bone.[20] Strontium washes out from normal bone with a half-life of 14 days but Blake et al.[21] have demonstrated that ^{89}Sr, once localized in the osteoblastic metastatic deposit, turns over less rapidly than in adjacent normal bone. ^{89}Sr remains deposited at the metastatic site for at least 100 days where most of the radiation effect is achieved. The absorbed doses to tumour have been calculated[22] giving a therapeutic ratio for metastases to red marrow of 10:1.[21]

Robinson et al.[23] carried out the first systematic investigation. Some 137 patients with metastatic cancer (prostate, $n = 100$; breast, $n = 28$; others, $n = 9$) received ^{89}Sr at doses between 1.1 and 1.5 MBq/kg. Response rates were evaluated over a period of 3 months by assessing a Karnofsky rating, need for pain medication, sleep patterns, mobility, ability to work, and

Table 12.3 Randomized controlled trials of strontium-89

Authors	Patient population	Control treatment	Experimental treatment	Primary palliative outcome	Palliative findings	Survival findings	Comments
Lewington et al., 1991[25]	Endocrine refractory patients	Placebo (n = 17)	150 MBq wk 1 150/MBq wk 6 (if needed) (n = 15)	Pain relief (measured by composite response score) at 5 weeks	Significantly higher proportion of ^{89}Sr patients experienced improvement in score	Not addressed	6 of 32 patients unevaluable Unvalidated pain relief scale
Buchali et al., 1988[26]	Endocrine-sensitive and refractory patients	Placebo (n = 24)	75 MBq each month for 3 months (n = 25)	Pain relief (binary) 1–3 years after treatment	No significant difference in proportion of patients with pain relief	Significantly improved 2-year survival in patients receiving ^{89}Sr	10 patients were excluded from the survival analysis
Quilty et al., 1994[30] Statum I	Endocrine refractory patients deemed suitable for local XRT	Involved field XRT (n = 72)	200 MBq (n = 76)	Pain relief 8–12 weeks after treatment	No significant difference in proportion of patients with relief at index sites Significantly more patients free of new pain after ^{89}Sr group Significantly fewer patients in ^{89}Sr required XRT	No difference in median survival	37 of 148 patients were unevaluable Unvalidated palliative assessment method
Quilty et al., 1994[30] Stratum II	Endocrine refractory patients deemed suitable for hemibody XRT	Hemibody XRT 6 Gy upper 8 Gy lower (n = 80)	200 MBq (n = 77)	As above	No significant difference in proportion of patients with relief at index sites Significantly more patients free of new pain sites after ^{89}Sr	As above	51 of 157 patients were unevaluable Unvalidated palliative assessment method
Porter et al., 1993[29]	Endocrine refractory patients deemed suitable for local XRT (n = 126)	Involved field XRT and placebo injection	Involved field XRT and 400 MBq injection	Pain from new sites over 6 months following treatment	Significantly fewer new pain sites/patient in ^{89}Sr group No significant differences in relief of pain at index sites Significant differences in favour of ^{89}Sr in need for analgesics, time to further XRT, and quality of life	No significant difference in median survival	RTOG pain assessment scale Unvalidated quality-of-life scale 2 of 126 patients were unevaluable

From Cancer Care Ontario Practice Guideline Initiative CPG 3–6 medication diaries. Symptom improvement was generally noted within 3 weeks of therapy with some symptom improvement reported by 80% of patients with 11% becoming pain free. When analysed by primary tumour site overall response rates of 80% and 89% and completely pain-free response rates of 10% and 18% were reported among prostate and breast cancer patients, respectively. Minimal haematologic effects were observed.

In 1991 the results of an open-label study were published.[24] Patients with metastatic prostate cancer and painful bone metastases in whom conventional treatment had failed received a single injection of 1.5 Mbq/kg or more. An overall response rate of 75% was achieved, as well as a complete response rate of 22% among the 83 patients assessed 3 months following treatment. Symptom improvement was reported to occur within 6 weeks of ^{89}Sr with an average duration of 6 months. Myelotoxicity was reported as mild and transient.

It is important to ensure that this apparent success of treatment with ^{89}Sr cannot be attributed to a placebo response. A double-blind study was carried out to compare the palliative effects of ^{89}Sr with placebo.[25] Some 26 patients with refractory metastatic prostate cancer were assessed after 5–6 weeks. Assessment was carried out using a graded five-point score ranging from 0 = no pain (at best) to 4 = most severe (at worst). The pain evaluation was completed at the same time each day. These scales along with the various performance scales were as for the open-label studies. A significantly higher clinical response rate was noted in the ^{89}Sr group compared with placebo at the first assessment ($p < 0.01$) and at all assessments ($p < 0.03$). Complete symptom relief was reported by 33% of patients whereas none showed a dramatic response after injection of placebo.

Buchali and colleagues[26] reported a double-blind comparison of ^{89}Sr with placebo in 49 patients. Treatment allocation was blinded for at least 1 year after therapy. Palliation was rated by patients' subjective reports for 41 who required analgesic therapy. Seven of 19 patients (37%) receiving ^{89}Sr reported relief of pain 1–3 years after therapy compared with 11 of 22 patients (50%) receiving placebo. This difference was not statistically significant. When treatment groups were combined and examined across strata, relief of pain was reported in a significantly higher proportion of patients with a disease history of less than 1 year (14 of 21) compared to a disease history of more than 1 year (4 of 20; $p < 0.01$). Both groups included patients with endocrine-sensitive disease. The interpretation of the palliative benefit of ^{89}Sr in this study is limited by the small number of patients, by the long interval between treatment and evaluation, and by the limited information provided about the subjective assessment scale used. The authors found significant differences in survival at 2 years (46% vs 4%; $p < 0.05$) in favour of the group receiving ^{89}Sr. The authors have, however, excluded 10 patients who died of disease in the first 3 months and included patients with hormone-sensitive disease. These details limit the interpretation of the survival benefit.

The majority of the patients in the studies described had prostate cancer but it also seems equally effective in relieving bone pain arising from metastatic breast cancer. In the biggest study to date, Dusing et al.[27] reported an 81% response in 51 patients with painful skeletal metastases although in a smaller recent study a response rate of 47% was recorded.[28]

In addition to its use as monotherapy, two prospective randomized studies involving a total of 410 patients with prostate cancer who relapsed from, or failed to respond to, hormonal treatment have been performed. Both studies were designed to compare ^{89}Sr with the radiotherapy regimen considered most appropriate for the patient.

The Trans-Canadian Study was a randomized phase-III placebo-controlled trial examining the efficacy of ^{89}Sr as an adjunct to local field radiotherapy in endocrine-resistant metastatic prostate cancer.[29] No significant differences in survival or in relief of pain were documented between the external beam irradiation/placebo group and the external beam irradiation/^{89}Sr group. Progression of pain as measured by sites of new pain or the requirement for radiotherapy showed statistically significant benefits between the two arms in favour of the [89]Sr. Tumour markers were also reduced by more than 50% in the ^{89}Sr group suggesting a tumouricidal effect. Quality-of-life indices indicated the overall superiority of [89]Sr. Myelotoxicity as expected was significantly greater in the ^{89}Sr group and there were three cases with haematological complications at a time of low platelet count.

The second study provided a direct comparison of ^{89}Sr therapy to external beam radiotherapy in 305 enrolled patients with prostate cancer and painful skeletal metastases.[30] Patients were first clinically assessed as eligible for either local ($n = 148$) or hemibody ($n = 157$) radiation. They were then randomized to receive either radiotherapy or 200 MBq of [89]Sr. Both comparisons (^{89}Sr vs local radiation and ^{89}Sr vs hemibody radiation) demonstrated essentially equivalent pain relief 3 months following treatment. However, both comparisons demonstrated that significantly fewer patients developed new painful sites after ^{89}Sr therapy as compared with radiotherapy (^{89}Sr vs local radiation, $p < 0.05$; ^{89}Sr vs hemibody radiation, $p < 0.05$). It was also observed that significantly fewer ^{89}Sr-treated patients needed radiotherapy to new sites of pain (3%) compared with patients in the local radiotherapy group (18%; $p < 0.01$). Toxicity analyses demonstrated a markedly higher incidence of adverse gastrointestinal tract effects among radiotherapy-treated patients (local radiotherapy, 27%; hemibody radiation, 43%) compared with those who received [89]Sr (10%). There was significant haematological toxicity in the ^{89}Sr group with grade III/IV platelet toxicity affecting 6.9% compared with radiotherapy (3.4%) while white cell toxicity was only seen in the ^{89}Sr group. The platelet count fell to 60–70% of baseline after 4–6 weeks, from which there was little recovery over the 3-month follow-up. No clear dose–response relationship exists with a response plateau at doses greater than 1.5 MBq/kg while a response threshold occurs at 1 MBq/kg, below which ^{89}Sr is ineffective.[9]

The major toxicity, as with most site-directed radioisotopes, is myelosuppression, the most sensitive indicator of which is the peripheral platelet count, which typically falls to 75% of pretreatment levels 4–6 weeks after treatment with slow partial recovery over the next 3–6 weeks.[9] Regular haematological monitoring is essential. The clinical response is rarely associated with radiological or scintigraphic evidence of bone healing nor is there often correlation with a decrease in biochemical markers such as alkaline phosphatase, acid phosphatase, or prostate specific antigen, suggesting the mechanism of pain relief may not be directly associated with tumour regression.[25]

Samarium-153

Samarium-153 ([153]Sm) is a beta emitter with a short physical half-life of 46.8 hours. A gamma emission of 103 keV can be used for post-treatment imaging, the quality of which is comparable to technetium-99m methylene diphosphonate scans.[31] In 1984, Goeckeler[32] complexed [153]Sm to several phosphonate ligands, including the tetraphosphonate ethylenediaminetetramethylenephosphonate (EDTMP). [153]Sm-EDTMP was found to have the most favourable *in vivo* biodistribution. The [153]Sm-EDTMP complex was stable and gave a single species (peak on high-performance liquid chromatography).[33] It has recently been approved by the US Food and Drug Administration for the relief of pain in patients with osteoblastic bone metastases.

Following intravenous injection, [153]Sm-EDTMP is cleared rapidly from the vascular compartment with a $t_{1/2}$ of 3.7 ± 0.5 hours. Approximately 50% is excreted unchanged in the urine within 8 hours of administration, the remaining activity concentrating in the skeleton. It actively seeks out bone invaded by tumour by bridging the hydroxyapatite with preferential uptake at sites of increased osteoblastic activity.[34] The lesion to bone uptake ratios have been calculated at 17:1.[33]

Early uncontrolled studies with [153]Sm-EDTMP reported pain relief in 61–90% of patients with bone metastases arising from a variety of primary malignancies.[35,36] Pain relief was experienced by 17 out of 26 patients (65%) treated in a dose-escalating study with a reported duration of pain relief of 3.8 months.[37,38] Myelotoxicity was mild with levels of platelets and leukocytes returning to baseline by 6–8 weeks post-treatment.

The largest open-label study to date involved 114 patients[39] with a variety of tumour types who received single doses of either 0.5 mCi/kg (55 pts) or 1.0 mCi/kg (59 pts). Patients' pain diaries revealed benefit in favour of the 1.0 mCi/kg dose but not the 0.5 mCi/kg dose during the first 4 weeks after administration. Among subsets of patients examined, female patients with breast cancer receiving 1.0 mCi/kg had the most noticeable improvement. Physician assessments judged that 45% of the patients in each dose group were experiencing some degree of pain relief by week 2. This value increased to 51% for the 0.5 mCi/kg group and 66% for the 1.0 mCi/kg group at week 4. Pain relief persisted until week 12 with the lower dose and until at least week 16 with the higher dose. More patients in the higher-dose group (54%) than in the lower-dose group (44%) completed the 16-week study. Predictably, dose-related marrow suppression was the only toxicity associated with ^{153}Sm-EDTMP treatment. Values for platelets and white blood cells reached nadirs at 3 or 4 weeks with both doses and recovered fully by 8 weeks. Long-term follow-up revealed significantly longer survival among breast cancer patients who had received the higher dose than among breast cancer patients who had received the lower dose. The short half-life means repeated treatments can be attempted and worthwhile pain remission has been achieved in patients receiving second doses.[36,39]

The first phase-III double-blind placebo-controlled study was recently reported by Serafini and colleagues[40] in 118 patients with bone metastases secondary to a variety of primary malignancies. Patients were randomized to receive ^{153}Sm-EDTMP 0.5 or 1.0 mCi/kg, or placebo. Treatment was unblinded for patients who did not respond by week 4, with those who had received placebo eligible to receive 1.0 mCi/kg of active drug in an open-label manner. Patient and physician evaluations were used to assess pain relief, as was concurrent change in opioid analgesia. Only the 1.0 mCi/kg dose was effective compared with placebo, with pain relief observed in 62–72% in the first 4 weeks and marked or complete pain relief noted in 31% by week 4. Persistence of pain relief was seen through to week 16 in 43% of patients who received the 1.0 mCi/kg ^{153}Sm-EDTMP. Onset of pain relief was noted between 1 and 2 weeks after treatment. Toxicity as expected was confined to bone marrow suppression, which generally was mild and reversible with no grade-4 toxicity observed. No trials have been reported comparing ^{153}Sm-EDTMP with other radioisotopes or with radiation.

Rhenium-186

Rhenium-186 (^{186}Re) is complexed to hydroxyethylidene diphosphonate (HEDP). Like ^{153}Sm-EDTMP it has a 9% gamma emission making it suitable for post-treatment imaging and has a short half-life of 3.8 days. Once injected it is rapidly cleared from blood and deposits in the skeleton with minimal uptake to other tissues.[17] Approximately 50% of ^{186}Re-HEDP injected is excreted through the kidneys into the urine.[41] Doses ranging from 33 to 35 mCi/kg have been used by Maxon and his group to treat the painful skeletal metastases of prostate, breast, and other cancers such as lung and colon.[42] Response rates were between 75% and 80%, with pain relief usually occurring within the first 2 weeks. The average duration of palliation (5 weeks)[42] appears shorter than that reported for ^{89}Sr or ^{153}Sm.

The therapeutic efficacy of ^{186}Re has been confirmed in a double-blind cross-over comparison with placebo which found a significantly greater decrease in pain with the active agent.[43] Like ^{153}Sm-EDTMP there is the option of giving repeat doses. The main toxicity is temporary myelosuppression beginning 2 weeks after treatment and peaking at 4–6 weeks and usually returning to normal within 8 weeks.

SIDE-EFFECTS

As well as myelotoxicity these radionuclides may also cause a 'flare' response with an increase in pain in 10–15% of patients who must be warned of this possibility and advised to increase their analgesic intake appropriately. The flare response may occur 24–48 hours after injection and often indicates subsequent good analgesic efficacy.

Myelosuppression is largely confined to thrombocytopenia and leukopenia with platelet counts dropping to 20–40% of pretreatment levels with the nadir occurring between 6 and 12 weeks after administration of ^{89}Sr and between 4 and 6 weeks after treatment with the shorter half-life radioisotopes. Levels generally return to normal and it is rare to have grade 3 or 4 toxicity.

COST BENEFITS OF RADIOISOTOPES

Cost effectiveness is an important issue in palliative treatment of patients with cancer. It is recognized that both overall costs and clinical outcome determine which therapies offer the greatest pharmacoeconomic benefits.

McEwan et al.[44] assessed the comparative cost effectiveness of ^{89}Sr therapy in 29 patients recruited into the Trans-Canada Trial (^{89}Sr, n = 14; placebo, n = 15). Estimates were made of the direct costs of treatment, i.e. drugs (analgesics and hormonal agents) and external radiotherapy, and the indirect costs (investigations, outpatient visits, and inpatient days). No difference was noted between the groups in indirect costs but meaningful differences in direct costs were apparent, with the group receiving ^{89}Sr showing a reduction over the whole survival time of CAN$1720/person compared with placebo.

FUTURE DIRECTIONS

Survival

Palliative treatment of bone metastases is not expected to prolong survival. However, Buchali et al.[26] demonstrated a significant prolongation in survival for patients randomly assigned to receive ^{89}Sr compared with those who received a placebo. In terms of pain response, however, there were no significant differences between the two groups and there is debate as to whether all patients entering the study were completely resistant to endocrine treatment.[15]

Collins et al.[45] noted a significantly longer survival in patients with metastatic prostate cancer receiving 2.5 mCi/kg ^{153}Sm-EDTMP than in those who received 1.0 mCi/kg (median of 9 vs 6 months), although this was not a randomized trial, while Resche et al.[39] have demonstrated an increased median survival for patients with metastatic breast cancer who received 1.0 mCi/kg compared with the group receiving 0.5 mCi/kg (median of 10 months vs 22 months).

There have been no survival differences in the two large randomized studies of ^{89}Sr.[29,30] Randomized controlled trials will be required to determine whether systemic radionuclide therapy offers any survival advantage over supportive care.

Enhancement of efficacy

The main toxicity of radioisotopes is their myelosuppressive effects. However, it is clear at least with the shorter-acting radioisotopes that there may be a dose–response effect, not just in terms of response but also possibly of survival (see above). This dose–response effect could be explored by the concomitant use of *growth factors* to ameliorate the dose-limiting marrow toxicity or possibly even peripheral blood stem cell rescue and chemotherapy in aggressive strategies that would have less to do with palliation of painful bone metastases than with tumour control and, ultimately, prolonged survival.

The use of *radiosensitizers* such as cisplatinum could enhance tumour cell kill. One such study[46] infused low-dose cisplatin in conjunction with one injection of ^{89}Sr. They found a pain relief rate no greater than using ^{89}Sr alone but 19% of patients with hormone refractory prostate cancer experienced a decrease in serum prostate specific androgen (PSA) of more than 50%, a result that was better than expected for either the radioisotope or the dose of cisplatin administered. Tu et al.[47] combined repeated injections of ^{89}Sr every

3 months with weekly 24-hour infusions of doxorubicin. A reduction of more than 50% in the PSA was noted in 32% of patients and a 57% pain-free palliation rate. There is a need for controlled randomized studies of combined therapy if the additional cost, increased toxicity, and inconvenience are to be justified in patients with hormone refractory prostate cancer.

The *bisphosphonates* reduce skeletal morbidity by inhibiting the increased osteoclast-mediated bone resorption seen in patients with skeletal metastases. If given in combination with a radionuclide, the bisphosphonates may enhance retention of the radioisotope at the site of metastases as well as having palliative effect in their own right. No trials using only beta emitting radionuclides and bisphosphonates have been published.

The use of radionuclides to date has been confined to those patients with advanced disease. Better results might be expected if these drugs were used at an earlier stage of their disease when disease burden is low. This may best be achieved in the adjuvant setting for 'high risk' patients with either breast or prostate cancer.

CONCLUSION

Systemic radionuclides are a useful adjunct for the treatment of patients with painful skeletal metastases. At the present time the evidence only supports the use of these agents in patients primarily with endocrine refractory prostate cancer who have multiple uncontrolled sites of metastases on both sides of the diaphragm not adequately controlled with analgesic therapy and in whom the use of multiple single fields of external beam irradiation is not possible. The overall importance of systemic radionuclides in the treatment of these patients remains uncertain. The uncertainty is partly the result of methodologic flaws in previous trials and the proliferation of other treatment strategies such as the use of the bisphosphonates and new chemotherapy regimens for patients with hormone refractory prostate cancer. New well designed studies with validated measures of effectiveness are needed to explore new strategies using radioisotopes to treat patients with metastatic bone disease.

REFERENCES

1. Foley KM. Analgesic management of bone pain. In Weiss LS, Gilbert HA (eds) *Bone Metastasis* (Boston, MA: Hall, 1981): 348–68.
2. Richards MA, Braysher S, Gregory WM, Rubens RD. Advanced breast cancer: use of resources and cost implications. *Br J Cancer* (1993) **67**: 856–60.
3. Coleman RE, Purohit OP. Osteoclast inhibition for the treatment of bone metastases. *Cancer Treat Rev* (1993) **19**: 79–103.
4. Coleman RE, Rubens RD. The clinical course of bone metastases from breast cancer. *Br J Cancer* (1987) **55**: 61–6.
5. Clain A. Secondary malignant disease of bone. *Br J Cancer* (1965) **19**: 15–29.
6. Levine AM, Bone metastasis. In Moosa AR, Schimpff SC, Robson MC (eds) *Comprehensive Textbook of Oncology* (2nd edn) (Baltimore, MD: Williams & Wilkins, 1991): 1638–52.
7. Friedel HL, Storaasli JP. The use of radioactive phosphorus in the treatment of carcinoma of the breast with widespread metastases to the bone. *Am J Roentgenol Rad Ther* (1950) **64**: 559–75.
8. Charbord P, L'heritier C, Cukerstein W *et al*. Radio-iodine treatment in differentiated thyroid carcinomas. Treatment of first local recurrences and of bone and lung metastases. *Ann Radiol* (1977) **20**: 783–6.
9. Lewington VJ. Targeted radionuclide therapy for bone metastases. *Eur J Nucl Med* (1993) **20**: 66–74.
10. Reinhard EH, Moore CV, Bierbaum OS *et al*. Radioactive phosphorus as a therapeutic agent. A review of the literature and analysis of the results of treatment of 155 patients with various blood diseases, lymphomas and other malignant neoplastic diseases. *J Lab Clin Med* (1946) **31**: 107–95.
11. Cabrejas ML, Mundez Falcon MA, Mran Margenstein Z *et al*. The intestinal absorption of phosphate in normal human subjects. *Int J Nucl Med Biol* (1979) **6**: 45–8.
12. Hertz S. Modifying effect of steroid hormone

therapy on human neoplastic disease as judged by radioactive phosphorus (p32). *J Clin Invest* (1950) **29**: 821.

13. Burnet NG, Williams G, Howard N. Phosphorus-32 for intractable bony pain from carcinoma of the prostate. *Clin Oncol* (1990) **2**: 220–3.

14. Tong ECK. Parahormone and P-32 therapy in prostatic cancer with bone metastases. *Radiology* (1971) **98**: 343–51.

15. Porter AT, Ben-Josef E, Davis L. Systemic administration of new therapeutic radioisotopes including phosphorus, strontium, samarium, and rhenium. *Curr Opin Oncol* (1994) **6**: 607–10.

16. Aziz H, Choi K, Sohn C et al. Comparison of 32P therapy and sequential hemibody irradiation (HBI) for bony metastases as methods of whole body irradiation. *Am J Clin Oncol* (1986) **9**: 264–8.

17. Holmes RA. Radiopharmaceuticals in clinical trials. *Semin Oncol* (1993) **20 (Suppl 2)**: 22–31.

18. Pecher C. Biological investigations with radioactive calcium and strontium. Preliminary report on the use of radioactive strontium in the treatment of metastatic bone cancer. *Uni Calif Pub Pharmacol* (1942) **2**: 117–49.

19. Schmidt CG, Firusian N. 89-Sr for the treatment of incurable pain in patients with neoplastic osseous infiltrations. *Int J Clin Pharmacol* (1974) **7(3)**: 199–205.

20. Blake GM, Zivanovic MA, McEwan AJ et al. Sr-89 therapy: strontium kinetics in disseminated carcinoma of the prostate. *Eur J Nucl Med* (1986) **12**: 447–54.

21. Blake GM, Zivanovic MA, Blaquiere RM et al. Strontium-89 therapy: measurement of absorbed dose to skeletal metastases. *J Nucl Med* (1988) **29**: 549–57.

22. Blake GM, Gray JM, Zivanovic MA et al. Strontium-89 radionuclide therapy: a dosimetric study using impulse response function analysis. *Br J Radiol* (1987) **60**: 685–92.

23. Robinson R, Spicer JA, Preston DF et al. Treatment of metastatic bone pain with strontium-89. *Nucl Med Biol* (1987) **14**: 219–22.

24. Laing AH, Ackery DM, Bayly RJ et al. Strontium-89 therapy for pain palliation in prostatic skeletal malignancy. *Br J Radiol* (1991) **64**: 816–22.

25. Lewington VJ, McEwan AJ, Ackery DM et al. A prospective randomised double blind crossover study to examine the efficacy of strontium-89 in pain palliation in patients with advanced prostate cancer metastatic to bone. *Eur J Cancer* (1991) **27**: 954–8.

26. Buchali K, Correns HJ, Schuerer M et al. Results of a double blind study of 89-strontium therapy of skeletal metastases of prostate carcinoma. *Eur J Nucl Med* (1988) **14**: 349–51.

27. Dusing RW, Preston DF, Baxter KG, Robinson RG. Strontium-89 for pain palliation in the skeletal metastases of breast cancer. *Clin Nucl Med* (1993) **19**: 624 (abst).

28. Berna I, Carrio I, Alonso C et al. Bone pain palliation with strontium-89 in breast cancer patients with bone metastases and refractory bone pain. *Eur J Nucl Med* (1995) **22**: 1101–4.

29. Porter AT, McEwan AJB, Powe JE et al. Results of a randomized phase III trial to evaluate the efficacy of strontium-89 adjuvant to local field external beam irradiation in the management of endocrine resistant metastatic prostate cancer. *Int J Radiat Oncol Biol Phys* (1993) **25**: 805–13.

30. Quilty PM, Kirk D, Bolger JJ et al. A comparison of the palliative effects of strontium-89 and external beam radiotherapy in metastatic prostate cancer. *Radiother Oncol* (1994) **31**: 33–40.

31. Podoloff DA, Kasi LP, Kim EE et al. Evaluation of Sm-153-EDTMP as a bone imaging agent during a therapeutic trial. *J Nucl Med* (1991) **32**: 918 (abst).

32. Goeckeler WF. Sm-153 complexes as radiotherapeutic bone agents. PhD dissertation, University of Missouri-Columbia, 1984.

33. Goeckeler WF, Edwards B, Volkert WA et al. Skeletal localisation of samarium153 chelates: potential therapeutic bone agents. *J Nucl Med* (1987) **28**: 495–504.

34. Kasi LP, Fossella F, Holoye P et al. Evaluation of multiple dose Sm-153-EDTMP for bone palliation in cancer patients. Proceedings of the Seventh International Symposium of Radiopharmacology, 1991, Boston, MA, p. 11.

35. Turner JH, Claringbold PG, Hetherington EL et al. A phase I study of samarium-153-EDTMP therapy for disseminated skeletal metastases. *J Clin Oncol* (1989) **7**: 1926–31.

36. Turner JH, Claringbold PG. A phase II study of treatment of multifocal skeletal metastases with single and repeated dose samarium-153-ethyl-enediaminetetramethyline phosphonate. *Eur J Cancer* (1991) **27**: 1084–6.

37. Farhangi M, Holmes RA, Volkert WA et al. Samarium-153-EDTMP pharmacokinetic toxicity and pain response using an escalating dose schedule in treatment of metastatic bone cancer. *J Nucl Med* (1992) **33**: 1451–8.

38. Holmes RA [153Sm]-EDTMP: a potential therapy

for bone cancer pain. *Semin Nucl Med* (1992) **22**: 41–5.
39. Resche I, Chatal JF, Pecking A *et al.* A dose-controlled study of 153Sm-EDTMP in the treatment of patients with painful bone metastases. *Eur J Cancer* (1997) **33**: 1583–91.
40. Serafini AN, Houston SJ, Resche I *et al.* Palliation of pain associated with metastatic bone cancer using samarium-153 lexidronam: a double-blind placebo controlled clinical trial. *J Clin Oncol* (1998) **16**: 1574–81.
41. Maxon HR, Schroder LE, Thomas SR *et al.* Re-186-HEDP for treatment of painful osseous metastases: initial clinical experience in 20 patients with hormone resistant prostate cancer. *Radiology* (1990) **176**: 155–9.
42. Maxon HR, Thomas SR, Hertzberg VS *et al.* Rhenium-186-HEDP for the treatment of painful osseous metastases. *Semin Nucl Med* (1992) **21**: 33–40.
43. Maxon HR, Schroder LE, Hertzberg VS *et al.* Rhenium-186-HEDP for treatment of painful osseous metastases: results of a double blind crossover comparison with placebo. *J Nucl Med* (1991) **32**: 1877–81.
44. McEwan AJB, Amyotte GA, McGowan DG *et al.* A retrospective analysis of the cost effectiveness of treatment with metastron in patients with prostate cancer metastatic to bone. *Eur Urol* (1994) **26 (Suppl 1)**: 26–31.
45. Collins C, Eary JF, Donaldson G *et al.* Samarium-153-EDTMP in bone metastases of hormone refractory prostate cancer: a phase I/II trial. *J Nucl Med* (1993) **34**: 1839–44.
46. Mertens WC, Porter AT, Reid RH *et al.* Strontium-89 and low dose infusion cisplatin for patients with hormone refractory prostate carcinoma metastatic to bone: a preliminary report. *J Nucl Med* (1992) **33**: 1437–43.
47. Tu SM, Delpassand ES, Jones D *et al.* Strontium-89 combined with doxorubicin in the treatment of patients with androgen-independent prostate cancer. *Urol Oncol* (1996) **2**: 191–7.

Firusian N, Mellin P, Schmidt GC. Results of 89-strontium therapy in patients with carcinoma of the prostate and incurable pain from bone metastases. A preliminary report. *J Urol* (1976) **116**: 764–8.

13

Pain – mechanisms, assessment, and management

Jana Portnow and Stuart A Grossman

Introduction • Mechanisms of pain • Assessment of cancer pain • Management of cancer pain • Specific issues in the management of bone pain from metastatic disease • Conclusion

INTRODUCTION

More than 70% of patients with cancer suffer from moderate to severe pain at some point during their illness, but only a small fraction of these patients receive sufficient pain control. Data suggest that the majority of cancer patients could obtain excellent pain relief through currently available pharmacological and surgical techniques.

Several reasons exist for the undertreatment of cancer pain. There is an overall lack of formal training of physicians in pain management. As a result, many physicians have not been taught the general principles of treating cancer pain. A physician who is not aware of a pain medication's half-life and maximum dosage may inadvertently undermedicate a patient.

Moreover, since pain is subjective, physicians often have difficulty determining the severity of pain patients are experiencing. In a study comparing medical personnel's assessment of patients' pain to patients' rating of their pain, there was little correlation between the medical personnel's and the patients' ratings.[1] The medical personnel consistently underestimated the amount of pain the patients were experiencing, particularly when the pain was more severe. Such inaccurate assessments of the severity of cancer pain can lead to undertreatment.

The reluctance of some patients to communicate to their physicians the intensity of their pain is another factor which interferes with the adequate treatment of cancer pain. Patients' reluctance may be due to a perceived cultural value of stoicism, fear of becoming addicted to opiates, or an unwillingness to acknowledge their pain for fear that this might represent progression of their cancer.

One of the greatest concerns of cancer patients is dying in pain. Although curing a patient's cancer is often impossible, most cancer pain can be well controlled. Thus it is imperative that medical personnel caring for cancer patients are knowledgeable about cancer pain management. This chapter will review the general principles of cancer pain management and address some specific issues related to bone pain secondary to metastatic disease.

MECHANISMS OF PAIN

Pain in cancer patients is generally classified as nociceptive or neuropathic pain. Nociceptive

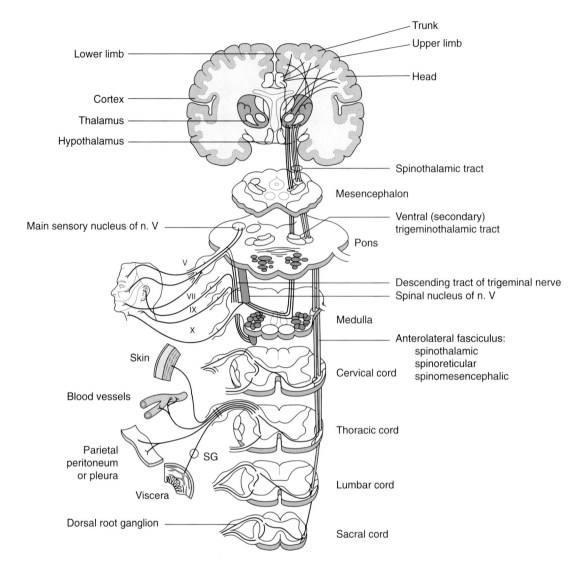

Fig. 13.1 Primary neural pathways for transmission of nociceptive information from various body structures to the brain. (*Source*: Grossman SA, Gregory RE.[37])

pain results from the activation of pain receptors in the skin and deeper tissues. When stimulated, these receptors transmit signals via peripheral nerves to the spinal cord. Most pain fibers cross to the other side of the spinal cord and continue in the anterolateral fasciculus. Modulation of this sensory input occurs at different levels in the central nervous system as the pain fibers ascend (Fig. 13.1).

Nociceptive pain can be subdivided into somatic and visceral pain. Somatic pain is usually well localized and associated with inflammation. Examples include a bone metastasis or a surgical incision. Somatic pain is often described as gnawing or aching pain. In contrast, visceral pain is frequently characterized as a vague, deep pressure. It tends to not be well localized, may present as referred pain, and is usually due to an infiltrative process such as tumor expansion causing distention of an organ. Pain from a bowel obstruction or distention of the capsule of the liver with referred right shoulder pain are common examples of visceral pain.

In contrast to nociceptive pain, which is mediated through peripheral pain receptors, neuropathic pain results from damage to the nerve itself. It is usually characterized by a burning, stinging, radiating pain which can persist even after tissue damage has resolved.[2] Neuropathic pain can occur as a result of direct nerve compression from a tumor or injury to nerves from chemotherapy, radiation, or surgery. Common examples include an apical lung tumor invading the brachial plexus or cisplatin-induced peripheral neuropathy. Of all pain syndromes, neuropathic pain is usually the least successfully treated. It is less responsive to opiates than nociceptive pain, and adjuvant analgesics, such as antidepressants and anticonvulsants, are often required. In cancer patients, many different types of pain typically coexist.

ASSESSMENT OF CANCER PAIN

Pain is subjective; there are no physiological or biochemical markers to determine objectively how much pain a patient is experiencing. Instead, all pertinent information must be provided by the patient. Therefore, a thorough history and physical examination, with special attention to the neurologic system, are essential. In addition to obtaining important details about a patient's pain such as the location, duration, quality, and any ameliorating or exacerbating factors, an attempt should also be made to quantify the pain. This can be achieved through the use of a pain intensity assessment scale. Figure 13.2 presents examples of validated pain intensity assessment scales. If patients cannot read or hold a pen, they may simply be asked to choose a number from 0, representing no pain, to 10, representing their idea of the most pain. Whatever method for quantifying pain is chosen, it should be consistently used, and the results should be recorded on bedside flow sheets. This serves to facilitate communication

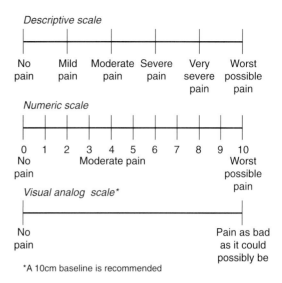

Fig. 13.2 Pain intensity assessment tools. (*Souce*: Grossman SA, Gregory RE.[37])

between patients and health-care providers and to evaluate the efficacy of pain treatments.

MANAGEMENT OF CANCER PAIN

Pharmacologic

In 1986, the World Health Organization (WHO) devised the analgesic ladder as a step-wise approach to cancer pain management (Fig. 13.3). The central idea is to begin with non-opiates, such as nonsteroidal anti-inflammatory drugs (NSAIDs) and acetaminophen for mild pain and proceed to 'weak' opiates in combination with acetaminophen for moderate pain, and then finally to 'strong' opiates for more severe pain. While this conceptual framework is useful as a starting point for organizing the various pain medications, it fails to address some important principles in cancer pain management which will be highlighted in the discussion below.

NSAIDs and acetaminophen

GENERAL PRINCIPLES OF ADMINISTRATION
NSAIDs and acetaminophen are on Step 1 of the WHO analgesic ladder and are indicated for the

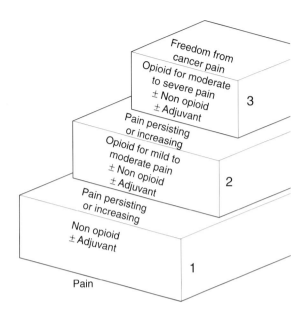

Fig. 13.3 World Health Organization analgesic ladder. (*Source*: WHO.[38])

relief of mild to moderate pain. NSAIDs produce analgesia through their anti-inflammatory properties. They decrease prostaglandins, mediators of inflammation, by inhibiting the enzyme cyclo-oxygenase which is responsible for prostaglandin synthesis. Prostaglandins make pain receptors more sensitive to stimulation and cause local swelling through vasodilation and increased blood flow. Because NSAIDs decrease inflammation, they are particularly effective in treating pain from bone metastases or soft tissue infiltration. When NSAIDs are contraindicated, acetaminophen is an alternative because it provides a similar degree of analgesia even though it lacks anti-inflammatory properties.

There is a maximum daily dosage for NSAIDs and acetaminophen beyond which toxicity increases without any gain in analgesia. The maximum daily dose for NSAIDs varies depending on which one is being used (Table 13.1). When administering an NSAID for pain relief, it should be titrated to its maximum therapeutic dose. If pain relief is insufficient, it may be worth while to try another NSAID because patients respond differently to different NSAIDs. The maximum daily dose of acetaminophen is 4–6 g per day.

SIDE-EFFECTS OF NSAIDS

In contrast to acetaminophen, hepatotoxicity usually occurs at doses beyond the maximum daily dose of 4–6 g, dangerous side-effects of NSAIDs can occur at therapeutic doses. These include peptic ulcer disease, platelet dysfunction, renal failure, fluid retention, and hepatic dysfunction.

NSAID-induced gastropathy is the most common of these adverse effects. Patients at high risk for this complication are those with at least two of the following: a history of peptic ulcer disease; an age greater than 60; a high dosage of NSAIDs; and a medication regimen of more than one NSAID at the same time.[3] Prophylactic treatment with misoprostol, a synthetic prostaglandin analogue, has been shown to reduce the risk of NSAID-induced gastropathy by 40% in patients with rheumatoid arthritis.[4]

The appropriate dose of misoprostol is 200 µg four times a day. The side-effects of this drug, such as diarrhea and abdominal cramping, can be avoided by starting with a dose of 100 µg twice a day and increasing the dose weekly. If a patient cannot tolerate misoprostol, high doses of omeprazole, a proton pump inhibitor, can be considered for prophylaxis of NSAID-induced gastropathy.[3,5] The prophylactic dose of omeprazole is 40 mg daily.

In contrast to other NSAIDs, choline magnesium trisalicylate does not interfere with platelet aggregation.[6] This can be helpful in cancer patients in whom chemotherapy-induced thrombocytopenia is anticipated. In addition, unlike other NSAIDs, this agent does not need to be stopped before surgical procedures.[7]

The development of a new class of NSAIDs, COX-2 inhibitors, resulted from the recent discovery that different forms of the enzyme cyclo-oxygenase exist. Cyclo-oxygenase-1 (COX-1) enzymes are present in most normal tissue, such as the gastrointestinal tract, heart, lung, kidneys, and brain. At these sites COX-1 enzymes produce prostaglandins that regulate homeostatic processes such as protection of the

Table 13.1 Selected nonopioid analgesics

Drug	Usual dose (mg)	Suggested maximum daily dose (mg)	Comments
Acetaminophen	650 q 4–6 h	4000–6000	Has no anti-inflammatory properties; therefore, should be considered after NSAIDs for the treatment of bone pain
Aspirin	650 q 4–6 h	6000	Tends to be less tolerated than NSAIDs
Choline magnesium trisalicylate	1000 q 12 h	3000	Does not inhibit platelet aggregation; safest NSAID to use in a thrombocytopenic patient
Diclofenac[a]	100 for 1st dose, then 50 q 8 h	150	
Etodolac[a]	400 for 1st dose, then 200–400 q 6–8 h	1200	
Ibuprofen[a]	600 q 6 h	3600	
Ketorolac[b]	(IV) 30 q 6 h (PO) 20 for 1st dose, then 10 q 4–6 h	120 40	The only NSAID which can be given IV; should not be used more than a total of 5 days, regardless of route
Nabumetone[a]	500 q 12 h	2000	
Naproxen[a]	500 for 1st dose, then 250 q 6–8 h	1250	

Notes:
[a]These NSAIDs appear to have a relatively low risk of causing NSAID-induced gastropathy compared to others.[39,40]
[b]If a patient is older than 65 years, has renal insufficiency, or weighs less than 50 kg, then the dose of ketorolac must be adjusted: 15 mg q 6 h IV with a maximum daily dose of 60 mg; 10 mg q 4–6 h PO (no initial loading dose) with a maximum daily dose of 40 mg.

gastric mucosa and renal function. In contrast, cyclo-oxygenase-2 (COX-2) enzyme levels are basically nonexistent in normal tissue. However, at sites of acute inflammation COX-2 enzymes are rapidly induced by cytokines resulting in production of the prostaglandins responsible for pain and inflammation.[8]

NSAIDs interfere with both COX-1 and COX-2 enzymes. However, the new selective COX-2 inhibitors should retain the analgesic and anti-inflammatory efficacy of current NSAIDs without the gastrointestinal, platelet, or renal toxicities. COX-2 inhibitors are approved for use in the treatment of rheumatoid arthritis. There is currently no data on their safety or efficacy in the treatment of cancer pain.

Opiates

Opiates are the mainstay of cancer pain management. They bind to receptors in the peripheral and central nervous systems and produce analgesia by inhibiting the transmission of pain signals. Before examining opiates in detail, it is important to understand basic principles regarding the prescribing of opiates and the difference between dependency and addiction.

GENERAL PRINCIPLES OF ADMINISTRATION

Opiates do not have a ceiling dose for producing analgesia. In contrast to NSAIDs, there is no maximum dose of an opiate beyond which no further increase in analgesia will occur – the larger the dose, the larger the analgesic effect. However, despite the continual increase in analgesia with incremental doses of opiates, the upper limit of dosing for opiates is determined by adverse side-effects, such as nausea, sedation, and respiratory depression. In practice this means that patients should receive as much opiate as they need to relieve pain until adverse side-effects interfere. The absolute number of milligrams administered is irrelevant. While most cancer patients' pain is controlled with conventional doses of opiates, if a patient has good analgesia with a very high dose and is not troubled by side-effects like oversedation or myoclonic jerks, then that is the appropriate dose for that patient.

Opiates should be administered around the clock, but extra doses of an opiate should be available for any additional pain. The goal of cancer pain treatment is to keep pain under control rather than 'rescue' the patient when severe pain recurs. Moreover, larger doses of medication are required to relieve pain once it has recurred than to prevent its recurrence. Therefore, when treating cancer pain, opiates should be given on an around the clock (ATC) schedule, *not just* on an as-needed (PRN) basis.

There is, however, a role for PRN opiate use in the treatment of breakthrough pain. As stated above, patients with chronic cancer pain should be placed on ATC doses of opiates. However, they should also have access to PRN opiates for pain that recurs, or breaks through, before it is time to give the next dose of regularly scheduled opiate. For example, if a patient is on a controlled-release morphine preparation, dosed every 12 hours, an immediate-release morphine preparation should be available for PRN use every 4 hours at a dose which is one third of the controlled-release dose. Frequent use of the PRN medication for breakthrough pain suggests that the patient's ATC dose of pain medication should be increased. Whenever the ATC dose is increased, the dose of the PRN immediate-release opiate should be increased as well to maintain its dose at one third of the dose of the controlled-release opiate.

If a patient requires additional analgesia, increase the dose of an oral opiate rather than increase the frequency of giving the dose. For example, if a patient is receiving 2 mg of hydromorphone every 4 hours, but the patient's pain recurs in 3 hours, then increase the 4-hourly dose to 4 mg or more, rather than administering the 2 mg of hydromorphone every 3 hours.

Whenever possible, use only one opiate at a time. As with NSAIDs, patients respond differently to different opiates. For example, a patient might experience more sedation with morphine than oxycodone or less nausea with morphine than hydromorphone. Using more than one opiate at the same time can make it difficult to determine which opiate is causing an intolerable side-effect. Therefore, it is better to do serial trials, rather than simultaneous ones.[7]

Always calculate equianalgesic doses when switching between opiates. Because patients respond differently to particular opiates, it is important to know how to switch patients to equivalent doses of different opiates. Table 13.2 lists the equianalgesic doses for several commonly used opiates. As the concept of equianalgesic dosing implies, no opiate is more effective than any other opiate. For example, while some opiates are less potent than morphine, such as codeine, or more potent, such as hydromorphone, no opiate is inherently more effective than morphine when an equianalgesic dose is administered. Thus, classifying opiates as 'weak' or 'strong' is misleading. With equianalgesic dosing ratios, any opiate can be dosed to deliver approximately the same amount of analgesia as another opiate. The most meaningful difference between opiates, what limits the use of one

Table 13.2 Equianalgesic doses of opioid analgesics used for the control of chronic pain[a]

Oral dose (mg)	Analgesic[b]	Parenteral (IV or SC) dose (mg)
150	Meperidine[c]	50
100	Codeine[c]	60
15	Hydrocodone[c,d]	—
15	MORPHINE[e,f]	5
10	Oxycodone	—
10	Methadone[g]	5
4	Hydromorphone[f]	1.5
—	Fentanyl (transdermal)[h]	—

Notes:
[a]Equianalgesic doses listed were obtained from a variety of sometimes conflicting studies and experiences and are meant only as guidelines for around-the-clock, standing-order, analgesic therapy of chronic pain.
[b]Dose interval: every 4 hours except for meperidine every 2 to 3 hours; controlled-released forms of morphine and oxycodone every 8 to 12 hours; transdermal fentanyl every 72 hours.
[c]Of little value in severe, chronic pain.
[d]Available only in combination with acetaminophen.
[e]No analgesic listed is superior orally to its equianalgesic dose of oral morphine.
[f]Rectal suppositories are available. Per rectum (PR) dose is equal to oral dose.
[g]Caution: risk of toxicity from delayed accumulation.
[h]Transdermal fentanyl μg/h dose: 1/2 × mg/d dose of oral morphine (one 100 μg/h patch every 3 days = 100 mg controlled-release morphine every 12 hours).
Source: Adapted from Levy.[7]

opiate versus another, is a particular opiate's side-effect profile, dosing interval, and/or route of administration.

Even when a patient's pain is well controlled, a change in opiates may be desired to reduce side-effects or to change from a short-acting opiate, such as hydrocodone, to an opiate which has a long-acting formulation, such as morphine. In this case, the initial dose of the new opiate should be 25–50% less than the calculated equianalgesic dose to allow for incomplete cross-tolerance among opiates.[9]

It is important to understand the difference between tolerance, physical dependence, and addiction to opiates. Tolerance is defined as the need for increasingly larger doses of a drug over time in order to maintain the same degree of analgesia. However, in patients with cancer, progression of disease rather than tolerance to opiates is usually responsible for increasing analgesic requirements.[7]

A patient receiving chronic opiates will develop a physical dependence on the opiate, manifested by development of withdrawal symptoms, such as nausea and diaphoresis, if the opiate is suddenly discontinued. Therefore, when an opiate can be stopped (such as after cordotomy eliminates a patient's lower extremity pain), the dose must be reduced gradually over several days.

While a patient can develop a physical dependence on an opiate, this does not mean that the

Table 13.3 General principles of opiate use for cancer pain

1) Patients should receive as much opiate as they need for pain relief until adverse side-effects interfere.
2) Opiates should be administered around the clock.
3) Patients should have access to PRN opiates for the treatment of breakthrough pain.
4) Increase the dose of an opiate, not the frequency of the dose if a patient needs more pain relief.
5) Whenever possible use only one opiate at a time.
6) Always calculate the equianalgesic dose of an opiate when changing opiates or routes of administration.
7) With equianalgesic dosing, no opiate is more effective than another opiate.
8) The most meaningful difference between opiates is a particular opiate's side-effect profile, dosing interval, and/or route of administration.
9) Taper opiates gradually to prevent withdrawal symptoms.

patient is addicted to the opiate. Addiction refers to a psychological dependence, which often leads to self-destructive behavior. Many patients, family members, and health-care providers are overly concerned about the possibility of cancer patients becoming addicted to opiates. However, studies have shown that it is very rare for cancer patients to become addicted to opiates.[10]

DIFFERENT TYPES OF OPIATES

Opiates such as codeine, hydrocodone, and oxycodone have traditionally been classified in Step 2 of the WHO analgesic ladder and are indicated for the treatment of moderate pain. These medications commonly come in fixed preparations with acetaminophen or aspirin, and thus these nonopioid analgesics set the maximum daily dosage for the fixed preparation.

Codeine is an opiate commonly used as a treatment for acute pain. It is less useful in chronic cancer pain management because many patients cannot tolerate the side-effects when it is given at higher doses. Patients may experience unacceptable nausea, dysphoria, and constipation at doses greater than 90 mg.[7] An equianalgesic dose of morphine, 13.5 mg, for example, often provides similar analgesia without the same side-effects. For the treatment of moderate pain, hydrocodone is an alternative to codeine with fewer side-effects. However, because hydrocodone is available only in a fixed preparation with acetaminophen, its use in chronic cancer pain management is also limited.

Oxycodone is available in a fixed combination with a nonopioid analgesic, or alone, either in an immediate-release or a controlled-release formulation. With oxycodone, the division between a Step 2 analgesic and a Step 3 analgesic is not so clear. When oxycodone is in a fixed combination the nonopioid analgesic sets the maximum dose, as with codeine and hydrocodone, and thus its use is limited to the treatment of moderate pain. However, it is actually slightly more potent than morphine and, because it is available as a single agent in both immediate-release and controlled-release forms, it is an excellent choice for the treatment of severe chronic cancer pain as well.

Morphine, hydromorphone, and fentanyl have traditionally been classified on the WHO analgesic ladder as Step 3 analgesics for the treatment of severe pain. Morphine is the paragon of these drugs: readily available, inexpensive, and well understood pharmacologically. It has been used successfully for decades in the treatment of cancer pain. Similar to oxycodone, morphine is available in both immediate-release and controlled-release forms.

Hydromorphone is also effective for the treatment of severe cancer pain. It is available in an immediate-release form, and a controlled-release form is being developed. Hydromorphone may be preferred over morphine when administered parenterally. Compared to morphine, hydromorphone is more soluble and more potent. Thus, less volume is needed for continuous subcutaneous or intravenous infusions of hydromorphone.

Fentanyl is a highly lipid soluble, synthetic opiate that provides alternative routes of administration for the treatment of severe pain. Fentanyl can be delivered transdermally for patients with stable pain who cannot take oral analgesics. In addition, a much more rapidly acting form of fentanyl has been recently developed that is administered via the buccal mucosa.[11]

In contrast to the opiates discussed above, meperidine and methadone are two opiates that are used infrequently for cancer pain management in the USA. Meperidine, a semisynthetic opiate, is a popular parenteral drug for the treatment of acute pain. However, meperidine has a shorter duration of analgesia than other opiates, requiring repeat dosing every 2–3 hours. This frequent dosing schedule is cumbersome for patients who require chronic, ATC pain medication. More importantly, meperidine has a toxic metabolite, normeperidine. Accumulation of this toxic metabolite can cause seizures, particularly in patients with renal insufficiency. As a result, it is recommended that meperidine not be used for more than 2 days.[12]

The use of methadone in the management of cancer pain is controversial. Methadone is an inexpensive opiate with a long pharmacologic half-life (varying from 15 to 25 hours). However, its duration of analgesia is only about 4 hours, requiring frequent repeat dosing.[13] More importantly, because of its long half-life, there is a risk of late respiratory depression from drug accumulation if the dose of methadone is increased more rapidly than every 3–5 days.

SIDE-EFFECTS OF OPIATES

While many clinicians are overly concerned about respiratory depression from opiates, the most common side-effects of these agents are constipation, nausea, and sedation. Opiates decrease bowel motility and prophylactic treatment of constipation is required in most patients. Roughage from fruits and vegetables, stool softeners, or bulk-forming laxatives such as methylcellulose and psyllium generally are ineffective against opioid-induced constipation. In order to maintain regular bowel movements, patients often need daily doses of bowel-stimulating laxatives such as senna or bisacodyl, osmotic laxatives such as lactulose, or enemas.

Nausea and sedation are also two frequent side-effects of opiates. However, unlike constipation, patients often develop tolerance to nausea and sedation. If tolerance does not develop, antiemetics, such as prochlorperazine, are useful. Other options are changing to a different opiate or attempting to reduce the dose of an opiate by using a coanalgesic or a pain-blocking procedure. Constipation may exacerbate the nausea associated with opioids, and thus strict adherence to the use of a laxative is important. When trying to prevent opioid-induced sedation, stimulants, such as methylphenidate or caffeine, may help. It may also be worth while to consider avoiding high-peak drug levels through the use of long-acting opiates or continuous infusions.

Less common side-effects of opiates include myoclonic jerks, seizures, and respiratory depression. Myoclonic jerks usually occur in patients receiving high doses of opiates. These can be treated, like nausea or sedation, by rotating opiates or by reducing their dose through the addition of coanalgesics. If these measures are not successful, clonazepam may be beneficial, though it may increase sedation.[14,15]

Seizures and respiratory depression usually occur with higher doses of opiates. However, they are relatively rare. Seizures are sometimes seen with high doses of parenteral morphine because the preservatives in the morphine preparation are neurotoxic in large amounts.[16] When a seizure occurs it can be treated with a benzodiazepine. It is important to look for causes of the seizure besides the opiate, such as the development of a brain metastasis. Respiratory depression usually occurs from a rapid increase in the dose of opiate or from the quick cessation of pain which leaves opioid sedative effects unopposed. Respiratory depression can be reversed with naloxone. However, this should be done slowly to prevent withdrawal symptoms.

It is very uncommon for a patient to be allergic to opiates. Symptoms such as dizziness or pruritis are due to opioid histamine release but are often mistaken for an allergic reaction. However, for the rare person who develops a true anaphylactic reaction to morphine there are safe alternatives. Fentanyl, methadone, and meperidine differ significantly from morphine in chemical structure, and so they may be administered to a morphine-allergic patient.[7]

ROUTES OF ADMINISTRATION OF OPIATES

Although oral administration is easiest and cheapest, if a patient cannot swallow or tolerate oral medications, other options are available. However, it is necessary to remember that opiates have different potencies depending on the route of administration. For example, orally administered morphine is incompletely absorbed and partially metabolized in the liver. In contrast, morphine administered subcutaneously directly enters the systemic circulation. Thus, parenteral morphine is 3–6 times more potent than oral morphine. Differences in dosage depending on the route of administration can be estimated using an opioid conversion table (Table 13.2).

The peak onset of analgesia occurs within 30–60 minutes with most orally administered immediate-release opiates and continues for about 4 hours. For controlled-release oral opiates, peak analgesia occurs in 2–3 hours, continuing for 12 hours. Opiates such as morphine and hydromorphone can be administered rectally with a bioavailability similar to oral administration.[17,18] However, rectal administration of opiates is not a reasonable long-term option because of the inconvenience and psychological distress it may cause the patient.

Another enteral route of opiate administration is sublingual or via the buccal mucosa. This requires a highly lipid soluble drug and bypasses the initial metabolism in the liver. Oral transmucosal fentanyl citrate (OTFC) produces an analgesic effect in 5–10 minutes, and the dose can be repeated every 15 minutes to achieve adequate pain relief. Because of its fast action, OTFC is a good treatment for breakthrough pain requiring immediate but short-lived relief.[19,20] The dosing of OTFC is difficult because its equianalgesic dosing with other opiates has not been calculated.

When patients cannot take opiates orally or when they need very rapid relief of uncontrolled pain, subcutaneous and intravenous administration of opiates are two common options. Subcutaneous administration provides pain relief in 10–15 minutes, lasting 3–4 hours. Intravenous administration produces analgesia within 5 minutes and has a duration of analgesia similar to subcutaneous administration. Intramuscular injections of opiates are not recommended because they are more painful, and not necessary given so many other possible, convenient routes of administration.

Just as pain relief with oral opiates can be maximized by patients with the use of oral PRN short-acting opiates, parenteral opiates can be titrated by the patient as well. Intravenous or subcutaneous infusion pumps can be used in the hospital or at home for patient-controlled analgesia (PCA). PCA pumps usually deliver a set amount of opiate each hour. In addition to that basal amount, patients with breakthrough pain can obtain extra preset doses of opiate by pressing a button. This feature allows patients to titrate the opiate dose for optimal pain relief as in the PRN use of oral medication. However, the fear of patients accidentally overdosing themselves is removed because the maximum hourly dose is preset.

Another parenteral method of administering opiates is transdermally with the use of a fentanyl patch. Unlike oral, subcutaneous, and intravenous routes, the transdermal approach does not provide a PRN mechanism. Thus a different route of administration is required for treatment of breakthrough pain. After applying the patch, a subcutaneous store of fentanyl is created, and the drug is continuously absorbed into systemic circulation. Analgesia initially occurs about 12 hours after placement of the patch. The patch should be changed every 72 hours. This is an excellent route of administration for chronic stable pain. However, the enteral route is preferred unless the patient cannot tolerate oral medication, since it is cheaper and also provides for PRN breakthrough opiates.

Opiates, in doses much smaller than required for oral or parenteral routes, can be administered spinally, either into the epidural or subarachnoid space. As these opiates are placed directly adjacent to the opiate receptors, a small dose produces excellent analgesia with minimal toxicity. As a general rule, one tenth of the dose of systemic opiates is given epidurally, and one tenth the epidural dose is administered intrathecally. Epidural opiates can be administered chronically using a soft catheter or subcutaneous injection port. This is sometimes used for patients who cannot tolerate the side-effects of large doses of systemic opiates. However, drawbacks to this route include the expense and invasiveness of the procedure, and the potential for introducing infection. Intrathecal administration requires a closed system to reduce the incidence of infections.

Opiates can also be administered intraventricularly, in doses even smaller than that used for intrathecal administration. Intraventricular opiates can be effective in treating intractable pain from head and neck cancers.

Coanalgesics

While opiates are the mainstay of cancer pain management, several other classes of medications function as coanalgesics. These medications can be beneficial for pain which is partially resistant to opiates, and may allow dose reduction of opiates.

TRICYCLIC ANTIDEPRESSANTS

Tricyclic antidepressants (TCAs) are indicated for the treatment of neuropathic pain. Patients are started on a small dose at bedtime, and this is increased slowly every few days to a maximally tolerated dose. Improvement in pain usually begins in about 2 weeks but TCA treatment should be continued for 1–2 months at full dose before concluding that the treatment is ineffective.[7]

Amitriptyline has been used the most for the treatment of neuropathic pain; however, many patients cannot tolerate the sedation and orthostatic hypotension it produces. Nortriptyline and desipramine are less sedating alternatives. Other common side-effects of TCAs include dry mouth, constipation, urinary retention, delirium, and tachyarrhythmias.

ANTICONVULSANTS

Anticonvulsants may be helpful as an addition or an alternative to TCAs in the treatment of neuropathic pain. They likely exert their effect through stabilization of nerve cell membranes. Of the anticonvulsants, carbamazepine is most often chosen for treating neuropathic pain. However, myelosuppression associated with carbamazepine may interfere with the ability to give chemotherapy to some patients. Gabapentin, a relatively new anticonvulsant, also may be effective in treating neuropathic pain. Several case reports have documented its efficacy in patients with neuropathic pain in whom previous therapies were either not effective or not tolerated.[21] Formal clinical trials are still in process. Gabapentin is more expensive than other anticonvulsants but has fewer side-effects. Thus gabapentin may be an alternative for a cancer patient who may experience myelosuppression or cannot tolerate other anticonvulsants.[22]

CORTICOSTEROIDS

Glucocorticoids are potent anti-inflammatory agents which are known to decrease peritumoral edema. Thus, they may be effective in the treatment of somatic pain (e.g. soft tissue infiltration), visceral pain (e.g. organ distention), and neuropathic pain (e.g. nerve compression). When administering steroids, a trial period of 5–7 days can be considered. If no beneficial effect is seen, the steroid can be discontinued.

Common side-effects of steroids include hyperglycemia, oral candidiasis, fluid retention, and gastritis. Perhaps the most debilitating long-term side-effect of steroid use is the development of proximal myopathy.

Invasive anesthetic and neurosurgical approaches

Because of the effectiveness in controlling cancer pain with opiates and coanalgesic medications, invasive anesthetic and neurosurgical procedures are not often needed. However, some patients who have pain that is not responsive to opiates, such as incident pain, or who cannot tolerate the side-effects of systemic opiates may be excellent candidates for these more invasive approaches.

Injection of a local anesthetic or a neurolytic agent is an excellent option for some patients with regional pain. For example, bupivacaine can be injected into an intercostal nerve to control pain from a rib metastasis, or into the hypogastric plexus to control pain in the pelvic area. The analgesia from a local anesthetic only lasts several hours. However, it is useful for diagnostic purposes. If the patient's pain is relieved by the local anesthetic without unacceptable toxicities, the area can then be injected with a neurolytic agent, such as alcohol or phenol, to achieve long-lasting pain relief.

Nerve fibers can be destroyed at different locations as they ascend to the brain. Neurolytic agents can be injected, under fluoroscopic guidance, either into the epidural space (targeting dorsal root ganglia) or the subarachnoid space (targeting dorsal rootlets). The resulting nerve damage is temporary but can result in analgesia that lasts for 2–4 months.[23] In contrast to intraspinal opiates which do not block sensory and motor function, intraspinal neurolytic agents cause nonselective nerve root destruction, sometimes resulting in loss of motor function. Because there is little risk of damaging major motor function by doing these procedures in the thoracic region, patients with pain on one side of the chest wall are generally best suited for spinal neurolysis. Spinal dorsal rhizotomy is an analogous neurosurgical procedure where, via laminectomy, posterior nerve roots are severed. Spinal dorsal rhizotomy can also be performed percutaneously with radiofrequency current. As with intraspinal neurolytics, spinal dorsal rhizotomy is mainly performed in the thoracic region to control chest wall pain.

Patients with pelvic pain that is resistant to other pain treatments may be well palliated with a commissural myelotomy. In this procedure pain fibers crossing in the anterior commissure of the spinal cord are severed. The potential complications include loss of bowel and bladder function.[22]

Although neuroablative procedures are rarely necessary to control cancer pain, the commonest of these procedures is cordotomy. Pain fibers of the spinothalamic tract in the anterolateral fasciculus of the spinal cord are severed with this procedure. Patients with cancer pain that is below the level of the shoulder and on one side of the body are best suited for cordotomy. In properly selected patients, cordotomies can produce good pain relief in 90% of patients. However, the efficacy decreases to about 50% by 1 year.[23] Cordotomy should only be performed on patients who have a limited life expectancy because many patients develop neuropathic pain within a year which may be very difficult to treat.

Cordotomies may be performed via a percutaneous procedure or an open procedure. In a percutaneous cordotomy radiofrequency current is used. In an open procedure the fibers are severed, generally through a T2–T3 laminectomy when the pain is in the pelvis or at the C1–C2 level for pain above the pelvis. Postoperatively, respiratory complications and bowel and bladder incontinence are not very frequent, but about 20% of patients will experience ipsilateral motor weakness. Fortunately, these motor deficits generally improve as spinal cord edema decreases.[23]

A final example of neuroablative procedures is cingulotomy. This stereotactic procedure uses radiofrequency to destroy the cingulum, which is located near the corpus callosum. This procedure is rarely done, but it can provide effective pain relief for patients with head and neck tumors.[24]

SPECIFIC ISSUES IN THE MANAGEMENT OF BONE PAIN FROM METASTATIC DISEASE

Metastatic cancer to bones is the most common cause of pain in patients with cancer.[25]

Furthermore, many patients with isolated bone metastases may live with these lesions for many years. Fortunately, there are many excellent treatment options for this type of pain.

Diagnosis

When a tumor infiltrates bone, it causes distension of the periosteum and causes an inflammatory reaction. Local nociceptors are stimulated by the release of prostaglandins, bradykinin, and other mediators of inflammation produced by osteoclasts and macrophages. Pain can also occur as a result of mechanical stresses on weakened, tumor-infiltrated bones.

Cancers which commonly metastasize to bone include breast, thyroid, lung, renal, and prostate cancer.[26] When they metastasize, these cancers most frequently spread to the spine, pelvis, and base of the skull. Metastases to the spine produce back and neck pain, whether or not cord compression is present. Metastases to the pelvis and femur may result in pain in the lower back and/or lower extremities. This pain is often accompanied by pathological fractures leading to problems with weight-bearing. Metastases to the base of the skull can cause headache and cranial nerve dysfunctions, such as pain, weakness, and sensory loss in the face, hoarse voice, and dysphagia.[27]

The evaluation of a cancer patient complaining of bone pain includes imaging studies such as plain radiographs and bone scans (see Chapters 7 and 8). A metastatic lesion must replace at least 30% of the bone before it becomes visible on a plain radiograph.[28] Bone scans are more sensitive than plain radiographs. However, a bone scan will not provide information about the risk of fracture, and thus plain radiographs are also needed.

Treatment of bone pain

NSAIDs and opiates

NSAIDs should be used when treating pain from bone metastases. These agents reduce the local mediators of inflammation that cause pain by sensitizing and stimulating nociceptors in bone. Even when a patient's bone pain is severe enough to require opiates, adding an NSAID to the opiate can be considered because of the NSAID's coanalgesic effect on bone pain.[29]

Radiation

External beam radiation is the most commonly used palliative treatment for metastatic bone pain (see Chapter 11). It works by producing a cytotoxic effect on the underlying tumor. However, even when there is no obvious cytoreduction of tumor, patients may experience pain relief with radiation therapy. Similar to NSAIDs, radiation may also inhibit bone cells from producing local inflammatory mediators which activate nociceptors in the bone.[25]

Radioisotope therapy

Radioisotopes can also be used to deliver radiation to painful bone metastases (see Chapter 12). For example, strontium-89 can provide pain relief in properly selected patients with osteoblastic bone metastases, such as those seen with prostate cancer. Because strontium-89, which emits beta particles, chemically resembles calcium, it is deposited like calcium in areas of osteoblastic activity. Once deposited, the metastatic lesions receive the short-range radiation, while the surrounding normal tissue is relatively unaffected. Because intravenously administered radioisotopes can treat many metastatic lesions simultaneously, it can complement or obviate the need for external beam radiation.

Treatment with strontium-89 is appropriate for patients with a life expectancy of greater than 3 months. It takes at least 4–6 weeks for pain relief to begin. Then the analgesic effect lasts, on average, 6 months.[30] Patients tolerate strontium-89 well, but the treatment can cause bone marrow suppression which may interfere with tolerance of future chemotherapy. Samarium-153 lexidronam is another bone-seeking radiopharmaceutical agent that can palliate painful bone metastases.[31]

Bisphosphonates

Bisphosphonates can provide pain relief to patients with bone metastases (see Chapters

14–16). This class of drugs inhibits osteoclasts from resorbing bone and are used to treat cancer-related hypercalcemia, reduce the incidence of pathologic fractures, and relieve pain. Several randomized, placebo-controlled clinical trials have confirmed the effectiveness of repeat infusions of bisphosphonates on patients with pain from metastatic bone disease.[28] However, additional analgesics may still be needed.

Chemotherapy

For certain tumors that are very sensitive to chemotherapy, treating the underlying tumor with systemic chemotherapy may provide effective treatment of bone pain. Analgesia may occur even before regression of the lesions is seen radiographically. Examples of chemosensitive tumors include breast cancer, small cell lung cancer, lymphoma, and multiple myeloma. Hormonal therapy can provide pain relief in patients with metastatic breast and prostate cancer.

Calcitonin

Calcitonin may also have a role in reducing bone pain from metastatic disease, although its analgesic efficacy remains uncertain. This hormone's physiologic function is similar to bisphosphonates in that it prevents calcium release from bone. It also inhibits production of local prostaglandins and increases the level of endogenous opiates in the brain. Which mechanism or mechanisms, if any, produce calcitonin's analgesic effect is not entirely clear. Many of the studies that initially suggested that calcitonin was effective in treating bone pain from metastases were not randomized or placebo-controlled. However, two of three small, double-blinded, randomized studies did show a modest effect of calcitonin on improving bone pain.[32–34]

Specific pain syndromes associated with metastatic bone disease

Incident pain

Many cancer patients have no pain or controllable pain at baseline, but experience temporary, often severe pain with voluntary movements, such as reaching for an object or walking, or with involuntary movements, such as swallowing or breathing. These brief exacerbations of pain are referred to as incident pain. In patients with bone metastases, the mechanical stimulation of nociceptors with movement is thought to be the underlying mechanism for this type of pain.

Incident pain is difficult to manage with oral analgesics because they neither act quickly enough to prevent the transient increase in pain nor briefly enough to prevent over-sedation during periods when the incident pain is not present. When a patient can anticipate the activities which produce pain, even routine acts as simple as getting out of bed, the use of oral transmucosal fentanyl citrate, which has a rapid onset of action of 5–10 minutes, or the use of a subcutaneous or intravenous PCA pump, may be adequate to prevent the incident pain. In general, however, incident pain is difficult to manage. The most successful long-term approach is to treat the underlying tumor with radiation or chemotherapy for susceptible tumors. Some patients may require orthopedic stabilization to treat pain and prevent pathologic fracture. Others may require an invasive anesthetic or neurosurgical procedure to relieve the pain.

Epidural spinal cord compression

Patients with metastatic bone disease who develop neck or back pain may have an epidural spinal cord compression. This possible complication must be investigated immediately. Pain may arise at the site of the metastasis or it may present as referred pain or radicular pain if the lesions compress adjacent nerve roots. Other symptoms which usually develop after the onset of pain include weakness, sensory loss, bowel and bladder incontinence, and paraplegia. A completely normal neurologic examination does not rule out epidural cord compression. In one study of cancer patients who had back pain, a normal neurologic examination, and abnormal plain films of the spine, 74% of those patients had spinal cord compression diagnosed by myelography.[35]

Early treatment is essential because a patient's functional status usually remains the same before and after treatment for a cord compression. Once patients develop neurologic deficits, they are rarely reversed. In other words, a patient who develops weakness and incontinence before treatment for the epidural cord compression will likely remain that way, even after aggressive treatment.

A thorough diagnostic work-up of possible epidural cord compression includes magnetic resonance imaging of the spine or, if magnetic resonance imaging is not available or contraindicated, a computed tomography scan with myelography. Epidural cord compression most commonly results from a direct extension of the metastasis from a vertebral body and may thus be seen on plain films or bone scans. However, in 10–15% of cases the tumor is located in a paravertebral space (reaching the epidural space via an intervertebral foramen) that can only be seen with an MRI or CT scan.[36] In most cases, only the symptomatic area of the spine needs to be imaged.

The preferred treatment for spinal cord compression is radiation with high-dose steroids. Steroids are administered along with the radiation to decrease edema around the cord, and thus relieve pressure until the radiation starts to become effective. If the tumor causing the cord compression is very chemosensitive, such as lymphoma, chemotherapy may be considered. Patients who have an unstable spine, bony compression of the spinal cord from collapsed vertebrae, or who have already received maximum radiation to the affected region, may require a surgical approach.

CONCLUSION

Pain will affect the majority of cancer patients at some point during the course of their illness. Fortunately, most cancer pain can be successfully treated with the many medications and procedures outlined in this chapter. Opiates remain the mainstay of cancer pain management. Therefore, clinicians must understand how to switch between opiates and routes of administration, how to treat and prevent opioid side-effects, and how and when to use coanalgesics, such as TCAs, anticonvulsants, and steroids. Opiates and coanalgesic medications can control pain in the majority of cancer patients. Invasive anesthetic and neuroablative procedures can be helpful in patients who have pain which is unresponsive to those medications or who cannot tolerate their side-effects.

Bone pain from metastatic disease is a common cause of morbidity among cancer patients. In addition to opiates, NSAIDs are particularly effective in treating musculoskeletal pain. Several other treatment options also exist for this type of pain: radiation, radioisotopes, bisphosphonates, chemotherapy, and possibly calcitonin. Pain-blocking procedures and orthopedic stabilization via surgery are possibilities as well.

Incident pain and epidural cord compression are two important complications of metastatic bone disease. Incident pain can be a particularly challenging problem to treat and may require the use of more than one of the options mentioned above. On the other hand, epidural cord compressions are usually relatively easy to treat once they are diagnosed. However, they are often diagnosed late, resulting in uncontrolled pain and rapid progression to irreversible paralysis and incontinence.

Successful management of cancer pain requires: 1) careful diagnostic evaluation; 2) trials of medications with frequent adjustments to ensure maximum efficacy and minimal toxicity; and 3) constant re-evaluation of new or progressive pain. These strategies usually result in excellent palliation of pain which is a key objective in the overall care of these patients.

REFERENCES

1. Grossman SA, Sheidler VR, Swedeen K et al. Correlation of patient and caregiver ratings of cancer pain. *J Pain Symptom Manage* (1991) **6**: 53–7.
2. Weinstein SM. New pharmacological strategies in the management of cancer pain. *Cancer Invest* (1998) **16**: 94–101.
3. Ament PW, Childers RS. Prophylaxis and treatment of NSAID-induced gastropathy. *Am Fam Physician* (1997) **55**: 1323–32.
4. Silverstein FE, Graham DY, Senior JR et al. Misoprostol reduces serious gastrointestinal complications in patients with rheumatoid arthritis receiving nonsteroidal anti-inflammatory drugs. *Ann Intern Med* (1995) **123**: 241–9.
5. Scheiman JM, Behler EM, Loeffler KM et al. Omeprazole ameliorates aspirin-induced gastroduodenal injury. *Dig Dis Sci* (1994) **39**: 97–103.
6. Stuart JJ, Pisko EJ. Choline magnesium trisalicylate does not impair platelet aggregation. *Pharmatherapeutica* (1981) **2**: 547–51.
7. Levy MH. Pharmacologic management of cancer pain. *Semin Oncol* (1994) **21**: 718–39.
8. Masferrer JL, Isakson PC, Seibert K. Cyclooxygenase-2 inhibitors. *Gastroenterol Clin North Am* (1996) **25**: 363–71.
9. Levy MH. Pharmacologic treatment of cancer pain. *N Engl J Med* (1996) **335**: 1124–32.
10. Foley KM. Controversies in cancer pain: medical perspectives. *Cancer* (1989) **63**: 2257–65.
11. Farrar JT, Cleary J, Rauck R et al. Oral transmucosal fentanyl citrate: randomized, double-blinded, placebo-controlled trial for treatment of breakthrough pain in cancer patients. *J Natl Cancer Inst* (1998) **90**: 611–16.
12. Acute Pain Management Panel. Acute pain management: operative or medical procedures and trauma. In *Clinical Practice Guideline. AHCPR pub no. 92-0032* (Rockville, MD: Agency for Health Care Policy and Research, Public Health Service, US Department of Health and Human Services, 1992).
13. Grochow L, Sheidler V, Grossman SA et al. Does intravenous methadone provide longer lasting analgesia than intravenous morphine? A randomized, double-blind study. *Pain* (1989) **38**: 151–7.
14. Ellison NM. Opioid analgesics for cancer pain: toxicities and their treatments. In Patt RB (ed) *Cancer Pain* (Philadelphia, PA: Lippincott, 1993): 185–94.
15. Eisele JH, Grigsby EJ, Dea G. Clonazepam treatment of myoclonic contractions associated with high dose opioids: case report. *Pain* (1992) **49**: 231–2.
16. Gregory RE, Grossman SA, Sheidler VR. Grand mal seizures associated with high-dose intravenous morphine infusions: incidence and possible etiology. *Pain* (1992) **51**: 255–8.
17. Bruera E, Ripamonti C. Alternate routes of administration of opioids for the management of cancer pain. In Patt RB (ed) *Cancer Pain* (Philadelphia, PA: Lippincott, 1993): 161–84.
18. Ellison NM, Lewis GO. Plasma concentrations following single doses of morphine sulfate in oral solution and rectal suppository. *Clin Pharmacol* (1984) **3**: 614–17.
19. Coluzzi PH. Cancer pain management: newer perspectives on opioids and episodic pain. *Am J Hosp Palliat Care* (1998) **15**: 13–22.
20. Christie JM, Simmonds M, Patt R et al. Dose-titration, multicenter study of oral transmucosal fentanyl citrate for the treatment of breakthrough pain in cancer patients using transdermal fentanyl for persistent pain. *J Clin Oncol* (1998) **16**: 3238–45.
21. Rosner H, Rubin L, Kestenbaum A. Gabapentin adjunctive therapy in neuropathic pain states. *Clin J Pain* (1996) **12**: 56–8.
22. Fisher K, McPherson ML. Gabapentin (Neurontin, Parke-Davis). *Am J Hosp Palliat Care* (1997) **14**: 311–12.
23. Rosen SM. Procedural control of cancer pain. *Semin Oncol* (1994) **21**: 740–7.
24. Long DM. *Contemporary Diagnosis and Management of Pain* (Newton, PA: Handbooks in Health Care, 1997).
25. Mercadante S. Malignant bone pain: pathophysiology and treatment. *Pain* (1997) **69**: 1–18.
26. Coleman RE. Skeletal complications of malignancy. *Cancer* (1997) **80 (Suppl 8)**: 1595–607.
27. Campa JA, Payne R. The management of intractable bone pain: a clinician's perspective. *Semin Nucl Med* (1992) **22**: 3–10.
28. Thurlimann B, de Stoutz ND. Causes and treatment of bone pain of malignant origin. *Drugs* (1996) **51**: 383–98.
29. Phillips LL. Managing the pain of bone metastases in the home environment. *Am J Hosp Palliat Care* (1998) **15**: 32–42.
30. Soffen EM, Greenberg AS, Baumann JC. Treating

symptomatic osseous metastases from prostate cancer. *New Jersey Med* (1997) **94**: 33–7.
31. Serafini AN, Houston SJ, Resche I *et al*. Palliation of pain associated with metastatic bone cancer using samarium-153 lexidronam: a double-blind placebo-controlled clinical trial. *J Clin Oncol* (1998) **16**: 1574–81.
32. Roth A, Kolaric K. Analgetic activity of calcitonin in patients with painful osteolytic metastases of breast cancer. *Oncology* (1986) **43**: 282–7.
33. Hindley AC, Hill EB, Leyland MJ *et al*. A double-blind controlled trial of salmon calcitonin in pain due to malignancy. *Cancer Chemother Pharmacol* (1982) **9**: 71–4.
34. Blomquist C, Elomaa I, Porkka L *et al*. Evaluation of salmon calcitonin treatment in bone metastases from breast cancer – a controlled trial. *Bone* (1988) **9**: 45–51.
35. Rodichok LD, Ruckdeschel JC, Harper GR *et al*. Early detection and treatment of spinal epidural metastases: the role of myelography. *Ann Neurol* (1986) **20**: 696–702.
36. Byrne TN. Spinal cord compression from epidural metastases. *N Engl J Med* (1992) **327**: 614–19.
37. Grossman SA, Gregory RE. Pain. In Kirkwood JM, Lotze MT, Yasko JM (eds) *Current Cancer Therapeutics* (Philadelphia, PA: Current Medicine, 1994).
38. World Health Organization. *Cancer Pain Relief and Palliative Care: Report of a WHO Expert Committee. Technical Report Series 804* (Geneva: WHO, 1990).
39. Rodriguez LAG, Hershel J. Risk of upper gastrointestinal bleeding and perforation associated with individual non-steroidal anti-inflammatory drugs. *Lancet* (1994) **343**: 769–72.
40. Lanza FL. Gastrointestinal toxicity of newer NSAIDs. *Am J Gastroenterol* (1993) **88**: 1318–23.

14

Mechanisms of action of bisphosphonates in tumor bone disease

Herbert Fleisch

Introduction • Chemistry • Physicochemistry • Effect on calcification • Effect on bone resorption • Effect on bone formation • Pharmacokinetics • Animal toxicology • Adverse side-effects in humans • Summary

INTRODUCTION

The bisphosphonates are a class of drugs that have been developed over the past three decades for diagnostic and therapeutic use in various diseases of bone and calcium metabolism. Although they have been known to chemists since the middle of the last century (the first bisphosphonate having been synthesized in Germany in 1865[1]), it is only relatively recently that it was discovered they could be useful in bone disease. This review, however, limits itself to the mechanisms of action involved in their use in tumor bone disease. For more extensive coverage, the reader may consult some of the more exhaustive reviews.[2-4]

CHEMISTRY

The bisphosphonates used clinically are compounds characterized by a P–C–P bond. They are therefore analogues of pyrophosphate with a carbon instead of an oxygen atom (Fig. 14.1). A large number of bisphosphonates with various structures have been synthesized. The ones listed in Fig. 14.2 are those that have been used for some indications in humans. Seven are commercially available, and five of them,

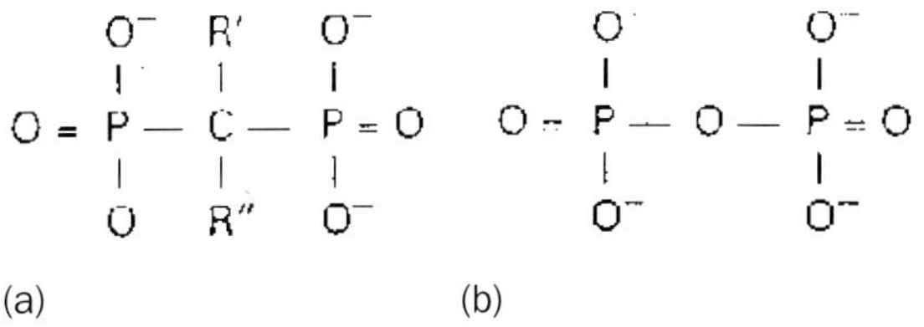

Fig. 14.1 Structure of (a) bisphosphonates and (b) pyrophosphate.

namely, alendronate, clodronate, etidronate, ibandronate, and pamidronate are used in tumor-induced bone disease.

PHYSICOCHEMISTRY

The P–C–P bond of the bisphosphonates is relatively stable when exposed to heat and to most chemical reagents, and is completely resistant to enzymatic hydrolysis. The physicochemical effects of most of the bisphosphonates are very similar to those of pyrophosphate and polyphosphates. Thus, many of the bisphosphonates inhibit the precipitation of calcium

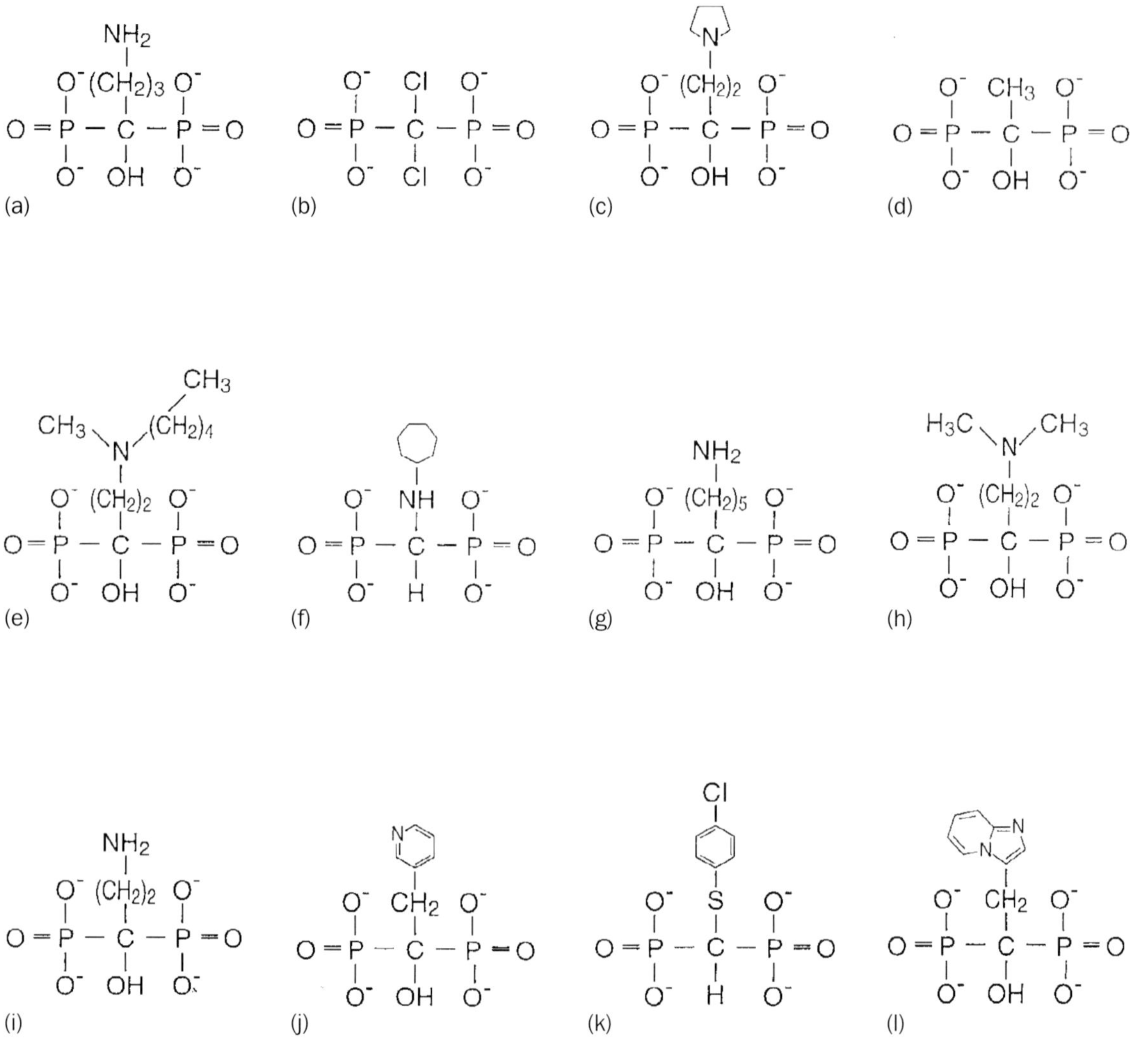

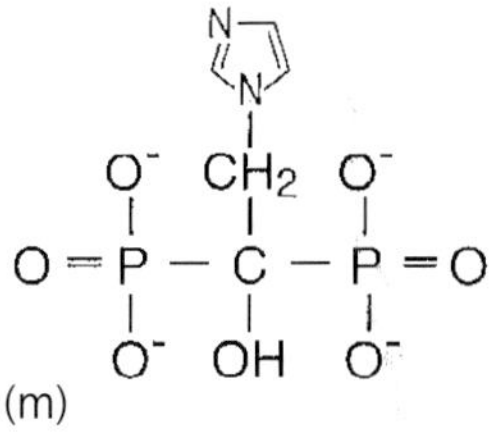

Fig. 14.2 Structure of the administered to humans[2']. (a) (4-amino-1-hydroxybutylidene)bisphosphonate alendronate*; (b) (dichloromethylene)-bisphosphonate clodronate*; (c) (1-hydroxy-3-(1-pyrrolidinyl)-prophylidene)bisphosphonate EB 1053; (d) (1-hydroxyethylidene)- bisphosphonate etidronate*; (e) (1-hydroxy-3-(methylpentylamino)propylidene)bisphosphonate ibandronate*; (f) ((cycloheptylamino)-methylene)bisphosphonate incadronate; (g) (6-amino-1-hydroxyhexylidene)bisphosphonate neridronate; (h) (3-(dihyethylamino)-1-hydroxypropylidene)bisphosphonate olpadronate; (i) (3-amino-1-hydroxypropylidene)bisphosphonate pamidronate*; (j) (1-hydroxy-2-(3-pyridinyl)-ethylidene)bisphosphonate risedronate; (k) (((4-chlorophenyl)thio)-methylene)bisphosphonate tiludronate; (l) (1-hydroxy-2-imidazo-(1,2-a)pyridin-3-ylethylidene)bisphosphonate minodronate; (m) (1-hydroxy-2-(1H-imidazole-1-yl)ethylidene)bisphosphonate zoledronate.
* Commercially available for tumor bone disease.

phosphate even at very low concentrations[5,6] and they also slow down the dissolution of these crystals.[7,8] All these effects appear to be related to the marked affinity of these compounds for solid-phase calcium phosphate, to which they bind by chemisorption on to calcium[9] and then act as crystal poisons on both growth and dissolution.

EFFECT ON CALCIFICATION

The bisphosphonates have been shown to prevent experimentally induced calcification of many soft tissues (amongst others, the arteries, kidneys, and skin) when given both parenterally and orally.[5,6] If administered in a sufficient dose, certain bisphosphonates, such as etidronate, can also impair the mineralization of normal calcified tissues, such as bone[10,11] and cartilage,[11] as well as dentine, enamel, and cement. This inhibition is eventually reversed after discontinuation of the drug.[12] It is of interest that the bisphosphonate has to be present continuously to produce this effect, both in vitro[13] and in vivo.[11] The inhibition of ectopic mineralization is most probably mainly, if not entirely, due to the physicochemical inhibition of crystal growth.[6,14]

EFFECT ON BONE RESORPTION

In vitro

The bisphosphonates block bone resorption induced by various means in organ cultures.[7,8,15,16] Inhibition can also be observed when the effect of isolated osteoclasts is investigated on various mineralized matrices in vitro,[17,18] where the osteoclasts form fewer erosion cavities of a smaller size.

In vivo

In growing rats and mice, the bisphosphonates block the degradation of both bone and cartilage and thus arrest the remodeling of the metaphysis, which becomes club shaped and radiologically more dense than normal.[11] This effect is often used as a model when studying the potency of new compounds.[19] The inhibition of endogenous bone resorption has also been documented in kinetic studies of ^{45}Ca and in hydroxyproline excretion,[20] and also in the release of radioactive tetracycline that was previously incorporated into the skeleton.[21] This effect occurs within 24–48 hours[21] and is therefore slower than that induced by calcitonin. The decrease in resorption is accompanied by an increase in the calcium balance[20] and in the mineral content of bone. This is possibly a result of an increase in the intestinal absorption of calcium,[20] consequent upon an elevation of 1, 25 (OH)$_2$ vitamin D. This increased balance is the medical rationale behind administering these compounds to patients suffering from osteoporosis.

The inhibition of bone resorption eventually achieves a steady plateau even if the compounds are given continuously.[22] The plateau achieved depends on the administered dose. There appears to be no accumulation effect with time, and it seems the bisphosphonate embedded in the bone is inactive, or at least inactive while it remains embedded in the bone.

In therapeutic doses there appears to be no danger over time of continuously decreasing bone turnover with a concomitant increase in bone fragility, as is observed in osteopetrosis. It is now clear that, if not given to excess, the bisphosphonates improve biomechanical properties, both in normal animals and in experimental models of osteoprosis. (For review, see ref. 4.)

The bisphosphonates also impair bone resorption induced experimentally by various means. Thus, they have been observed to blunt the effect of various enhancers of bone resorption, such as parathyroid hormone,[7,8] retinoids,[23] and others. Their effect on retinoids is also an excellent way to test the anti-resorbing effect of new bisphosphonates. The bisphosphonates also prevent various forms of osteoporosis, among others, those induced by immobilization,[24] corticosteroids,[25] and ovariectomy.[26] All the bisphosphonates that had previously been found to inhibit bone resorption in other systems were active (among others, alendronate, clodronate, etidronate, ibandronate, incadronate, olpadronate, pamidronate, and risedronate).

Tumor-induced bone resorption

The bisphosphonates also inhibit tumoral bone resorption very effectively, both *in vitro* and *in vivo*. In culture, they inhibit the bone-resorbing effect of the supernatants of various cancers on mice calvaria *in vitro*.[27,28] Activity has also been observed when the bisphosphonates were injected into the mice before explanation of the calvaria.[28]

In vivo, the first studies performed used humoral hypercalcemia induced by subcutaneously implanted Leydig[29] or Walker 256 carcinoma cells. In both models, increased calcemia and calciuria could be presented either partially or entirely. The effect was generally more pronounced in calciuria than in calcemia. This could be explained by the fact that hypercalcemia is often due to the systemic production of PTH-related peptide, which increases not only bone resorption but also tubular reabsorption of calcium. Since the bisphosphonates act only on the former, they are more effective in hypercalciuria that is caused only by bone resorption – hypercalcemia is also caused by renal reabsorption.[30] This also explains why the bisphosphonates are more effective in the hypercalcemia of tumors that only affect the bone, such as myeloma.

The bisphosphonates also prevent or slow down bone resorption that is a consequence of actual tumor invasion, as has been shown in numerous experiments. The first investigation injected Walker carcinosarcoma cells into the iliac artery of the rat. A procedure that induced the cells to spread into the bone.[31] A similar effect can also be obtained if tumor cells are implanted directly into the bone[32] or are implanted into the muscle adjacent to bone.[33] Many kinds of tumor cells have been used, such as bladder tumor, rat mammary adenocarcinoma, prostate adenocarcinoma, myeloma, and melanoma. Experiments have recently been improved through the use of nude mice.[34,35] In all these investigations, bone reabsorption has been decreased by the bisphosphonates.

One of the questions under investigations is whether the bisphosphonates can decrease the skeletal tumor burden. While earlier results showed no effect or possibly even an increased effect on burden of the bisphosphonates,[36] newer studies have demonstrated a decrease in burden.[35] In contrast, although one study showed an increase, in the other ones the bisphosphonates had no effect on the development of the tumors in the soft tissues. Similarly, the osteoblastic process initiated by prostate tumor cells is not blocked by the bisphosphonates.[37]

In general, the effects of bisphosphonates can be seen when the compounds are administered during metastases, but also before the implantation, no drug being given during the growth of the tumor.[38]

Structure effect of the various bisphosphonates

Individual bisphosphonates vary greatly in their effect.[8,39] For etidronate, the first bisphosphonate to be used in clinical practice, the amount necessary to inhibit bone resorption is very close to that needed to induce a block in normal mineralization. Therefore, one of the aims of bisphosphonate research has been to find compounds that have a higher anti-resorptive activity without a consequent higher inhibition of mineralization. This has proved possible – today there are compounds that have ten thousand times the amount of anti-resorptive activity than etidronate. Clodronate, for example, is about ten times more potent than etidronate.[7,8] Adding a hydroxyl group to the carbon atom at position 1 increases anti-resorbing potency.[39] Derivatives that have an amino group at the end of the alkyl side-chain are extremely active. The first of these compounds to be described was pamidronate,[22,40] which is about ten times more active than clodronate. The length of the side-chain is also important. Among the compounds with a primary amine, the highest activity has been found in those with an alkyl chain of four carbons (alendronate), a compound that is again ten times more active than pamidronate.[19] More recently it has been shown that if the nitrogen is not primary, as in pamidronate, but is tertiary, then efficacy is increased. This occurs if the nitrogen atom of pamidronate is dimethylated, as in olpadronate.[41]

Activity is increased still further when a methyl and a pentyl group are added to the nitrogen, such as in ibandronate.[42] Nitrogen also greatly increases efficacy if it is within a heterocyclic ring. Some of the most active compounds described so far, such as risedronate,[43] zoledronate,[16] and minodronate, belong to this class, having five to ten thousand times higher activity than etidronate. The effect of nitrogen is very intriguing and, as yet, has not been explained. A three-dimensional structural requirement appears to be involved, with the nitrogen atom having to be at the correct place. However, although no clear-cut structure–activity relationship has yet been worked out, it appears that both the P–C–P structure and the two side-chains are of importance. One of the side-chains seems to be necessary for binding to the apatite through a tridentate hook, while both of them,[44] together with the P–C–P structure, are needed for cellular activity.

The rankings of the potencies of the various bisphosphonates used in humans are shown in Fig. 14.3. This is the same as that seen in rats, although the range between the most and the least potent is about 1000 in humans as opposed to 10,000 observed in the rat.

Mechanisms of action in inhibiting bone resorption

The mechanism involved in inhibiting bone resorption is till not clear. There is, however, general agreement that the final target of bisphosphonate action is the osteoclast. Action on this cell appears to be mediated through cellular mechanisms and not through an inhibition of crystal dissolution as initially postulated. These cellular mechanisms can be divided into three levels of action, namely, tissue, cellular, and molecular. Furthermore, the action can go through the intermediary of other cells.

Etidronate*
Tiludronate
Clodronate*
Pamidronate*
Neridronate
EB 1053
Incadronate
Olpadronate
Alendronate*
Risedronate
Ibandronate*
Minodronate
Zoledronate

Fig. 14.3 Anti-resorbing properties of the various bisphosphonates in increasing order of potency.[2]
* Commercially available for tumor bone disease.

Tissue level

The main effect of the bisphosphonates is a decrease in bone turnover, which is secondary to the inhibition of bone resorption. This effect is due to a decrease in the number of osteoclasts actively destroying bone, which leads to a decrease in the number of new BMUs. Furthermore, the bisphosphonates act at the individual BMU level by decreasing the depth of the resorption site. Since the amount of new bone formed in the BMU is not decreased, but possibly even increased,[45,46] the local and consequently the whole-body balance will be less negative or possibly even positive.

Cellular level

Four mechanisms appear to be involved: 1) inhibition of osteoclast recruitment; 2) inhibition of osteoclastic adhesion; 3) shortening of the lifespan of osteoclasts; and 4) inhibition of osteoclast activity. The former three will lead to a decrease in the number of osteoclasts. All four effects could be due either to a direct action on the osteoclast or its precursors, or indirectly through action on cells which modulate the osteoclast.

Several bisphosphonates inhibit osteoclast formation in various culture systems of both cells[47] and bones.[48] Part of this effect is probably directly on the osteoclast precursors, part indirectly through osteoblasts.[49–52] One recent study has shown that the bisphosphonates decrease osteoclastic adhesion to the mineralized matrix.[53]

It was originally proposed that osteoclast lifespan might be shortened because of a toxic effect of the bisphosphonates on these cells after the bisphosphonates had engulfed them. Recently, however, it has been reported that the bisphosphonates induce osteoclast programmed cell death (apoptosis), both *in vitro* and *in vivo*.[54] This effect is seen with simple non-nitrogen-containing bisphosphonates such as clodronate, as well as with those containing a nitrogen atom. The ranking of the effectiveness of clodaronate, pamidronate, and risedronate was the same as seen *in vivo* on bone resorption.

It is generally accepted that the bisphosphonates also inhibit osteoclast activity after uptake in these cells. Indeed, they induce numerous morphological changes in these cells, which include alterations in the cytoskeleton (among others, in actin and vinculin[18,55–57] as well as in the ruffled border[11,56,57]). This is possible because the bisphosphonates can enter cells[58] (perhaps by endocytosis), particularly those cells of the macrophage lineage, such as osteoclasts.[57] The bisphosphonates can attain very high concentration values, not only within the cells[58] but also under the osteoclasts, possibly up to 100–1000 μM or more. This occurs partly because they deposit preferentially under these cells,[57] and partly because they are released during the resorption process from the mineral at the acid pH prevailing at this location.

Molecular level
The low concentrations necessary for activity suggest either some sort of 'receptor' or some sort of cellular binding site, which induces a cellular transduction mechanism. This site could be either on the cell membrane or within the cell and might be an enzyme, a pump, or some other intracellular protein involved in the signaling cascade. AS yet, however, no such active receptor or binding site has been identified.

It has been known for some time that the bisphosphonates decrease the acid production of various cells[59] and of calvaria.[60] Recently, the bisphosphonates were shown to decrease the extrusion of acid through a sodium-independent mechanism by osteoclasts.[61] Part of this effect is possibly due to a decrease of proton transport by the vascular-type proton ATPase, which is inhibited by tiludronate. Surprisingly, this is not induced by other bisphosphonates.[62] However, no correlation has as yet been discovered between the effect *in vitro* on acid production and *in vivo* on bone resorption. Some bisphosphonates, such as pamidronate or long-chain bisphosphonates (especially in high concentrations), actually increase lactic acid production.[39] This is possibly due to a toxic action. They also inhibit prostaglandin synthesis by bone cells or calvaria, both *in vitro* and *in vivo*.[63] This mechanism may be relevant in certain tumors.

Bisphosphonates can in inhibit lysosomal enzymes *in vitro*,[64] in cultured calvaria, or when given *in vivo*. In view of the homology between pyrophosphate and bisphosphonates, various enzymes involving pyrophosphates or ATP have been examined. Phosphatases and pyrophosphatases were influenced only at relatively high concentrations or not influenced at all.[65] PTPε, PTPδ and PTPmeg1, however (protein-tyrosine phosphatases present in osteoclasts), are inhibited *in vitro* by various bisphosphonates with an IC_{50} of only a few μM.[65–67] These effects might be relevant since protein-tyrosine phosphorylation is important in the signal transduction pathways that control cell growth, differentiation, and activity. Unfortunately, the potency to inhibit the PTPs of the various bisphosphonates tested so far has demonstrated no relationship to their pharmacological potency.

It has been demonstrated recently that the various bisphosphonates might be classified into two major groups according to their different modes of action. One group comprises those that resemble closely pyrophosphate, such as etidronate, tiludronate, and clodronate. These can be incorporated into the phospshate chain of ATP-containing compounds so they become nonhydrolysable.[68,89] For example, clodronate will form adenosine 5'-(βγdichloromethylene) triphosphate. This incorporation is brought about by aminoacyl-tRNA synthetases[70] and occurs in various mammalian cells, including osteoclasts. The new P–C–P analogues inhibit cell function and may lead to cell death. It has been suggested that this mechanism is at least part of the cause of the apoptosis induced by bisphosphonates.

The second group comprises the N-containing compounds and these have the ability to inhibit the mevalonate pathway.[71] This leads to a decrease in the formation of isoprenoid lipids such as farnesyl- and geranylgeranyldiphosphates. These are required for the post-translation prenylation of proteins, including the GTP-binding proteins Ras, Rho, Rac, and Rab. Since these compounds are important for many cell functions, a lack of them will lead to a series of changes in cells (including osteoclasts) that result in decreased activity and apoptosis.[72] It seems that the enzymes involved in this inhibition are not prenyl transferases but more likely isopentenylpyrophosphate isomerase or farnesylpyrophosphate synthase.[73]

Many mechanisms that could be involved in the inhibition of bone resorption have therefore been described. However, it is not yet clear which of them is the most relevant *in vivo*. It is possible more than one or two mechanisms are involved, and that their relevance varies from one compound to another. The various cellular modes of action are summarized in Fig. 14.4.

Other cells

It is likely that the bisphosphonates act – at least in part – through other cells. One likely candidate is the macrophages, which release many cytokines that are able to modulate the osteoclasts and that are influenced by the bisphosphonates. Another candidate is the osteoblasts. It is now generally accepted that cells of osteoblastic lineage control the recruitment and activity of osteoclasts. One of the modulators involved in this mechanism appears to be the bisphosphonates. Indeed, these compounds induce them to synthesize an inhibitory activity of osteoclast recruitment and therefore of bone resorption.[49–52]

Mechanisms of action in tumoral bone resorption

As described earlier, the bisphosphonates inhibit tumoral bone destruction as well as the development of new metastases induced by various tumors. The most generally accepted explanation for this has been that this effect is secondary to the inhibition of bone resorption: since less bone is destroyed, room for tumoral expansion is limited. However, another explanation is that, as a consequence of a decrease in bone resorption, the release of matrix or osteoclastic cytokines which would stimulate the multiplication of tumor cells (such as TGFβ and IGFs) is decreased (the 'seed and soil' hypothesis)[74,75] (Fig. 14.5).

Recent evidence has shown that the bisphosphonates can also inhibit the adhesion of tumor cells *in vitro*.[76,77] This effect is specific to mineralized matrices, and the potency of the various

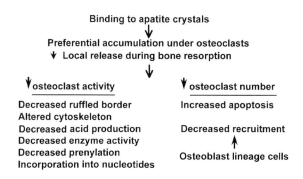

Fig. 14.4 Mechanisms of action of the inhibition of bone resorption.[2]

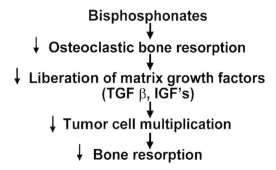

Fig. 14.5 Effect of the bisphosphonates through the 'seed and soil' mechannisms.

bisphosphonates correlates well with the potency to inhibit bone resorption *in vivo*. Lastly, bisphosphonates have been shown to induce apoptosis in various tumor cells, including myeloma cells.[78–80] The effect is thought to be mediated by the inhibition of prenylation.[80] These last three effects might, in part, explain the bisphosphonate-induced decrease in the development of tumor burden in animals.[35]

EFFECT ON BONE FORMATION

Until recently, the bisphosphonates were considered not to affect bone formation itself but to increase bone balance merely by inhibiting bone resorption. However, recent results suggest this may not be entirely the case. Morphological data suggest a possible increase in formation at the BMU level, implying that some stimulating effect on bone formation might possibly be present.[45,46] Furthermore, the bisphosphonates have been shown to increase the proliferation of osteoblasts and the formation of mineralized nodules,[81] as well as the biosynthesis of collagen and osteocalcin[81,82] *in vitro*. The possibility of an increase in bone formation, although as yet far from established, is of enough potential interest to warrant further research.

PHARMACOKINETICS

The bisphosphonates have a very low bioavailability – from a few percent in those given in larger amounts to below 1% in the newer ones that are given in lower amounts. This is partly explained by their low lipophilicity (which hampers transcellular transport) and their high negative charge (which hampers paracellular transport, probably the main route).[83] Paracellular transport is controlled by calcium, which tightens the junctional complex. This possibly explains why high doses of bisphosphonates (which also chelate calcium) will lead to an increase in their own absorption.[84] Furthermore, in the gut the bisphosphonates are partly in an insoluble form due to their chelation to calcium. For unknown reasons orange juice and coffee decrease absorption.[85]

Once in the blood, the bisphosphonates disappear very rapidly, mostly to bone.[86] On average about 50% go into the skeleton, the remainder being excreted in the urine, the repartition varying according to the compounds. This skeletal affinity is explained by the strong binding to hydroxyapatite crystals.[9] Consequently, soft tissues are exposed to these compounds for only short periods, which explains their low toxicity.

It was generally considered that the bisphosphonates were deposited in those locations within the bone where new bone is formed. Recently, however, they have also been found to deposit under osteoclasts.[57] The amount deposited at bone formation and bone resorption sites depends upon the amount of the bisphosphonate administered.[87] When small amounts are given, they deposit mostly under the osteoclasts, while larger amounts go to both bone-forming and bone-resorbing sites.

Once the bisphosphonates are in the skeleton, they will be released only when the bone is destroyed during the course of bone turnover. The skeletal half-life of the various bisphosphonates is between 3 months and one year for mice and rats, but much longer, sometimes over 10 years, for humans.[88] The bisphosphonates do not usually deposit in soft tissues. However, some – when administered in very large doses paterenterally – can at times deposit in other organs, such as the stomach, liver, spleen, and kidney as a result of the formation of insoluble aggregates.

The stability of the P–C–P bond to enzymatic hydroylsis explains why the bisphosphonates have not been found to be metabolized *in vivo*, all compounds investigated so far having been excreted unaltered. However, it is quite possible that, in the future, some compounds will be metabolized in their side-chain (especially in the gut), so that it cannot be stated categorically that the bisphosphonates are not metabolized *in vivo*.

ANIMAL TOXICOLOGY

Acute, subacute, and chronic administration of the bisphosphonates has, in general, shown little toxicity. This is explained by their rapid incorporation into calcified tissues and, hence, their short duration in the circulation. Acute toxicity is mostly the result of hypocalcemia, which is induced by the formation of complexes or aggregates with calcium, leading to a decrease in ionized calcium.

Nonacute toxicity like many phosphates, usually first manifests itself in the kidney.[89,90] This occurs, however, only at doses substantially larger than those administered in humans. At still higher doses other organs show cellular alterations. The mechanisms leading to these changes are not known. In the skeleton and in teeth, an inhibition of normal mineralization occurs, usually at parenteral doses of approximately 10 mg/kg daily.[10,11,91] This inhibition is explained by a physicochemical impairment of crystal growth. Very large doses of bisphosphonates can inhibit bone destruction to such an extent that the lower bone turnover achieved can lead to increased fragility and to fractures.[12]

ADVERSE SIDE-EFFECTS IN HUMANS

Studies in humans have revealed only a few significant adverse side-effects. Caution must be taken with all intravenous administrations of large amounts of bisphosphonates, since rapid intravenous injection has led to renal failure,[92] possibly because the bisphosphonate transforms into a solid phase when in the blood which is then held back in the kidney. Such events will not occur if all bisphosphonates given intravenously in large amounts are administered by slow infusion with plenty of fluid.

The oral administration of bisphosphonates (especially those with a primary amine) can be accompanied by esophageal and gastrointestinal side-effects, such as nausea, dyspepsia, vomiting, gastric pain and diarrhea, and sometimes even ulceration.[93–95] These adverse effects can be reduced if the drug is taken with plenty of water and with the patient not lying down, which will minimize esophageal reflux.

As has been observed in animals, etidronate, when given at daily oral doses of 400–800 mg, can produce an inhibition of normal skeletal mineralization that leads to a clinical and histological picture of osteomalacia.[96,97] This condition regresses after discontinuation of therapy. Similar results have been seen in Paget's disease with pamidronate, when given intravenously at doses equal to or higher than 180 mg per year.[98,99]

The last commonly encountered side-effect to be observed is after the intravenous administration of the various, more potent bisphosphonates that contain a nitrogen atom. (This is not, however, observed with etidronate, clodronate, or tiludronate.) A transient pyrexia of, usually 1–2°C (sometimes more), accompanied by flu-like symptoms, may occur. This is at its maximum within 24–48 hours and disappears after approximately 3 days, in spite of continued treatment. It is usually observed once only, even if treatment is continued and restarted later.[100] The mechanism of these changes, which resemble an acute-phase response, seems to involve the release by macrophages of IL-6 and TNFα.

Most of the other adverse side-effects are only seen occasionally, and there is no proof any of them are actually related to the drugs being administered.

SUMMARY

The bisphosphonates are a class of drugs characterized by a P–C–P bond. They bind strongly to hydroxyapatite crystals, which explains their preferential deposition in bone. Their main effect is to inhibit bone resorption. This is seen both *in vitro* in normal animals and in animals with experimentally induced resorption. Thus they prevent bone destruction induced by several tumor models in animals as well as in human tumor bone disease.

The inhibition of bone resorption is mediated by an effect on osteoclasts. These are decreased in number as a result of an inhibition of their recruitment and/or as a result of accelerated apoptosis. Furthermore, osteoclasts are less active because of a direct effect after they have engulfed the bisphosphonates.

The cellular mechanisms which lead to these changes are complex. Reduced recruitment can be a consequence of a direct effect on precursor cells as well a consequence of indirect action on the osteoblasts, which are stimulated to produce an inhibitor to this process. The direct effect on the osteoclasts appears to differ according to the compounds involved. The bisphosphonates without nitrogen may act, at least in part, through the formation of a bisphosphonate containing analogues of adenyl compounds. In contrast, those containing nitrogen appear to act on the mevalonate pathway where they prevent the formation of intermediates necessary for prenylation and therefore for the activity of GTP-ATPase. This leads to disruption of many cellular processes, some of which are necessary for osteoclast formation, survival, and activity.

The effect of tumor-induced bone destruction was once thought to be mediated only by the inhibitory effect on bone resorption. However, other mechanisms have recently been observed that may possibly come into play. Thus, the bisphosphonates inhibit the adhesion of the tumor cells on to bone matrix. Furthermore, they favor apoptosis of tumor cells. Lastly, there may also be a secondary inhibitory effect on the proliferation of tumor cells because of reduced liberation from bone of cytokines that activate tumor growth (such as TGFb, IGFs, and others) as a consequence of the reduced osteolysis (the 'seed and soil' concept).

Acute, subacute, and chronic administration have demonstrated little toxicity. In large doses, the first nonosseous alterations are observed in the kidney, as is the case for many phosphates. In the skeleton, large doses can induce an inhibition of calcification, and very large doses can lead to an excessive decrease in bone resorption with an increase in fragility.

In humans, only a few significant adverse side-effects are seen. Very rapid intravenous administrations of large concentrated doses may lead to renal failure but this is avoided if the drug is infused slowly and in sufficiently diluted measures. Oral administration of nitrogen-containing bisphosphonates, especially those with a primary amine, can induce gastrointestinal side-effects if taken with too little water. Nitrogen-containing bisphosphonates provoke, when given intravenously, a transient acute phase-like response. Lastly, large doses of eitdronate can inhibit normal skeletal mineralization.

REFERENCES

1. Menschutkin N. Ueber die Einwirkung des Chloracetyls auf phosphorige Säure. *Ann Chem Pharm* (1865) **133**: 317–20.
2. Fleisch H. *Bisphosphonates in Bone Disease. From the Laboratory to the Patient* (3rd edn) (New York: Parthenon, 1997).
3. Fleisch H. Bisphosphonates: mechanisms of action and clinical use. In Bilezikian JP, Raisz LG, Rodan GA (eds) *Principles of Bone Biology* (San Diego, CA, and London: Academic Press, 1996): 1037–52.
4. Fleisch H. Bisphosphonates: mechanisms of action. *Endocrine Rev* (1998) **19**: 80–100.
5. Francis MD, Russell RGG, Fleisch H. Diphosphonates inhibit formation of calcium phosphate crystals *in vitro* and pathological calcification *in vivo*. *Science* (1969) **165**: 1264–6.
6. Fleisch H, Russell RGG, Bisaz S, Mühlbauer RC, Williams DA. The inhibitory effect of phosphonates on the formation of calcium phosphate crystals *in vitro* and on aortic and kidney calcification *in vivo*. *Eur J Clin Invest* (1970) **1**: 12–18.
7. Fleisch H, Russell RGG, Francis MD. Diphosphonates inhibit hydroxapatite dissolution *in vitro* and bone resorption in tissue culture and *in vivo*. *Science* (1969) **165**: 1262–4.
8. Russell RGG, Mühlbauer RC, Bisaz S, Williams DA, Fleisch H. The influence of pyrophosphate, condensed phosphates, phosphonates and other phosphate compounds on the dissolution of hydroxyapatite *in vitro* and on bone resorption induced by parathyroid hormone in tissue culture and in thyroparathyroidectomised rats. *Calcif Tissue Res* (1970) **6**: 183–96.
9. Jung A, Bisaz S, Fleisch H. The bind of pyrophosphate and two diphosphonates by hydroxyapatite crystals. *Calcif Tissue Res* (1973) **11**: 269–80.
10. King WR, Francis MD, Michael WR. Effect of disodium ethane-1-hydroxy-1, 1-diphosphonate on bone formation. *Clin Orthop* (1971) **78**: 251–70.
11. Schenk R, Merz WA, Mühlbauer R, Russell RGG, Fleisch H. Effect on ethane-1-hydroxy-1, 1-diphosphonate (EHDP) and dichloromethylene diphosphonate (Cl_2MDP) on the calcification and resorption of cartilage and bone in the tibial epiphysis and metaphysis of rats. *Calcif Tissue Res* (1973) **11**: 196–214.
12. Flora L, Hassing GS, Parfitt AM, Villanueva AR. Comparative skeletal effects of two diphosphonates in dogs. *Metab Bone Dis Rel Res* (1980) **2**: 389–407.

13. Van Beek E, Hoekstra M, van de Ruit M, Löwik C, Papapoulos S. Structural requirements for bisphosphonate actions *in vitro*. *J Bone Miner Res* (1994) **9**: 1875–82.
14. Trechsel U, Schenk R, Bonjour JP, Russell RGG, Fleisch H. Relation between bone mineralization, Ca absorption, and plasma Ca in phosphonate-treated rats. *Am J Physiol* (1977) **232**: E298–E305.
15. Reynolds JJ, Minkin C, Morgan DB, Spycher D, Fleisch H. The effect of two diphosphonates on the resorption of mouse calvaria *in vitro*. *Calcif Tissue Res* (1972) **10**: 302–13.
16. Green JR, Müller K, Jaeggi KA. Preclinical pharmacology of CGP 42'446, a new, potent, heterocyclic bisphosphonate compound. *J Bone Miner Res* (1994) **9**: 745–51.
17. Flanagan AM, Chambers TJ, Dichoromethylenebisphosphonate (Cl$_2$MBP) inhibits bone resorption through injury to osteoclasts that resorb Cl$_2$MBP-coated bone. *Bone Miner* (1989) **6**: 33–43.
18. Sato M, Grasser W. Effects of bisphosphonates on isolated rat osteoclasts as examined by reflected light microscopy. *J Bone Miner Res* (1990) **5**: 31–40.
19. Schenk R, Eggli P, Fleisch H, Rosini S. Quantitative morphometric evaluation of the inhibitory activity of new aminobisphosphonates on bone resorption in the rat. *Calfic Tissue Int* (1986) **38**: 342–9.
20. Gasser AB, Morgan DB, Fleisch HA, Richelle LJ. The influence of two diphosphonates on calcium metabolism in the rat. *Clin Sci* (1972) **43**: 31–45.
21. Mühlbauer RC, Fleisch H. A method for continual monitoring of bone resorption in rats: evidence for a diurnal rhythm. *Am J Physiol* (1990) **259**: R679–R89.
22. Reitsma PH, Bijvoet OLM, Verlinden-Ooms H, van der Wee-Pals LJA. Kinetic studies of bone and mineral metabolism during treatment with (3-amino-1-hydroxy-propylidene)-1, 1- bisphosphonate (APD) in rats. *Calcif Tissue Int* (1980) **32**: 145–57.
23. Trechsel U, Stutzer A, Fleisch H. Hypercalcemia induced with an arotinoid in thyroparathyroidectomized rats. A new model to study bone resorption *in vivo*. *J Clin Invest* (1987) **80**: 1679–86.
24. Mühlbauer RC, Russell RGG, Williams DA, Fleisch H. The effects of diphosphonates, polyphosphates and calcitonin on 'immobilisation osteoporosis' in rats. *Europ J Clin Invest* (1971) **1**: 336–44.
25. Jee WSS, Black HE, Gotcher JE. Effect of dichloromethane diphosphonate on cortisol-induced bone loss in young adult rabbits. *Clin Orthop* (1981) **156**: 39–51.
26. Wronski TJ, Dann LM, Scott KS, Crooke LR. Endocrine and pharmacological suppressors of bone turnover protect against osteopenia in ovariectomized rats. *Endocrinology* (1989) **125**: 810–16.
27. Galasko CSB, Samuel AW, Rushton S, Lacey E. The effect of prostaglandin synthesis inhibitors and diphosphonates on tumour-mediated osteolysis. *Br J Surg* (1980) **67**: 493–6.
28. Jung A, Mermillod B, Barras C, Baud M, Courvoisier B. Inhibition by two diphosphonates of bone lysis in tumor conditioned media. *Cancer Res* (1981) **41**: 3233–7.
29. Martodam RR, Thornton KS, Sica DA, D'Souza SM, Flora L, Mundy GR. The effects of dichloromethylene diphosphonates on hypercalcemia and other parameters of the humoral hypercalcemia of malignancy in the rat Leydig cell tumor. *Calcif Tissue Int* (1983) **35**: 512–19.
30. Rizzoli R, Caverzasio J, Fleisch H, Bonjour JP. Parathyroid hormone-like changes in renal calcium and phosphate reabsorption induced by Leydig cell tumor in thyroparathyroidectomized rats. *Endocrinology* (1986) **119**: 1004–9.
31. Jung A, Bormaud J, Mermillod B, Edouard C, Meunier PJ. Inhibition by diphosphonates of bone resorption induced by the Walker tumor of the rat. *Cancer Res* (1984) **44**: 3007–11.
32. Guaitani A, Polentarutti N, Filippeschi S *et al*. Effects of disodium etidronate in murine tumor models. *Eur J Cancer Clin Oncol* (1984) **20/5**: 685–93.
33. Guaitani A, Sabatini M, Coccioli G, Cristina S, Garattini S, Bartosek I. An experimental rat model for local bone cancer invasion and its responsiveness to ethane-1-hydroxy-1, 1-bis (phosphonate). *Cancer Res* (1985) **45**: 2206–9.
34. Nemoto R, Sato S, Nishijima Y, Miyakawa I, Koiso K, Harada M. Effects of a new bisphosphonate (AHBuBP) on osteolysis induced by human prostate cancer cells in nude mice. *J Urol* (1990) **144**: 770–4.
35. Sasaki A, Boyce BF, Story B *et al*. Bisphosphonate risedronate reduces metastatic human breast cancer burden in bone in nude mice. *Cancer Res* (1995) **55**: 3551–7.
36. Kostenuik PJ, Orr FW, Suyama K, Singh G. Increased growth rate and tumor burden of

spontaneously metastatic Walker 256 cancer cells in the skeleton of bisphosphonate-treated rats. *Cancer Res* (1993) **53**: 5452–7.

37. Pollard M, Luchert PH, Scheu J. Effects of diphosphonate and X-rays on bone lesions induced in rats by prostate cancer cells. *Cancer* (1988) **61**: 2027–32.

38. Krempien B, Wingen F, Eichmann T, Müller M, Schmähl D. Protective effects of a prophylactic treatment with the bisphosphonate 3-amino-1-hydroxypropane-1, 1-bisphosphonic acid on the development of tumor osteopathies in the rat: experimental studies with the Walker carcinosarcoma 256. *Oncology* (1988) **45**: 41–6.

39. Shinoda H, Adamek G, Felix R, Fleisch H, Schenk R, Hagan P. Structure–activity relationships of various bisphosphonates. *Calcif Tissue Int* (1983) **35**: 87–99.

40. Bijvoet OLM, Frijlink WB, Jie K et al. APD in Paget's disease of bone. Role of the mononuclear phagocyte system? *Arth Rheum* (1980) **23**: 1193–204.

41. Boonekamp PM, Löwik CWGM, van der Wee-Pals LJA, van Wijk-van Lennep MLL, Bijvoet OLM. Enhancement of the inhibitory action of APD on the transformation of osteoclast precursors into resorbing cells after dimethylation of the amino group. *Bone Miner* (1987) **2**: 29–42.

42. Mühlbauer RC, Bauss F, Schenk R et al. BM 21.0995, a potent new bisphosphonate to inhibit bone resorption. *J Bone Miner Res* (1991) **6**: 1003–11.

43. Sietsema WK, Ebetino FH, Salvagno AM, Bevan JA. Antiresorptive dose–response relationships across three generations of bisphosphonates. *Drugs Exp Clin Res* (1989) **15**: 389–96.

44. Van Beek E, Löwik C, Oue I, Papapoulos S. Dissociation of binding and antiresorptive properties of hydroxybisphosphonates by substitution of the hydroxyl with an amino group. *J Bone Miner Res* (1996) **10**: 1492–7.

45. Balena R, Toolan BC, Shea M et al. The effects of 2-year treatment with the aminobisphosphonate alendronate on bone metabolism, bone histomorphometry, and bone strength in ovariectomized nonhuman primates. *J Clin Invest* (1993) **92**: 2577–86.

46. Boyce RW, Paddock CL, Gleason JR, Sletsema WK, Eriksen EF. The effects of risedronate on canine cancellous bone remodeling: three-dimensional kinetic reconstruction of the remodeling site. *J Bone Miner Res* (1995) **10**: 211–21.

47. Hughes DE, MacDonald BR, Russell RGG, Gowen M. Inhibition of osteoclast-like cell formation by bisphosphonates in long-term cultures of human bone marrow. *J Clin Invest* (1989) **83**: 1930–5.

48. Boonekamp PM, van der Wee-Pals LJA, van Wijk-van Lennep MML, Thesing CW, Bijvoet OLM. Two modes of action of bisphosphonates on osteoclastic resorption of mineralized matrix. *Bone Miner* (1986) **1**: 27–39.

49. Sahni M, Guenther HL, Fleisch H, Collin P, Martin TJ. Bisphosphonates action rat bone resorption through the mediation of osteoblasts. *J Clin Invest* (1993) **91**: 2004–11.

50. Vitté C, Fleisch H, Guenther HL. Bisphosphonates induce osteoblasts to secrete an inhibitor of osteoclast-mediated resorption. *Endocrinology* (1996) **137**: 2324–33.

51. Nishikawa M, Akatsu T, Katayama Y et al. Bisphosphonates act on osteoblastic cells and inhibit osteoclast formation in mouse marrow cultures. *Bone* (1996) **18**: 9–14.

52. Nishikawa M, Yamamoto M, Murakami T, Akatsu T, Kugai N, Nagata N. A third generation bisphosphonate, YM175, inhibits osteoclast formation in murine cocultures by inhibiting proliferation of precursor cells via supporting cell-dependent mechanisms. *J Bone Miner Res* (1998) **13**: 986–95.

53. Colucci S, Minielli V, Zambonin G, Grano M. Etidronate inhibits osteoclast adhesion to bone surface but does not interfere with their specific recognition of single bone proteins. *Ital J Miner Electroklte Metab* (1995) **9**: 159–64.

54. Hughes DE Wright KR, Uy HL et al. Bisphosphonates promote apoptosis in murine osteoclasts *in vitro* and *in vivo*. *J Bone Miner Res* (1995) **10**: 1478–87.

55. Selander K, Lehenkari P, Väänänen HK. The effects of bisphosphonates on the resorption cycle of isolated osteoclasts. *Calcif Tissue Int* (1994) **55**: 368–75.

56. Murakami H, Takahashi N, Sasaki T et al. A possible mechanism of the specific action of bisphosphonates on osteoclasts: tiludronate preferentially affects polarized osteoclasts having ruffled borders. *Bone* (1995) **17**: 137–44.

57. Sato M, Grasser W, Endo N et al. Bisphosphonate action. Alendronate localization in rat bone and effects on osteoclast ultrastructure. *J Clin Invest* (1991) **88**: 2095–105.

58. Felix R, Guenther HL, Fleisch H. The subcellular distribution of [^{14}C] dichloromethylenebisphos-

59. Fast DK, Felix R, Dowse C, Neuman WF, Fleisch H. The effects of diphosphonates on the growth and glycolysis of connective-tissue cells in culture. *Biochem J* (1978) **172**: 97–107.
60. Morgan DB, Monod A, Russell RGG, Fleisch H. Infuence of dichloromethylene diphosphonate (Cl$_2$MDP) and calcitonin on bone resorption, lactate production and phosphatase and phyrophosphatase content of mouse calvaria treated with parathyroid hormone *in vitro*. *Calcif Tissue Res* (1973) **13**: 287–94.
61. Zimolo Z, Wesolowski G, Rodan GA. Acid extrusion is induced by osteoclast attachment to bone: inhibition by alendronate and calcitonin. *J Clin Invest* (1995) **96**: 2277–83.
62. David P, Nguyen H, Barbier A, Baron R. The bisphosphonate tiludronate is a potent inhibitor of the osteoclast vacuolar H$^+$-ATPase. *J Bone Miner Res* (1996) **11**: 1498–507.
63. Ohya K, Yamada S, Felix S, Fleisch H. Effect of bisphosphonates on prostaglandin synthesis by rat bone cells and mouse calvaria in culture. *Clin Sci* (1985) **69**: 403–11.
64. Felix R, Russell RGG, Fleisch H. The effect of several diphosphonates on acid phosphohydrolases and other lysosomal enzymes. *Biochim Biophys Acta* (1976) **429**: 429–38.
65. Schmidt A, Rutledge SJ, Endo N *et al*. Protein-tyrosine phosphatase activity regulates osteoclast formation and function: inhibition by alendronate. *Proc Natl Acad Sci USA* (1996) **93**: 3068–73.
66. Endo N, Rutledge SJ, Opas EE, Vogel R, Rodan GA, Schmidt A. Human protein tyrosine phosphatase-σ: alternative splicing and inhibition by bisphosphonates. *J Bone Miner Res* (1996) **11**:535–43.
67. Opas EE, Rutledge SJ, Golub E *et al*. Alendronate inhibition of protein-tyrosine phosphatase-Meg1. *Biochem Pharmacol* (1997) **54**: 721–7.
68. Frith JC, Mönkkönen J, Blackburn GM, Russell RGG, Rogers MJ. Clodronate and liposome-encapsulated clodronate are metabolised to a toxic ATP analog, adenosine 5′ (βΓ-dichloromethylene) triphosphate, by mammalian cells *in vitro*. *J Bone Miner Res* (1996) **12**: 1358–67.
69. Auriola S, Frith J, Rogers MJ, Koivuniemi A, Mönkkönen J. Identification of adenine nucleotide-containing metabolites of bisphosphonates drugs using ion-pair liquid chromatography-electrospary mass spectrometry. *J Chromatogr* (1997) **704**: 187–95.
70. Rogers MJ, Brown RJ, Hodkin V, Russell RGG, Watts DJ. Bisphosphonates are incorporated into adenine nucleotides by human aminoacyl-tRNA synthetase enzymes. *Biochem Biophys Res Commun* (1996) **224**: 863–9.
71. Luckman SP, Hughes DE, Coxon FP, Russell RGG, Rogers MJ. Nitrogen-containing bisphosphonates inhibit the mevalonate pathway and prevent post-translational prenylation of GTP-binding proteins, including Ras. *J Bone Miner Res* (1998) **13**: 581–9.
72. Luckman SP, Coxon FP, Ebetino FH, Russell RGG, Rogers MJ. Heterocycle-containing bisphosphonates cause apoptosis and inhibit bone resorption by preventing protein prenylation: evidence from structure–activity relationships in J774 macrophages. *J Bone Miner Res* (1998) **13**: 1668–78.
73. Van Beek E, Pieterman E, Cohen L, Löwik C, Papapoulos S. Nitrogen-containing bisphosphonates inhibit isopentenyl pyrophosphate isomerase/farnesyl pyrophosphate synthase activity with relative potencies corresponding to their antiresorptive potencies *in vitro* and *in vivo*. *Biochem Biophys Res Comm* (1999) **255**: 491–4.
74. Mundy GR, Yoneda T. Facilitation and suppression of bone metastasis. *Clin Orthop Relat Res* (1995) **312**: 34–44.
75. Guise TA, Mundy GR. Cancer and bone. *Endocr Rev* (1998) **19**: 18–54.
76. Van der Pluijm G, Vloedgraven H, van Beek E, van der Wee-Pals L, Löwik C, Papapoulos S. Bisphosphonates inhibit the adhesion of breast cancer cells to bone matrices *in vitro*. *J Clin Invest* (1996) **98**: 698–705.
77. Boissier S, Magnetto S, Frappart L *et al*. Bisphosphonates inhibit prostate and breast carcinoma cell adhesion to unmineralized and mineralized bone extracellular matrices. *Cancer Res* (1997) **57**: 3890–4.
78. Shipman CM, Rogers MJ, Apperley JF, Russell RGG, Croucher PJ. Bisphosphonates induce apoptosis in human myeloma cells; a novel anti-tumor activity. *Brit J Haematol* (1997) **98**: 665–72.
79. Aparicio A, Gardner A, Tu Y, Savage A, Berenson J, Lichtenstein A. *In vitro* cytoreductive effects on multiple myeloma cells induced by bisphosphonates. *Leukemia* (1998) **12**: 220–9.

80. Shipman CM, Croucher PI, Russell RGG, Helfrich MH, Rogers MJ. The bisphosphonate incadronate (YM175) causes apoptosis of human myeloma cells *in vitro* by inhibiting the mevalonate pathway. *Cancer Res* (1998) **58**: 5294–7.
81. Tsuchimoto M, Azuma Y, Higuchi O *et al.* Alendronate modulates osteogenesis of human osteoblastic cells *in vitro*. *Jpn J Pharmacol* (1994) **66**: 25–33.
82. Guenther HL, Guenther HE, Fleisch H. The effects of 1-hydroxyethane-1, 1-diphosphonate and dichloromethanediphosphonate on collagen synthesis by rabbit articular chondrocytes and rat bone cells. *Biochem J* (1981) **196**: 293–301.
83. Boulenc X, Marti E, Joyeux H, Roques C, Berger Y, Fabre G. Importance of the paracellular pathway for the transport of a new bisphosphonate using the human CACO-2 monolayers model. *Biochem Pharmacol* (1993) **46**: 1591–600.
84. Boulenc X, Roques C, Joyeux H, Berger Y, Fabre G. Bisphosphonates increase tight junction permeability in the human intestinal epithelial (CaCo-2) model. *Int J Pharmacol* (1995) **123**: 13–24.
85. Gertz BJ, Holland SD, Kline WF *et al.* Studies of the oral bioavailability of alendronate. *Clin Pharmacol Ther* (1995) **58**: 288–98.
86. Bisaz S, Jung A, Fleisch H. Uptake by bone on pyrophosphate, diphosphonates and their technetium derivatives. *Clin Sci Mol Med* (1978) **54**: 265–72.
87. Masarachia P, Weinreb M, Balena R, Rodan GA. Comparison of the distribution of ^{3}H-alendronate and ^{3}H-etidronate in rat and mouse bones. *Bone* (1996) **19**: 281–90.
88. Kasting GB, Francis MD. Retention of etidronate in human, dog, and rat. *J Bone Miner Res* (1992) **7**: 513–22.
89. Alden CL, Parker RD, Eastman DF. Development of an acute model for the study of chloromethanediphosphonate nephrotoxicity. *Toxicol Pathol* (1989) **17**: 27–32.
90. Cal JC, Daley-Yates PT. Disposition and nephrotoxicity of 3-amino-1-hydroxypropylidene-1, 1-bisphosphonates (APD) in rats and mice. *Toxicology* (1990) **65**: 179–97.
91. Larsson A. The short-term effects og high doses of ethylene-1-hydroxy-1, 1-diphosphonates upon early dentin formation. *Calcif Tissue Res* (1974) **16**: 109–27.
92. Bounameuax HM, Schifferli J, Montani JP, Jung A, Chatelanat F. Renal failure associated with intravenous diphosphonates. *Lancet* (1983) **1**: 471.
93. Van Bruekelen FJM, Bijvoet OLM, Frijlink WB, Sleeboom HP, Mulder N, van Oosterom AT. Efficacy of amino-hydroxypropylidene bisphosphonate in hypercalcemia: observations on regulation of serum calcium. *Calcif Tissue Int* (1982) **34**: 321–7.
94. Lufkin EG, Argueta R, Whitaker MD *et al.* Pamidronate: an unrecognized problem in gastrointestinal tolerability. *Osteoporosis Int* (1994) **4**: 320–2.
95. De Groen PC, Lubbe DF, Hirsch LJ *et al.* Esophagitis associated with the use of alendronate. *N Engl J Med* (1996) **355**: 1016–21.
96. Jowsey J, Riggs BL, Kelly PJ, Hoffman DL, Bordier P. The treatment of osteoporosis with disodium ethane-1-hydroxy-1, 1-diphosphonate. *J Lab Clin Med* (1971) **78**: 574–84.
97. Boyce BF, Smith L, Fogelman I, Johnston E, Ralston S, Boyle IT. Focal osteomalacia due to low-dose diphosphonate therapy in Paget's disease. *Lancet* (1984) **1**: 821–4.
98. Adamson BB, Gallacher SJ, Byars J, Ralston SH, Boyle IT, Boyce BF. Mineralization defects with pamidronate therapy for Paget's disease. *Lancet* (1993) **342**: 1459–60.
99. Liens D, Delmas PD, Meunier PJ. Long-term effects of intravenous pamidronate in fibrous dysplasia of bone. *Lancet* (1994) **343**: 953–4.
100. Adami S, Bhalla AK, Dorizzi R *et al.* The acute-phase response after bisphosphonate administration. *Calcif Tissue Int* (1987) **41**: 326–31.

15

Management of myeloma bone disease

James R Berenson

Introduction • Biology of myeloma bone disease • Assessment of myeloma bone disease • Treatment of myeloma bone disease • Summary

INTRODUCTION

Multiple myeloma is a malignancy of B-cells characterized by the accumulation of terminally differentiated plasma cells in the bone marrow. Despite sensitivity to a number of chemotherapeutic agents, the median survival of 30 months remains unchanged over the past two decades.[1] The major clinical manifestation of this malignancy is related to the osteolytic bone destruction.[2] Even patients responding to chemotherapy may have progression of skeletal disease,[3,4] and recalcification of osteolytic lesions is rare. The bone disease can lead to pathologic fractures, spinal cord compression, hypercalcemia, and pain, and is a major cause of morbidity and mortality in these patients.[5] These patients frequently require radiation therapy or surgery. These complications result from asynchronous bone turnover wherein increased osteoclastic bone resorption is not accompanied by a comparable increase in bone formation. The increase in osteoclast activity in multiple myeloma is mediated by the release of osteoclast-stimulating factors.[6,7] These factors are produced locally in the bone marrow microenvironment by cells of both tumor nontumor origin.[7,8] Bisphosphonates are specific inhibitors of osteoclastic activity and are effective in the treatment of hypercalcemia associated with malignancies.[9–11] These agents have been evaluated alone and as adjunctive therapy to primary anti-cancer treatment in patients with cancers involving the bone, including multiple myeloma.[12–16] Bisphosphonates have been evaluated in several large randomized trials in myeloma patients also receiving chemotherapy. Oral etidronate given daily showed no clinical benefit,[3] while the use of oral clodronate daily has produced variable clinical results in three randomized trials.[12,17] Oral administration of pamidronate was ineffective in reducing the skeletal complications of these patients.[18] A large randomized double-blind study was conducted in which Stage III multiple myeloma patients received either pamidronate (90 mg) or placebo as a 4-hour infusion every 4 weeks for 21 cycles in addition to anti-myeloma chemotherapy.[19,20] This intravenously administered bisphosphonate significantly reduced the development of skeletal complications. Although survival was not different between the pamidronate group and placebo group overall, patients receiving pamidronate who had failed first-line chemotherapy lived longer than those receiving placebo. The patients who received pamidronate also had significant decreases in bone pain, did not increase analgesic usage unlike the placebo group, and showed a better quality of life. Ongoing studies are evaluating newer more potent bisphosphonates.

BIOLOGY OF MYELOMA BONE DISEASE

Much progress has been made over the past few years to define the biological basis of bone loss in myeloma patients better. Using bone histomorphometry, increased bone resorption with both increased eroded surfaces and mean erosion depth has been clearly demonstrated in myeloma patients.[21,22] This excessive bone resorption has been shown to occur in the proximity of the tumor cells themselves even in patients without obvious lytic bone disease.[23] Patients in remission and the uninvolved marrow of patients with solitary plasmacytomas do not show this excessive bone resorption.[8] This observation suggests the importance of the bone marrow microenvironment in leading to the local destruction of myeloma bone, and that this may be mediated by a direct intercellular means as well as local release of bone-resorbing factors. Even patients presenting with early myeloma show this phenomenon. In patients with monoclonal gammopathy of undetermined significance (MGUS), the presence of increased bone resorption is associated with a greater likelihood of developing overt multiple myeloma.[24] Although osteoclast size appears to be normal in these patients, there appears to be increased recruitment, survival, and activation of these cells.[25]

Obviously, enhanced osteoclastic activity would not be associated with enhanced bone loss if there was not an accompanied loss in bone formation.[8,23] This uncoupling bone process (i.e. increased bone resorption in the presence of a reduction in bone formation) is the hallmark of multiple myeloma patients with osteolytic bone disease. Interestingly, in the one fourth of patients who present without these lesions, this uncoupling process has not been observed.[26] These patients often have both enhanced bone resorption and bone formation. In addition, osteocalcin, a marker of bone formation activity, has been shown to be decreased in patients with lytic bone disease whereas those patients without evidence of lytic disease had higher osteocalcin levels.[27] In support of the important relationship of bone disease to overall outcome in these patients, serum osteocalcin levels have been shown to be inversely related to survival.[28]

Bone-resorbing factors

The landmark studies of Mundy and colleagues suggested the presence of osteoclast activating factors in the supernatants derived from cultures of both human myeloma cell lines and freshly obtained myeloma bone marrow.[29] Although early work suggested that interleukin-1β (IL-1β) and lymphotoxin (tumor necrosis factor (TNF) β) were these factors, other factors have been implicated from more recent studies including interleukin-6 (IL-6), transforming growth factor-β (TGF-β), macrophage colony stimulating factor (M-CSF), hepatocyte growth factor (HGF), metalloproteinases (MMPs), as well as not yet fully characterized novel proteins (Alsina) (Table 15.1).

IL-1β

Controversy exists as to the importance of IL-1β in myeloma bone resorption as well as the cells which produce this cytokine in the myeloma microenvironment. Although IL-1β is clearly increased in supernatants from unseparated fresh myeloma bone marrow samples,[30] recent attempts to determine whether the malignant cells themselves were producing this factor have produced conflicting results.[31–35] The role of IL-1β in stimulating bone resorption has been shown in some studies using bone organ cultures, and this activity has been blocked by antibodies to this cytokine.[31–33] The inhibitors of IL-1β function, the soluble IL-1 receptor and IL-1 receptor antagonist, have been shown to be able completely to inhibit the bone resorption generated by supernatants derived from unfractionated myeloma bone marrow.[36] However, other workers have not confirmed the importance of IL-1β in stimulating bone resorption in myeloma patients.[37]

Table 15.1 Cytokines in myeloma bone disease

Cytokine	Source	Effect on:		
		Growth	Apoptosis	Bone disease
IL-1β	stroma/?tumor			+++
TNFα	stroma			+
IL-6	stroma/occ tumor	++	—	+
HGF	tumor	++		++
TGF-β	stroma			+
M-CSF	?			+
MMPs	stroma/tumor			+
Sydecan-1	tumor	—	+	—

TNFs
Early studies suggested that lymphotoxin was the important factor in enhancing bone resorption in these patients.[31,38] However, more recent studies have failed to confirm these initial studies, and have not even shown increased secretion of this cytokine from bone marrow cells derived from these patients.[30] TNFα has been shown to be an important bone-resorbing cytokine,[7] and has been found in increased amounts in the supernatants from unfractionated myeloma bone marrow,[30] and recent studies have also suggested its production by the malignant cells.[35] The importance of this cytokine in stimulating myeloma bone resorption remains to be determined.

IL-6
IL-6 has been shown to be a critical factor in stimulating growth and preventing apoptosis of the malignant cells in myeloma.[39] Although early studies suggested IL-6 was produced by tumor cells in myeloma,[40] most studies have shown that IL-6 is highly produced by the bone marrow stromal cells and its production is enhanced by adhesion of tumor cells.[41] In addition, this cytokine has been shown to play a major role in bone disease.[42] IL-6 has been shown to inhibit bone formation.[43] IL-6 stimulates the development of osteoclasts[42] but also has been shown to promote osteoblasts. Interestingly, IL-6 is produced in large quantities by both these cell types.[42,44] The use of anti-IL-6 antibodies clinically has demonstrated the importance of this cytokine in stimulating bone loss in myeloma patients.[45] It has also been shown that both IL-1 and TNF stimulate IL-6,[46] and that IL-6 is capable of synergizing with IL-1 in the stimulation of osteoclasts.[47] In addition to IL-6, its soluble receptor, GP180, also is important in this process. Specifically, when GP180, which is present in large amounts in the myeloma bone marrow, becomes associated with IL-6, it stimulates myeloma growth[48] as well as osteoclast formation.[49] Thus, IL-6 and its soluble receptor GP180 together provide dual roles in both increasing tumor burden as well as bone loss in myeloma patients.

TGF-β
Recently, TGF-β has been shown to be produced by both the tumor cells and stromal cells in myeloma bone marrow.[50] Recently, this cytokine has been shown to play an important role in the pathogenesis of metastatic bone disease in breast cancer.[51] The cytokine in the bone milieu is capable of stimulating parathyroid thyroid hormone releasing peptide (PTHRP) release from breast cancer cells which in turn stimulates bone resorption and more TGF-β release from

the bone microenvironment. In myeloma, TGF-β has been shown to stimulate IL-6 production by tumor cells and stromal cells which may similarly enhance bone resorption in addition to stimulating tumor growth.[50]

Other factors

M-CSF is present in increased amounts in the serum of myeloma patients and correlates with tumor load.[52,53] This cytokine is capable of attracting osteoclast precursors as well as enhancing survival of osteoclasts.[54–56] A recent study has shown that HGF is produced by myeloma cells[57] and higher serum levels portend a poor outcome.[58] This protein is a potent stimulator of bone resorption.[59,60] MMPs have been shown to have an increasingly important role in stimulating bone resorption because their inhibitors, called TIMPs, can prevent bone resorption.[61–63] Specifically, MMP-9 has been shown to be expressed by the tumor cells in myeloma patients whereas the bone marrow stromal cells produce MMP-1 and MMP-2.[64] In addition, coculture of stromal cells with myeloma cells upregulates MMP-1 secretion.[64] These specific MMPs have been shown to play a critical role in directly degrading matrix and promoting metastasis.[65]

Syndecan-1, a heparan sulfate proteoglycan, has recently been shown to be expressed on the surface of myeloma cells.[66] This molecule is actively released from the cell surface of the tumor cells, and has been demonstrated both to reduce tumor burden as well as bone destruction in animal and *in vitro* myeloma models.[66,67] Syndecan-1 inhibits osteoclast differentiation while stimulating osteoblast formation, and SCID mice injected with the human myeloma cell line ARH-77 transfected with this gene were less likely to develop lytic bone disease.[67]

ASSESSMENT OF MYELOMA BONE DISEASE

Plain radiographs and bone scans

Because the major clinical manifestations of myeloma are related to bone disease, the impor-

Table 15.2 Assessing myeloma bone disease

- Plain radiographs – skeletal survey
- Bone scan
- Magnetic resonance imaging
- Bone densitometry
- ^{99m}Tc-MIBI scan (experimental)
- Bone resorption markers: pyridinoline, deoxypyridinoline, ICTP, N-telopeptide
- Bone formation markers: alkaline phosphatase, osteocalcin, PINP

ICTP = C-terminal telopeptide of Type I collagen; PINP = amino-terminal propeptide of Type I procollagen.

tance of assessing its status cannot be overestimated. A variety of techniques have been used to evaluate myeloma patients' bone disease (Table 15.2). Early detection of lesions at risk of fracture or that could lead to cord compression allows prompt use of prophylactic surgery or radiotherapy. In addition, determination of changes in bone disease is an important part of assessing the patient's response to systemic treatment. The gold standard has been the use of plain radiographs of the skull, spine, pelvis, and long bones of the upper and lower extremities. One study has suggested that patients without either osteoporosis or lytic bone disease have the worst survival whereas patients with minimal lytic changes have the longest survival.[68] Although older studies suggest that the lytic lesions which make up myeloma bones are not well demonstrated using bone scans,[69,70] recent studies suggest that this modality may be useful especially in lesions in the ribs, vertebral bodies, and sternum.[71] On the other hand, the skull, extremities, and pelvic bones were better evaluated with plain radiographs in this study. In most cases, bone scans are really unnecessary as part of the routine evaluation of myeloma bone disease.

Bone histomorphometry

Although bone histomorphometry may be effective in assessing the extent of bone loss at individual sites,[8] its usefulness is limited by both the invasiveness of the procedure and the heterogeneous nature of bone involvement in these patients. The expertise of an experienced bone pathologist is required for interpretation of the results.

Bone densitometry

In order to gain a better idea of general bone status in these patients, use of dual energy X-ray absorptiometry (DEXA) has now been evaluated in some centers.[72,73] This technique has clearly provided important information in patients with osteoporosis with respect to risk of fractures and response to therapeutic interventions.[74] Early studies in myeloma patients have shown marked bone loss, and have suggested that changes in bone density correlate with clinical stage and risk of fractures.[72,73] Although treatment with oral glucocorticoids effectively lowers tumor burden in these patients, its use has also been shown to be associated with loss of bone mineral density.[73] DEXA has recently been used to assess changes in bone density in myeloma patients treated with bisphosphonates, and show marked increases in patients receiving intravenous pamidronate alone as their anti-myeloma therapy in an ongoing Phase II trial.[75] Whether it will be predictive of the efficacy of bisphosphonate treatment or of the risk of developing skeletal complications during the course of an individual's disease remains to be determined.

Magnetic resonance imaging (MRI)

MRI techniques have become increasingly used in assessing myeloma patients. These procedures are much more sensitive in detecting lesions which are not identified by plain radiographs. In the small subset of patients (approximately 20%) with normal MRI scans, the clinical features suggest earlier stage disease and the prognosis appears to be better.[76] When the MRI scan is abnormal, it generally demonstrates three patterns including diffuse involvement without the appearance of normal marrow signal, nodular or focal areas of replacement of normal marrow, or multiple tiny areas of replacement.[77] Studies demonstrate that patients with diffuse involvement have the worst outlook, with decreased hemoglobin and increased plasma cell loads.[76] Recent studies by Moulopoulos *et al.* show that MRI may be particularly useful in determining which patients with early myeloma will develop active disease.[78] Approximately 2% of patients with plasma cell dyscrasias present with a solitary bony lesion. Although radiotherapy may effectively eliminate this tumor, most patients eventually develop multiple myeloma.[79] It is in these patients that MRI may be especially useful in predicting outcome. The presence of other bone lesions on the MRI scan is associated with an earlier progression to multiple myeloma than in those patients without other abnormalities.[80] However, no studies have shown that additional interventions at the time of diagnosis in this group of patients changes the clinical outcome for these individuals.

In patients with more advanced myeloma, MRI is particularly useful in the evaluation of spinal cord compression but its role as a routine procedure in these patients has not been well established. However, the presence of more than 10 focal lesions or diffuse involvement in the spine predicted the earlier development of vertebral compression fractures in these patients.[81,82] Other studies, on the other hand, show a lack of correlation between MRI-identified lesions and risk of vertebral fractures.[83]

With the increasing use of MRI in evaluating myeloma patients at diagnosis, the modality has also been used to assess response to treatment. Despite effective chemotherapy, most MRI scans remain abnormal although there does appear to be some improvement in their appearance in responding patients.[81,84] However, until the cost of this procedure is reduced, it is unlikely to gain widespread use in the routine follow-up of myeloma patients.

Other radionuclide scans

Recently, a new radionuclide tracer has been shown to predict overall disease status in these patients. Patterns of uptake of the tracer, technetium-99m 2-methoxyisobutylisonitrile (^{99m}Tc-MIBI), have been shown useful in predicting the stage of disease and current clinical status of myeloma patients.[85,86]

Markers of bone resorption and bone formation

A variety of markers of bone resorption and formation have been used to assess bone disease in myeloma patients. Patients with multiple myeloma show the expected increases in bone resorption markers such as C-terminal telopeptide of Type I collagen, pyridinoline and deoxypyridinoline and decreases in bone formation markers such as osteocalcin.[27,28,87,88] In addition, a decrease in osteocalcin level or higher ICTP (C-terminal telopeptide of Type I collagen) concentrations predict a shortened survival in myeloma. In a recent placebo-controlled randomized Finnish clinical trial involving oral clodronate,[89] higher baseline levels of the amino-terminal propeptide of Type I procollagen (PINP) – a product of growing osteoblasts – ICTP, and alkaline phosphatase (AP) were associated with a worse survival. PINP and ICTP levels decreased dramatically during clodronate treatment. Similarly, treatment with oral risedronate reduced urinary pyridinoline/creatinine and deoxypyridinoline/creatinine ratios as well as the bone formation markers AP and osteocalcin plasma levels.[90] Monthly administration of intravenous pamidronate is also associated with a decrease in both bone resorption and bone formation markers.[16] In the Finnish clodronate trial, a decrease in these markers during clodronate therapy was associated with a better survival. In current clinical trials evaluating newer bisphosphonates, it is being determined whether baseline values or changes in these markers predict for either the development of new skeletal complications or whether these agents will be clinically effective in individual cases.

TREATMENT OF MYELOMA BONE DISEASE

Until the early 1950s, radiotherapy and surgery were the only treatment modalities available to the myeloma patient. Although both modalities could effectively palliate the majority of patients, these interventions had little impact on the overall course of the disease. With the development of effective chemotherapy, the role of these other modalities became of secondary importance in the overall management of the myeloma patient. With the recent use of hemibody irradiation, total body irradiation, and bone-seeking radionuclides as part of high-dose therapy regimens, radiation treatment may become recognized as an important part of the systemic management of these patients' disease.

The treatment of bone disease in these patients has been greatly changed by the effective use of bisphosphonates. These drugs have become part of standard treatment for myeloma patients with bony involvement.

Radiation therapy

Early studies showed the exquisite sensitivity of myeloma cells to irradiation.[91] This treatment modality may be curative in some patients with solitary plasmacytoma of bone or extramedullary sites although the majority of these patients will eventually progress to multiple myeloma. Most patients with multiple myeloma will require radiotherapy at some time in the course of their disease. The most common indication for radiotherapy is a painful lesion.[92,93] The vast majority of patients achieved pain relief with local radiotherapy at a dose of approximately 3000 cGy given in 10–15 fractions.[91] Occasional patients with more extensive bone pain may benefit from more extensive hemibody irradiation.[94,95] Other indications for radiotherapy may include treatment of impending or actual pathologic fractures, spinal cord compression, tumor, causing local neurologic problems, and large soft-tissue plasma cell tumours.[93] Approximately 10% of patients with multiple myeloma will develop spinal cord compression and the immediate use of systemic glucocorticosteroids and radiotherapy is important to prevent the development of a permanent neurological deficit. Radiotherapy has also been evaluated in preventing the development of new vertebral fractures in myeloma patients with neurologic complications.[96] In this small nonrandomized study, there was some suggestion that fewer vertebral fractures occurred in irradiated vertebrae than in nonirradiated ones as assessed by MRI. However, caution must be used in the application of radiotherapy since this will result in permanent bone marrow damage in the treated areas. The importance of this point cannot be overemphasized in a patient whose overall clinical status depends upon chemotherapeutic agents which cause loss of bone marrow function. A recently published study showed that radiation of the entire shaft of the long bone is probably not necessary in most cases.[97] Even in the few cases showing recurrence outside the previously irradiated field, palliation with radiotherapy was effective.

Surgery

Surgical intervention may be required in patients with an impending or actual fracture or a destabilized spine. Several recent reports suggest that this modality is underutilized in myeloma patients with either long bone or vertebral fractures. In some patients, the presence of myeloma not evident radiographically in areas adjacent to the surgical site may impede the success of the procedure. Most patients also require radiotherapy in conjunction with the surgical procedure. Importantly, consideration must be given to the patient's overall clinical status in decisions regarding the timing of surgery.

Drug therapy

Earlier attempts to reduce the skeletal complications of myeloma involving large randomized trials with sodium fluoride either alone or in combination with calcium, and androgenic steroids, proved unsuccessful.[4,98,99] In addition, gallium nitrate was evaluated in one published study which suggested both a decrease in bone pain and loss of total body calcium with this treatment but this trial was open label involving only 13 patients.[100]

Bisphosphonates

Most of the recent studies have evaluated whether a variety of bisphosphonates administered either orally or intravenously have an impact on skeletal disease as well as its clinical manifestations. Bisphosphonates are specific inhibitors of osteoclastic activity and are effective in the treatment of hypercalcemia associated with malignancies.[10,11]

Pharmacology of bisphosphonates

Pyrophosphates are natural compounds which contain two phosphonate groups bound to a common oxygen and are potent inhibitors of bone resorption *in vitro*. However, when used *in vivo*, this compound is readily hydrolyzed and ineffective at reducing bone resorption.[10,11] By simply substituting the oxygen with a carbon, the molecule becomes resistant to hydrolysis and yet remains active as an inhibitor of bone resorption. With the carbon substitution, these synthetic compounds known as bisphosphonates contain two additional chains of variable structure (called R_1 and R_2) which have given rise to a large number of different drugs (Fig. 15.1). Most bisphosphonates contain a hydroxyl group at R_1 which allows high affinity for calcium crystals and bone mineral. Marked differences in anti-resorptive potency result from differences at the R_2 site.

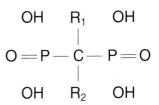

Fig. 15.1 Backbone chemical structure of a bisphosphonate

Table 15.3 Randomized long-term studies of bisphosphonates in multiple myeloma

Drug	No. of patients[a]	Dose	Route	Duration	SEs	Fx	RT	Lesions	Pain	QOL	Survival	Ref.
Etidronate[b]	166	5 mg/kg/d	PO	until death	0	0	NE	NE	0	NE	–	3
Clodronate[b]	336	2400 mg/d	PO	24 months	0	0	NE	+	0	0	0	12
Clodronate[c]	157	1600 mg/d	PO	12 months	0	0	NE	0	+	0	0	17
Clodronate[b]	536	1600 mg/d	PO	until prognosis	0	+	0	NE	+/0	+/0	0	101
Pamidronate[b]	300	300 mg/d	PO	until death	0	0	0	NE	+/0	0	0	18
Pamidronate[b]	377	90 mg/4 wk	IV	21 months	+	+	+	0	+	+	+	19,20

a = number of patients randomized; b = placebo controlled; c = no placebo used in control arm.
PO = by mouth; IV = intravenously; SEs = skeletal events; Fx = pathological fractures; RT = radiation therapy; QOL = quality of life.
0 = no significant difference; – = worse in bisphosphonate group; + = better in bisphosphonate group; NE = not evaluated.

These drugs are poorly absorbed orally (usually < 1%) and are also poorly tolerated orally with significant gastrointestinal toxicity, particularly esophagitis and esophageal ulcers. The bisphosphonates are almost exclusively eliminated through renal excretion and significant nephrotoxicity can occur with these compounds. Because bisphosphonates have high affinity for bone mineral, the drug is highly concentrated in bone. Once the drug becomes a part of the bone, which is not remodeling, it is biologically inactive. As a result, continued administration of bisphosphonates is required to achieve the desired lasting inhibition of bone resorption.

Bisphosphonates in myeloma bone disease
These agents have been evaluated alone and as adjunctive therapy to primary anti-cancer treatment in patients with cancers involving the bone including multiple myeloma.[3,10–20] Recent large placebo-controlled clinical trials have shown the efficacy of bisphosphonates in reducing skeletal complications in myeloma patients, and suggested that these agents may also alter the overall course of the disease.

Although early studies involving bisphosphonates in myeloma patients suggested a reduction in bone pain and healing of lytic lesions, the trials involved relatively few patients.[13,14] Six large randomized trials of long-term bisphosphonate use have now been published (Table 15.3), and involved the use of either the first-generation bisphosphonates etidronate or clodronate or the second-generation aminobisphosphonate pamidronate.[12,17–20,101]

Etidronate
In the Canadian study involving etidronate,[3] 173 newly diagnosed patients all received intermittent oral melphalan and prednisone as primary chemotherapy, and 166 were then randomized to receive either daily oral etidronate (5 mg/kg) or placebo until death or stopping the treatment die to side-effects. Although significant height loss occurred in both placebo and etidronate-

treated patients, no difference was found between the two arms. Similarly, the other outcome measures (new fractures, hypercalcemic episodes, and bone pain) showed no differences between the two arms. Survival was actually worse in patients receiving etidronate.

Clodronate

In a small study involving only 13 patients, use of daily oral clodronate was associated with a reduction in bone pain and lack of progression of bone lesions in contrast to the clinical deterioration which occurred in the patients treated with placebo.[102] Histomorphometric analysis of bone biopsies showed decreases in osteoclast numbers with clodronate treatment whereas patients receiving placebo showed a slight increase in these cells. Intravenously administered clodronate was evaluated in a randomized Italian study which involved only 30 patients with active bone disease.[103] There was a reduction in new lytic lesions and pathological fractures with the bisphosphonate therapy.

Three large randomized trials have been published using oral clodronate in myeloma patients. In the Finnish trial,[12] 350 previously untreated patients were entered, and 336 randomized to receive either clodronate (2.4 g) or placebo daily for 2 years. All patients were also treated with intermittent oral melphalan and prednisolone. Only a little more than half of patients had radiographs completed at both study entry and 2 years. Given this limitation, the proportion of patients with progression of lytic lesions was less in the clodronate-treated group (12%) than in the placebo group (24%). However, the progression of overall pathological fractures, as well as both vertebral and nonvertebral fractures, was not different between the arms. In addition, the number of patients developing hypercalcemia was similar in the two arms. Changes in pain index and use of analgesics were similar in both arms.

Clodronate has also been evaluated in an open-label randomized German trial.[101] In this study, 170 previously untreated patients were randomized to receive either no bisphosphonate or oral clodronate (1.6 g) daily for 1 year. All patients were also treated with intermittent intravenous melphalan and oral prednisone. Unfortunately, premature termination occurred in more than half of the patients despite the short length of the study (1 year). The results showed no difference in progression of bone disease as assessed by plain radiographs in the two arms. However, there was a trend toward a reduction in the number of new progressive sites in the clodronate-treated group after 6 and 12 months although this did not reach statistical significance. Although patients without pain and those not using analgesics were higher in number in the clodronate group, the open-label design of his trial makes it difficult to interpret these findings.

Recently, the Medical Research Council (MRC) has published the results of a large randomized trial involving 536 recently diagnosed myeloma patients randomized to receive either oral clodronate 1.6 g or placebo daily in addition to alkylator-based chemotherapy.[17] The primary end-points of the trial were unclear. However, after combining the proportion of patients developing either nonvertebral fractures or severe hypercalcemia, including those leaving the trial due to severe hypercalcemia, there were fewer clodronate-treated patients experiencing these combined events than placebo patients. However, the number of patients developing hypercalcemia was similar between the two arms. The number of patients experiencing nonvertebral fractures was lower in the clodronate group. Although vertebral fractures reportedly occurred in significantly fewer clodronate-treated patients than placebo patients, only half of patients obtained at least one post-baseline radiograph. Back pain and poor performance status were not significantly different between the two groups except at one time point (24 months). The proportion of patients requiring radiotherapy was similar between the two arms. There was no difference in time to first skeletal event or overall survival.

Pamidronate

In multiple myeloma patients, results of small open-label trials lasting up to 24 months

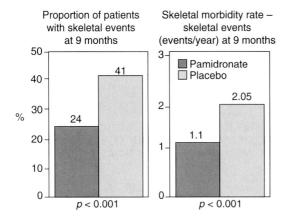

Fig. 15.2 Time to first skeletal-related event and a mean number of skeletal events/year in multiple myeloma patients treated with intravenous pamidronate or placebo (intent-to-treat patients)

suggested that pamidronate disodium might be effective in reducing skeletal complications of multiple myeloma.[13,14] Thus, a large, randomized, double-blind study was conducted to determine whether monthly 90 mg infusions of pamidronate compared to placebo for 21 months reduced skeletal events in patients with multiple myeloma who were receiving chemotherapy.[19,20]

This study included 392 patients with Durie–Salmon Stage III multiple myeloma and at least one osteolytic lesion. Unlike the etidronate and clodronate trials, which involved untreated patients, patients were required to receive an unchanged chemotherapy regimen for at least 2 months before enrollment. Patients were stratified according to their anti-myeloma therapy at trial entry: stratum 1, first-line chemotherapy; stratum 2, second-line or greater chemotherapy. The primary end-point, skeletal events (pathologic fractures, spinal cord compression associated with vertebral compression fracture, surgery to treat or prevent pathologic fracture or spinal cord compression associated with vertebral compression fracture, or radiation to bone), and secondary end-points (hypercalcemia, bone pain, analgesic drug use, performance status, and quality of life), were assessed monthly. Importantly, although the chemotherapeutic regimen was not uniform at study entry, the types and numbers of chemotherapeutic regimens in the two groups were similar at study entry and during the trial.

At the preplanned primary end-point after nine cycles of therapy,[10] the proportion of myeloma patients having any skeletal event was 41% in patients receiving placebo but only 24% in pamidronate-treated patients (Fig. 15.2). In

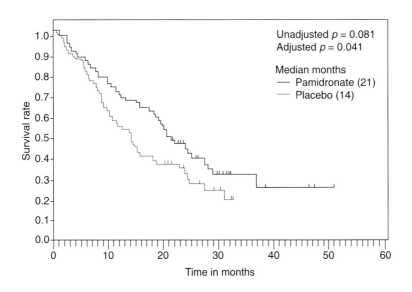

Fig. 15.3 Kaplan–Meier estimates of survival in stratum 2 patients with multiple myeloma treated with intravenous pamidronate or placebo. Survival was measured from randomization date to 1 February 1995. There was a median survival of 21 and 14 months in pamidronate ($n = 66$) and placebo ($n = 65$) patients, respectively. Log-rank test was adjusted for ECOG performance status and beta 2-microglobulin, which were the only two prognostic variables significantly influencing survival.

addition, the number of skeletal events/year was half in the patients treated with pamidronate. The proportion of pamidronate-treated patients with skeletal events was lower in both stratum 1 (first-line therapy) and stratum 2 (≥ second-line therapy). The patients who received pamidronate also had significant decreases in bone pain, no increase in analgesic usage, and showed no deterioration in performance status and quality of life at the end of 9 months. In contrast, patients receiving placebo showed increases in bone pain and analgesic use and deterioration in both performance status and quality of life. Similar to the results after nine cycles of therapy, the proportions of patients developing any skeletal event and the skeletal morbidity rate continued to remain significantly lower in the pamidronate group than the placebo group during the additional 12 cycles of treatment.[16] However, there were no differences between the treatment groups in the percentage of patients with healing or progression of osteolytic lesions. Although overall survival in all patients was not significantly different between the two treatment groups, in stratum 2 the median survival time was 21 months for pamidronate patients compared to 14 months for placebo patients (Fig. 15.3).

In a double-blind randomized trial, a Danish–Swedish co-operative group evaluated daily oral pamidronate (300 mg/day) compared to placebo in 300 newly diagnosed myeloma patients also receiving intermittent melphalan and prednisone.[18] After a median duration of 18 months, there was no significant reduction in the primary end-point defined as skeletal-related morbidity (bone fracture, surgery for impending fracture, vertebral collapse, or increase in number and/or size of lytic lesions), hypercalcemic episodes, or survival between the arms. Fewer episodes of severe pain and less height loss were observed in the oral pamidronate-treated patients, however.

SUMMARY

These results show that the benefit of adjunctive use of bisphosphonates in addition to chemotherapy is superior to chemotherapy alone in patients with Stage III multiple myeloma with respect to bone complications. Bisphosphonate treatment should now be considered for all patients with multiple myeloma and at least one osteolytic lesion. The three large randomized studies with clodronate show inconsistent results with oral administration of this first-generation bisphosphonate.[12,17,101] Curiously, the Finnish trial using a larger daily dose[12] shows less effect than the

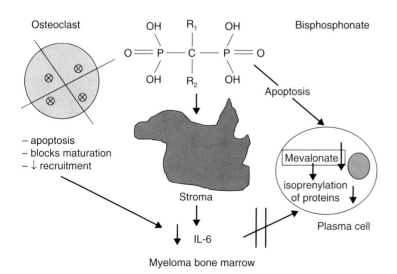

Fig. 15.4 Possible mechanisms of the anti-tumor effect of bisphosphonates in myeloma bone marrow

MRC trial using a smaller amount of clodronate.[17] In addition, in the latter trial, although the drug had some effect on reducing fractures and severe hypercalcemia in these patients, the drug did not affect the time to first skeletal event or use of radiotherapy. Similarly, oral pamidronate has not been effective either.[18] Given the clinical results and the poor tolerability of oral agents, this route of administration for bisphosphonates is unlikely to be of much benefit in these patients. Clearly, intravenous pamidronate both reduces the skeletal complications and improves the quality of life of these patients.[19,20] Although 90 mg monthly is efficacious, the optimal duration and dose of pamidronate are unknown, but patients should receive at least 21 months of treatment based on the results of the published trial. Whether this drug is effective in earlier-stage disease or in patients without bone disease is unknown. The role of this agent in myeloma may go beyond simply inhibiting bone resorption and the resulting skeletal complications. Some studies suggest the drug may have an antimyeloma effect either directly or indirectly (Fig. 15.4). Using the murine 5T2 multiple myeloma mode, Radl and colleagues suggested that pamidronate may reduce tumor burden in treated mice.[104] Recent *in vitro* studies also suggest pamidronate may possess anti-myeloma properties as demonstrated by its ability to induce apoptosis of myeloma cells[105,106] and to suppress the production of IL-6 (an important myeloma growth factor) by bone marrow stromal cells from myeloma patients.[107] A recent *in vitro* study may help explain the induction of apoptosis by these compounds.[108] These drugs inhibit the mevalonate pathway and, as a result, decrease the isoprenylation of proteins such as ras.[102] In addition to the survival advantage observed in relapsing patients in the large randomized Berenson *et al.* trial,[20] two myeloma patients treated with pamidronate alone were recently reported to show reductions in myeloma tumor cell burden.[109] Current ongoing trials involving higher doses of pamidronate given to patients in relapse without chemotherapy may provide further clinical evidence for the anti-tumor effect of these agents.[75]

Third-generation bisphosphonates (e.g. zoledronate and ibandronate), which appear to be more than 100 times more potent than second-generation aminobisphosphonates, have recently entered clinical trials. Very small doses of these agents effectively restore normocalcemia in patients with tumor-induced hypercalcemia.[110] This newer class of drugs may not only be more effective in palliating the devastating effects of bone disease in these patients but may hold the promise of being able to improve the overall survival of these patients while maintaining their quality of life.

REFERENCES

1. Alexanian RH, Dimopoulos MA. Management of multiple myeloma. *Semin Hematol* (1995) **32**: 20–30.
2. Mundy GR, Bertoline DR. Bone destruction and hypercalcemia in plasma cell myeloma. *Semin Oncol* (1986) **13**: 291–9.
3. Belch AR, Bergsagel DE, Wilson K *et al*. Effect of daily etidronate on the osteolysis of multiple myeloma. *J Clin Oncol* (1991) **9**: 1397–402.
4. Kyle RA, Jowsey J, Kelly PJ *et al*. Multiple myeloma bone disease. The comparative effect of sodium fluoride and calcium carbonate or placebo. *N Engl J Med* (1975) **293**: 1334–8.
5. Kyle RA. Multiple myeloma, review of 869 cases. *Mayo Clin Proc* (1975) **50**: 29–40.
6. Stashenko P, Dewhirst FE, Peros WJ *et al*. Synergistic interactions between interleukin 1, tumor necrosis factor, and lymphotoxin in bone resorption. *J Immunol* (1987) **138**: 1464–8.
7. Mundy GR. Mechanisms of osteolytic bone destruction. *Bone* (1991) **12 (Suppl 1)**: S1–S6.
8. Bataille R, Chappard D, Basle M. Excessive bone resorption in human plasmacytomas: direct induction by tumor cells *in vivo*. *Br J Haematol* (1995) **90**: 721–4.
9. Coleman RE, Purohit OP. Osteoclast inhibition for the treatment of bone metastases. *Cancer Treat Rev* (1993) **19**: 79–103.

10. Kanis JA, McCloskey EV, Taube T et al. Rationale for the use of bisphosphonates in bone metastases. Bone (1991) **12 (Suppl 1)**: S13–S18.
11. Fleisch H. Bisphosphonates: a new class of drugs in diseases of bone and calcium metabolism. In Brunner KW, Fleisch H, Senn H-J (eds) Recent Results in Cancer Research. Vol. 116. Bisphosphonates and Tumor Osteolysis (Berlin and Heidelberg: Springer-Verlag, 1989): 1–28.
12. Lahtinen R, Laakso M, Palva I et al. Randomized, placebo-controlled multicentre trial of clodronate in multiple myeloma. Lancet (1992) **340**: 1049–52.
13. Man Z, Otero AB, Rendo P et al. Use of pamidronate for multiple myeloma osteolytic lesions. Lancet (1990) **335**: 663.
14. Thiebaud D, Leyuraz S, Von Fliedner V et al. Treatment of bone metastases from breast cancer and myeloma with pamidronate. Eur J Cancer (1991) **27**: 37–41.
15. Purohit OP, Anthony C, Radstone CR et al. High-dose intravenous pamidronate for metastatic bone pain. Br J Cancer (1994) **70**: 554–8.
16. van Holten-Verzantvoort AATM, Kroon HM, Bijvoet OLM et al. Palliative treatment in patients with bone metastases from breast cancer. J Clin Oncol (1993) **11**: 491–8.
17. McCloskey EV, MacLennan CM, Drayson MT et al. A randomized trial of the effect of clodronate on skeletal morbidity in multiple myeloma. Br J Haematol (1998) **101**: 317–25.
18. Brincker H, Westin J, Abildgarrd et al. Failure of oral pamidronate to reduce skeletal morbidity in multiple myeloma: a double-blind placebo-controlled trial. Br J Haematol (1998) **101**: 280–6.
19. Berenson JR, Lichtenstein A, Porter L et al. Efficacy of pamidronate in reducing the skeletal events in patients with advanced multiple myeloma. N Engl J Med (1996) **334**: 488–93.
20. Berenson J, Lichtenstein A, Porter L et al. Long-term pamidronate treatment of advanced multiple myeloma patients reduces skeletal events. J Clin Oncol (1998) **16**: 593–602.
21. Bataille R, Chappard D, Alexandre C et al. Importance of quantative histology of bone changes in monoclonal gammapathy. Br J Cancer (1986) **53**: 805–10.
22. Valentin-Opran A, Charhon SA, Meunier PJ et al. Quantitative histology of myeloma-induced bone changes. Br J Haematol (1982) **52**: 601–10.
23. Taube T, Beneton MNC, McCloskey EV et al. Abnormal bone remodelling in patients with myelomatosis and normal biochemical indices of bone resorption. Eur J Haematol (1992) **49**: 192–8.
24. Bataille R, Chappard D, Basle M. Quantifiable excess of bone resorption in monoclonal gammopathy is an early symptom of malignancy: a prospective study of 87 biopsies. Blood (1996) **87**: 4762–9.
25. Chappard D, Rossi JF, Bataille R et al. Cytomorphometry of osteoclasts demonstrates an abnormal population in B-cell malignancies but not in multiple myeloma. Calcif Tissue Int (1991) **48**: 13–17.
26. Bataille R, Chappard D, Marcelli C et al. Mechanism of bone destruction in multiple myeloma. The importance of an unbalanced process in determining the severity of myeloma. J Clin Oncol (1989) **7**: 1909–14.
27. Bataille R, Delmas PD, Chappard D, Sany J. Abnormal serum bone Gla protein levels in myltiple myeloma. Cancer (1990) **66**: 167–72.
28. Carlson K, Ljunghall S, Simonsson B et al. Serum osteocalcin concentrations in patients with multiple myeloma – correlation with disease stage and survival. J Intern Med (1992) **231**: 133–7.
29. Mundy GR, Raisz LG, Cooper RA et al. Evidence for the secretion of an osteoclast stimulating factor in myeloma. N Engl J Med (1974) **291**: 1041–6.
30. Lichtenstein A, Berenson J, Norman D et al. Production of cytokines by bone marrow cells obtained from patients with multiple myeloma. Blood (1989) **74**: 1266–73.
31. Cozzolino F, Torcia M, Aldinucci D et al. Production of interleukin-1 by bone marrow myeloma cells. Blood (1989) **74**: 380–7.
32. Kawano M, Yamamoto I, Iwato K et al. Interleukin-1 beta rather than lymphotoxin as the major bone resorbing activity in human multiple myeloma. Blood (1989) **73**: 1646–9.
33. Yamamoto I, Kawano M, Sone T et al. Production of interleukin-1β, a potent bone resorbing cytokine, by cultured human myeloma cells. Br J Haematol (1989) **49**: 4242–6.
34. Bakkus MHC, Bakel-Van Peer KMJ, Adriaansen HJ et al. Detection of interleukin-1β and interleukin-6 in human multiple myeloma by fluorescent in situ hybridisation. Leuk Lymphoma (1991) **4**: 389–95.
35. Sati HIA, Greaves M, Apperley JF et al. Expression of Il-1β and TNFα mRNA by neoplastic plasma cells, detected by dual colour

fluorescence *in situ* hybridisation. *Bone* (1997) **20 (Suppl)**: 63S.
36. Torcia M, Lucibello M, Vannier E *et al.* Modulation of osteoclast-activating factor activity of multiple myeloma bone marrow bone marrow cells by different interleukin-1 inhibitors. *Exp Hematol* (1996) **24**: 868–74.
37. Alsina M, Boyce B, Devlin RD *et al.* Development of an in vivo model of human multiple myeloma bone disease. *Blood* (1996) **87**: 1495–501.
38. Garrett IR, Durie BGM, Nedwin GE *et al.* Production of lymphotoxin, a bone-resorbing cytokine, by cultured human myeloma cells. *N Engl J Med* (1987) **317**: 526–32.
39. Klein B, Zhang XG, Lu Z-Y, Bataille R. Interleukin-6 in multiple myeloma. *Blood* (1995) **85**: 863–72.
40. Kawano M, Hirano T, Matsuda T *et al.* Autocrine generation and requirement of BSF-2/IL-6 for human multiple myelomas. *Nature* (1988) **332**: 83–5.
41. Uchiyama H, Barut BA, Mohrbacher A *et al.* Adhesion of human myeloma-derived cell lines to bone marrow stroma stimulates IL-6 secretion. *Blood* (1993) **82**: 3712–20.
42. Ishimi Y, Mijaura C, Jin CH *et al.* IL-6 is produced by osteoblasts and induces bone resorption. *J Immunol* (1990) **145**: 3297–303.
43. Hughes FJ, Howells GL. Interleukin-6 inhibits bone formation in vitro. *Bone Miner* (1993) **21**: 21–8.
44. Linkhart TA, Linkhart SG, McCharles DC *et al.* Interleukin-6 messager RNA expression and interleukin-6 protein secretion in cells isolated from normal human bone: regulation by interleukin-1. *J Bone Miner Res* (1991) **6**: 1285–94.
45. Bataille R, Barlogie B, Lu ZY *et al.* Biologic effects of anti-interleukin-6 murine monoclonal antibody in advanced multiple myeloma. *Blood* (1995) **86**: 685–91.
46. Dinarello CA. The biology of interleukin-1 and comparison to tumor necrosis factor. *Immunol Lett* (1987) **16**: 227–32.
47. Lacey DL, Grosso LE, Moser SA *et al.* IL-1-induced murine osteoblast IL-6 production is mediated by the type 1 IL-1 receptor and is increased by 1,25 dihydroxyvitamin D_3. *J Clin Invest* (1993) **91**: 1731–42.
48. Gaillard JP, Bataille R, Brailly H *et al.* Increased and stable levels of functional soluble interleukin-6 receptor in sera of patients with monoclonal gammopathy. *Eur J Immunol* (1993) **23**: 820.
49. Tamura T, Udagawa N, Takahashi N. *et al.* Soluble interleukin-6 receptor triggers osteoclast formation by interleukin-6. *Proc Natl Acad Sci U S A* (1993) **90**: 11 924–8.
50. Urashima M, Ogata A, Chauhan D *et al.* Transforming growth factor-β1: differential effects on multiple myeloma versus normal B cells. *Blood* (1996) **87**: 1928–38.
51. Yoneda T. Cellular and molecular mechanisms of breast and prostate cancer metastasis to bone. *Eur J Cancer* (1998) **34**: 240–25.
52. Nakamura M, Merchav S, Carter A *et al.* Expression of a novel 3–5-kb macrophage colony-stimulating factor transcript in human myeloma cells. *J Immunol* (1989) **143**: 3543–7.
53. Janowska-Wieczorek A, Belch AR, Jacobs A *et al.* Increased circulating colony-stimulating factor-1 in patients with preleukemia, leukemia, and lymphoid malignancies. *Blood* (1991) **77**: 1796–803.
54. MacDonald BR, Mundy GR, Clark S *et al.* Effects of human recombinant CSF-GM and highly purified CSF-1 on the formation of multinucleated cells with osteoclast characteristics in long-term marrow cultures. *J Bone Miner Res* (1986) **1**: 227–33.
55. Sarma U, Flanagan AM. Macrophage colony-stimulating factor induces substantial osteoclast generation and bone resorption in human bone marrow cultures. *Blood* (1996) **88**: 2531–40.
56. Fuller K, Owens JM, Jagger CJ, Wilson A, Moss R, Chambers TJ. Macrophage colony-stimulating factor stimulates survival and chemotactic behaviour in isolated osteoclasts. *J Exp Med* (1993) **189**: 1733–44.
57. Borset M, Hjorth-Hansen H, Seidel C *et al.* Hepatocyte growth factor and its receptor c-Met in multiple myeloma. *Blood* (1996) **88**: 3998–4004.
58. Seidel C, Borset M, Turesson I, Abildgaard N, Sundan A, Waage A. Elevated serum concentrations of hepatocyte growth factor in patients with multiple myeloma. *Blood* (1998) **91**: 806–12.
59. Fuller K, Owens J, Chambers TJ. The effect of hepatocyte growth factor on the behaviour of osteoclasts. *Biochem Biophys Res Commun* (1995) **212**: 334–40.
60. Grano M, Galimi F, Zambonin G *et al.* Hepatocyte growth factor is a coupling factor for osteoclasts in vitro. *Proc Natl Acad Sci U S A* (1996) **93**: 7644–8.
61. Conway JG, Wakefield JA, Brown RH *et al.* Inhibition of cartilage and bone destruction in

adjuvant arthritis in the rat by a matrix metalloproteinase inhibitor. *J Exp Med* (1995) **182**: 449.
62. Hill PA, Docherty AJP, Bottomley KMK *et al*. Inhibition of bone resorption in vitro by selective inhibitors of gelatinase and collagenase. *Biochem J* (1995) **308**: 167.
63. Yoneda T, Sasaki A, Dunstan C *et al*. Inhibition of osteolytic bone metastasis of breast cancer by combined treatment with the bisphosphonate ibandronate and tissue inhibitor of the matrix metalloproteinase-2. *J Clin Invest* (1997) **99**: 2509–17.
64. Barille S, Akhoundi C, Collette M *et al*. Metalloproteinases in multiple myeloma: production of matric metalloproteinase-9 (MMP-9), activation of proMMP-2, and induction of MMP-1 by myeloma cells. *Blood* (1997) **90**: 1649–55.
65. Ray J, Stetler-Stevenson W. Gelatinase A activity modulates melanoma cell adhesion and spreading. *EMBO J* (1995) **19**: 15–29.
66. Ridley RC, Xiao H, Hata H *et al*. Expression of syndecan regulates human myeloma plasma cell adhesion to type I collagen. *Blood* (1993) **81**: 767–74.
67. Dhodapkar MV, Abe E, Theus A *et al*. Syndecan-1 is a multifunctional regulator of myeloma pathobiology: control of tumor cell survival, growth, and bone cell differentiation. *Blood* (1998) **91**: 2679–88.
68. Smith DB, Scarffe JH, Eddelston B. The prognostic significance of X-ray changes at presentation and reassessment in patients with multiple myeloma. *Hematol Oncol* (1988) **6**: 1–6.
69. Bataille R, Chevalier J, Rossi M *et al*. Bone scintigraphy in plasma-cell myeloma. *Radiology* (1982) **145**: 801–4.
70. Woolfenden JM, Pitt MJ, Durie BGM, Moon TE. Comparison of bone scintigraphy and radiography in multiple myeloma. *Radiology* (1980) **134**: 723–8.
71. Agren B, Lonnqvist B, Bjorkstrand B *et al*. Radiography and bone scintigraphy in bone marrow transplant multiple myeloma patients. *Acta Radiologica* (1997) **38**: 144–50.
72. Abildgarrd N, Brixen K, Kristensen JE *et al*. Assessment of bone involvement in patietns with multiple myeloma using bone densitometry. *Eur J Haematol* (1996) **57**: 370–6.
73. Diamond T, Levy S, Day P *et al*. Biochemical, histomorphometric and densitometric changes in patients with multiple myeloma: effects of glucocorticoid therapy and disease activity. *Br J Haematol* (1997) **97**: 641–8.
74. Cummings SR, Black DM, Thompson DE *et al*. Effect of alendronate on risk of fracture in women with low bone density but without vertebral fractures. *JAMA* (1998) **280**: 2077–82.
75. Berenson J, Webb I *et al*. A phase II dose-ranging trial of single-agent pamidronate for relapsed/refractory multiple myeloma. *Blood* (1998) **92**: 107A.
76. Kusumoto S, Jinnai I, Itoh K. Magnetic resonance imaging patterns in patients with multiple myeloma. *Br J Haematol* (1997) **99**: 649–55.
77. Moulopoulos LA, Dimopoulos MA. Magnetic resonance imaging of the bone marrow in hematologic malignancies. *Blood* (1997) **90**: 2127–47.
78. Moulopoulos LA, Dimopoulos MA, Smith TL *et al*. Prognostic significance of magnetic resonance imaging in patients with asymptomatic multiple myeloma. *J Clin Oncol* (1995) **13**: 251–6.
79. Frassica DA, Frassica FJ, Schray MF *et al*. Solitary plasmacytoma of bone: Mayo clinic experience. *Int J Radiat Oncol Biol Phys* (1989) **16**: 43–8.
80. Moulopoulos LA, Dimopoulos MA, Weber D *et al*. Magnetic resonance imaging in the staging of solitary plasmacytoma of bone. *J Clin Oncol* (1993) **11**: 1311–15.
81. Rahmouni A, Divine M, Mathieu D *et al*. MR appearance of multiple myeloma of the spine before and after treatment. *AJR* (1993) **160**: 1053–5.
82. Agren B, Rudberg U, Isberg B *et al*. MR imaging of multiple myeloma patients with bone-marrow transplants. *Acta Radiologica* (1998) **39**: 36–42.
83. Lecouvet FE, Vande Berg BC, Michaux L. Development of vertebral fractures in patients with multiple myeloma: does MRI enable recognition of vertebrae that will collapse? *J Comp Assist Tomog* (1998) **22**: 430–6.
84. Moulopoulos LA, Dimopoulos MA, Alexian R *et al*. Multiple myeloma: MR patterns of response to treatment. *Radiology* (1994) **193**: 441–6.
85. Tirovola EB, Biassoni L, Britton KE *et al*. The use of ^{99m}Tc-MIBI scanning in multiple myeloma. *Br J Cancer* (1996) **74**: 1815–20.
86. Pace L, Catalano L, Pinto A *et al*. Different patterns of technetium-99m sestamibi uptake in multiple myeloma. *Eur J Nucl Med* (1998) **25**: 714–20.
87. Nawawi H, Samson D, Apperley J *et al*.

Biochemical bone markers in patients with multiple myeloma. *Clinica Chimica Acta* (1996) **253**: 61–77.

88. Abildgaard N, Bentzen SM, Nielsen JL *et al*. Serum markers of bone metabolism in multiple myeloma: prognostic significance of the carboxy-terminal telopeptide of type 1 collagen (ICTP). *Br J Haematol* (1997) **96**: 103–10.

89. Elomaa I, Risteli L, Laakso M *et al*. Monitoring the action of clodronate with type I collagen metabolites in multiple myeloma. *Eur J Cancer* (1996) **32A**: 1166–70.

90. Roux C, Ravaud P, Cohen-Solal M *et al*. Biologic, histologic and densitometric effects of oral risedronate on bone in patients with multiple myeloma. *Bone* (1994) **15**: 41–9.

91. Rowell NP, Tobias JS. The role of radiotherapy in the management of multiple myeloma. *Blood Rev* (1991) **5**: 84–9.

92. Bosch A, Frias Z. Radiotherapy in the treatment of multiple myeloma. *Int J Radiat Oncol Biol Phys* (1988) **15**: 1363–9.

93. Adamietz IA, Schober C, Schulte RWM *et al*. Palliative radiotherapy in plasma cell myeloma. *Radiother Oncol* (1991) **20**: 111–16.

94. Rostom AY. A review of the place of radiotherapy in myeloma with emphasis on whole body irradiation. *Hematol Oncol* (1988) **6**: 193–8.

95. Giles FJ, McSweeney EN, Richards JDM *et al*. Prospective randomised study of double hemibody irradiation with and without subsequent maintenance recombinant alpha 2b interferon on survival in patients with relapsed multiple myeloma. *Eur J Cancer* (1992) **28A**: 1392–5.

96. Lecouvet F, Richard F, Vande Berg B *et al*. Long-term effects of localized spinal radiation therapy on vertebral fractures and focal lesions appearance in patients with multiple myeloma. *Br J Haematol* (1997) **96**: 743–5.

97. Catell D, Kogen Z, Donahue B *et al*. Multiple myeloma of an extremity: must the entire bone be treated? *Int J Radiat Oncol Biol Phys* (1998) **40**: 117–19.

98. Cohen HJ, Silberman HR, Tornyos K *et al*. Comparison of two long-term chemotherapy regimens, with or without agents to modify skeletal repair, in multiple myeloma. *Blood* (1984) **63**: 639–48.

99. Acute Leukemia Group B, Eastern Cooperative Oncology Group B. Inffectiveness of fluoride therapy in multiple myeloma. *N Engl J Med* (1972) **286**: 1283–8.

100. Warrell RP, Lovett D, Dilmanian A *et al*. Low-dose gallium nitrate for prevention of osteolysis in myeloma: results of a pilot randomized study. *J Clin Oncol* (1993) **11**: 2443–50.

101. Heim ME, Clemens MR, Queisser W *et al*. Prospective randomized trial of dichloromethylene bisphosphonate (clodronate) in patients with multiple myeloma requiring treatment. A multicenter study. *Onkologie* (1995) **18**: 439–48.

102. Delmas PD, Charhon S, Chapuy MC *et al*. Long-term effects of dichloromethylene diphosphonate (C12MDP) on skeletal lesions in multiple myeloma. *Metab Bone Dis Rel Res* (1982) **4**: 163–8.

103. Merlini G, Parrinello GA, Piccinini L *et al*. Long-term effects of parenteral dichloromethylene bisphosphonate (C12MDP) on bone disease myeloma patients treated with chemotherapy. *Hem Oncol* (1990) **90**: 2127–47.

104. Radl J, Croese JW, Zurcher C *et al*. Influence of treatment with APD-bisphosphonate on the bone lesions in the mouse 5T2 multiple myeloma. *Cancer* (1985) **55**: 1030–40.

105. Aparicio A, Gardner A, Tu Y *et al*. In vitro cytoreductive effects on multiple myeloma cells induced by bisphosphonates. *Leukemia* (1998) **12**: 220–9.

106. Shipman CM, Rogers MJ, Apperley JF *et al*. Bisphosphonates induce apoptosis in human myeloma cell lines: a novel anti-tumour activity. *Br J Haematol* (1997) **98**: 665–72.

107. Savage AD, Belson DJ, Vescio RA *et al*. Pamidronate reduces IL-6 production by bone marrow stroma from multiple myeloma patients. *Blood* (1996) **88**: 105A.

108. Shipman CM, Croucher PI, Russell GG *et al*. The bisphosphonate incadronate (YM175) causes apoptosis of human myeloma cells in vitro by inhibiting the mevalonate pathway. *Cancer Res* (1998) **58**: 5294–7.

109. Dhodapkar MV, Singh J, Mehta J *et al*. Anti-myeloma activity of pamidronate in vivo. *Br J Haematol* (1998) **103**: 530–2.

110. Percherstorfer M, Hermann Z, Body • *et al*. Randomized phase II trial comparing different doses of bisphosphonate ibandronate in the treatment of hypercalcemia of malignancy. *J Clin Oncol* (1996) **14**: 268–76.

16

Bisphosphonates in breast cancer and other solid tumors

Jean-Jaques Body

Why use bisphosphonates in patients with bone metastases from solid tumors? • Mechanisms of action of bisphosphonates • Bisphosphonates in breast cancer • Bisphosphonates in other solid tumors

WHY USE BISPHOSPHONATES IN PATIENTS WITH BONE METASTASES FROM SOLID TUMORS?

The osteotropism of breast and prostate neoplasms is a well known phenomenon although it remains poorly understood. It is interesting to note that both types of neoplasms are hormone-dependent tumors and that, at least for breast cancer, steroid hormone receptor-positive tumors are more likely to develop bone metastases than hormone receptor-negative tumors. The relevance of these clinical observations to the pathophysiology of tumor-induced osteolysis has surprisingly been little studied although it has been shown several years ago that estrogen-receptor positive breast cancer cells in primary culture produce more osteolytic prostaglandins (PGE2 and PGF2a) than estrogen-receptor negative cells.[1]

Deposits into the skeleton can be due to the attraction of tumor cells by chemotactic factors released by the normal and, even more, the pathological remodeling of bone matrix. These factors include fragments of Type I collagen and of osteocalcin, and of several growth factors.[2,3] Moreover, preferential access of prostate cancer cells to the axial skeleton has been attributed to passage through the vertebral venous plexus of Batson which is a low-pressure, high-volume system of vertebral veins running adjacent to the spine.

The importance of direct osteolytic effects of metastatic cancer cells, including the effects of collagenases, is uncertain although possible in the late stages of tumor-induced osteolysis (TIO). Cancer cells appear to induce osteoclast differentiation of hematopoietic stem cells and/or activate mature osteoclasts already present in bone. We and other authors have reported that specific markers of bone matrix resorption, such as the collagen cross-links pyridinoline (Pyr) and deoxypyridinoline (DPyr), are markedly increased in normocalcemic patients with bone metastases from breast cancer.[4] The increased differentiation and activation of osteoclasts at metastatic sites have been nicely demonstrated by morphological studies in several animal models of TIO as well as in human specimens.[5] The osteoclast number has been quantified in bone biopsies of normocalcemic women with breast cancer and predominantly lytic bone metastases, whether in bone adjacent to tumor or directly in the invaded bone, confirming that increased bone resorption in metastatic breast cancer is essentially mediated by the osteoclasts and not directly by the tumor cells themselves.[6]

Immune cells and osteoblasts could also be important target cells for tumor secretory products in the bone microenvironment.[2] We have observed that breast cancer cells secrete factors that inhibit the proliferation of osteoblast-like cells, of normal human osteoblasts, and that they increase their second messenger response to osteolytic agents.[7] Osteoblasts could thus keep in the process of TIO the central role they have in the physiological regulation of osteoclast resorption activity.

Several studies have established the essential pathogenic role of parathyroid hormone-related protein (PTHrP) in most types of tumor-induced hypercalcemia (TIH).[8] The nature of the tumor-derived factor(s) responsible for osteoclastic activation in the process of TIO remains unknown, but recent data indicate that PTHrP could play an important role. PTHrP-like substances are expressed by about 60% of human breast cancers, and breast tumors which spread to the skeleton appear to produce PTHrP more frequently than tumors metastasizing to non-bone sites.[9] Similarly, increased PTHrP gene expression, as quantitated by PCR, has also been shown in the primary tumors of patients who will subsequently recur in bone as compared to patients without metastases or with extraskeletal metastases.[10] PTHrP and other factors would stimulate osteoclastic bone resorption, leading to the release of bone matrix degradation products which may be chemotactic and growth stimulatory for cancer cells. PTHrP can also increase the invasive capacity of tumor cells, partly through the secretion of various enzymes, and can exert positive autocrine effects.[11]

The propensity of breast cancer cells to metastasize and proliferate in bone could thus be explained by a 'seed and soil' concept.[2] Breast cancer cells (the 'seed') appear to secrete factors, such as PTHrP, potentiating the development of metastases in the skeleton which constitute a fertile 'soil' rich in cytokines and growth factors that stimulate breast cancer cells' chemotaxis and growth. Local production of PTHrP and of other osteolytic factors such as TGF-α by cancer cells in bone would stimulate osteoclastic bone resorption, partly through the osteoblasts, the proliferation of which may also be inhibited. Such factors probably induce osteoclast differentiation from hematopoietic stem cells and activate mature osteoclasts already present in bone. Increased osteoclast number and activity would then cause local foci of osteolysis, which could further stimulate cancer cell proliferation.[2] As an example of this vicious cycle, we have shown that 2 out of 13 breast cancer cell lines, MDA-MB-231 and Hs578T, express the cytokine IL-11 at both the protein and the mRNA levels. It is important to note that MDA-MB-231 cells constitute the classical animal model of bone metastases, thanks to their aggressive osteolytic properties, and that IL-11 is a potent stimulator of osteoclast formation. The production of IL-11 was markedly enhanced by TGF-β which is an abundant constituent of bone matrix.[12]

Although skeletal metastases from prostate cancer are typically osteoblastic, histomorphometric and biochemical studies have shown unequivocal evidence for an osteoclast-mediated increase in bone resorption. The levels of the collagen cross-link DPyr are thus increased about threefold in patients with bone metastases from prostate cancer, as compared to patients with localized prostate cancer or to healthy subjects,[13] and there is an excellent correlation between Alk Phos and hydroxyproline levels in patients with metastatic bone disease from prostate cancer.[14] Prostate cancer cells stimulate osteoclast activity probably through the osteoblasts. The precise nature of the responsible factor is unknown as various substances have been implicated, notably TGF-β, bone morphogenetic proteins, IGFs, urokinase, and PTHrP.[15]

The data summarized above indicate that bone-resorbing cells are a logical target for the treatment and perhaps the prevention of bone metastases.[16]

MECHANISMS OF ACTION OF BISPHOSPHONATES

The structure of all bisphosphonates comprises a P–C–P bond which promotes their binding to the mineralized bone matrix and their subsequent inhibitory effects on bone resorption. The rest of the bisphosphonate molecule varies according to the structural modification of the side chain, the features which determine their relative potency, side-effects, and their precise mechanisms of action. The mode of action of bisphosphonates is undoubtedly complex and variable to some extent from one compound to another.

Bisphosphonates localize preferentially to sites of active bone remodeling. They can act directly on mature osteoclasts, decreasing their bone resorption activity, notably by lowering H$^+$ and Ca^{++} extrusion and modifying the activity of various enzymes.[17] Alternatively, recent findings suggest that osteoblasts, or at least those lining the bone surface, could also be essential target cells for bisphosphonates with secondary effects on the osteoclasts, probably by increasing the secretion of an inhibitor of osteoclast recruitment.[18] Moreover, bisphosphonates can induce osteoclast apoptosis and this effect could also be mediated through the osteoblasts. The relative importance of the osteoblast-dependent inhibitory activity of bisphosphonates compared with a direct inhibition of osteoclast activity or secretory capacity remains a subject of controversy. Clodronate, but not the aminobisphosphonates, can be metabolized to an ATP analog which is toxic for macrophages and probably for osteoclasts as well.[19] On the other hand, enzymes of the mevalonate pathway constitute molecular targets for nitrogen-containing bisphosphonates, such as pamidronate or alendronate, which seem to inhibit bone resorption, at least partly, by preventing protein prenylation in osteoclasts.[20]

Whatever their precise mechanism(s) of action on bone resorption, it was a postulate until recently that bisphosphonates did not exert any direct effects on cancer cells. It has recently been shown that bisphosphonates could also inhibit the adherence of cancer cells to the bone matrix. Bisphosphonate pretreatment of cortical bone slices partially inhibits breast cancer cells' adhesion[21] whereas pretreatment of breast and prostate carcinoma cells with bisphosphonates inhibits tumor cell adhesion to osteoblastic extracellular matrices in a dose-dependent

Table 16.1 Indications for bisphosphonates in breast cancer metastatic to the skeleton

Tumor-induced hypercalcemia
  90 mg iv pamidronate or
  1500 mg iv clodronate or
  4–6 mg ibandronate
  Success rate: 75–95%

Metastatic bone pain
  (60)–90 mg iv pamidronate every 3–4 weeks
  1500 mg iv clodronate every 2 weeks?
  Success rate: ≥ 50% (function of the degree of bone resorption?)

Long-term prevention of the complications of metastatic bone disease

- Oral clodronate 1600 mg/d for life: decreases the combined rate of SREs by 28%, especially hypercalcemia and vertebral fractures

- Intravenous pamidronate 90 mg monthly infusions for ≥ 1–2 years: decreases the skeletal morbidity rate (number of SREs/year) by 36%; the number of nonvertebral pathological fractures and the proportion of patients having radiation to bone or surgery on bone are reduced by 45–60%

Unresolved issues:
  Optimal therapeutic schemes?
  When to start therapy?
  How to monitor and change therapy?

Prevention of bone metastases
  Only in the framework of clinical trials

SREs = skeletal-related events (= major complications of metastatic bone disease).

manner.[22] Recent findings also indicate that bisphosphonates can under certain circumstances induce direct tumor cell apoptosis.

Bisphosphonates constitute one of the most important advances of the last decade in the area of supportive care in cancer. Their therapeutic potential is probably even larger than what is currently believed and the data summarized below indicate that their spectrum of use has become wider and wider (Table 16.1).

BISPHOSPHONATES IN BREAST CANCER

Tumor-induced hypercalcemia

Hypercalcemia can be observed with any type of solid tumor, but breast and lung carcinomas are the two most frequently encountered causes. Secretion of humoral and paracrine factors by the tumor cells stimulates osteoclast activity and proliferation, as exemplified by a marked increase in collagen cross-links excretion.[23] Moreover, osteoblast activity is often inhibited, leading to a characteristic uncoupling between bone resorption and bone formation.[24] This causes a rapid rise in serum calcium, in contrast to the relatively stable levels of serum calcium seen in primary hyperparathyroidism where bone coupling is usually maintained. The ratio between deoxypyridinoline and osteocalcin is thus normal in primary hyperparathyroidism but markedly increased in both types of TIH, whether of humoral or of local osteolytic origin.[25] Several studies have established the essential role of PTHrP in most types of cancer hypercalcemia.[8] Circulating PTHrP levels are thus elevated in almost all patients with humoral hypercalcemia of malignancy (HHM) and in about two thirds of the patients with bone metastases.[8] Cytokines, such as IL-6, are probably responsible for the inhibition of osteoblast activity.[26]

Rehydration has generally mild and transient effects on calcium levels, effecting a median decrease of only 1 mg/dl,[27] but it improves the clinical status and interrupts the vicious cycle of TIH by inhibiting the increased tubular reabsorption of calcium. Bisphosphonates have become the standard treatment for TIH and they have supplanted all other drugs except corticosteroids for hypercalcemia of multiple myeloma. Clodronate and pamidronate are most often used.

A single-day 1500 mg infusion of clodronate is as efficient as daily 300 mg infusions for 5 days and this therapy achieves normocalcemia in approximately 80% of the cases.[28] Clodronate can also be given by subcutaneous infusion. At a dose of 1500 mg administered over 4–30 hours, mild site toxicity has been observed in 29% of 45 infusions and a definite hypocalcemic activity was demonstrated in 12 evaluable episodes. This mode of administration can be particularly useful in the palliative setting.[29] Pamidronate was first administered as repeated daily 15 mg, 2-hour infusions. In a multicenter trial, 90% of 132 patients treated in this manner became normocalcemic after a mean interval of 3–4 days.[30] Such a therapeutic scheme is, however, cumbersome and it was later shown that pamidronate could be given as a single infusion over 2–24 hours. Large studies indicate that a dose of 90 mg achieves normocalcemia in more than 90% of patients.[31] At these dose levels, the effects on either serum calcium or calcium excretion are not influenced by the tumor type or by the presence of bone metastatic involvement. These doses are thus higher than what is currently recommended by the manufacturer and other authors have also found that such recommended doses are too low for patients with moderate hypercalcemia.[32] The response to lower doses of pamidronate will thus be less in patients with HHM compared with patients with bone metastases as the importance of PTHrP will become more evident.

The superiority of pamidronate over clodronate in patients with TIH has been demonstrated in a randomized trial involving 41 patients, not significantly so in terms of success rate, but quite evidently in the duration of normocalcemia. The median duration of action of clodronate was 2 weeks compared with 4 weeks for pamidronate.[33] Pamidronate is well tolerated, the only clinically detectable side-effect being transient fever and a flu-like syndrome in about one quarter of the cases. Oral clodronate is often prescribed after successful intravenous therapy but the efficacy of this strategy is not proven.

Newer and more potent bisphosphonates, such as ibandronate and zoledronate, are currently being studied. A dose escalation trial with ibandronate has been conducted in 147 patients with Ca levels of ≥ 3.0 mmol/l (= 12 mg/dl) after rehydration, 125 of whom were evaluable for response. The success rate was 50% in the 2 mg group, which was significantly lower than the responses in the 4 and 6 mg dose groups, 76% and 77%, respectively. A logistic regression analysis indicated that the response rate was also dependent on the initial Ca level and on the tumor type because the group of patients with breast cancer or myeloma responded better than patients with other tumors. The drug was well tolerated, and the only noticeable side-effect was drug-induced fever in 13% of the cases.[34] A phase-I dose finding study in 30 hypercalcemic cancer patients has shown that very low doses of zoledronate (0.02 and 0.04 mg/kg, i.e. 1.2 and 2.4 mg for a 60 kg individual) administered by a short-time infusion (30 minutes) constitute a quite effective treatment of TIH.[35] These newer compounds will simplify the current treatment for TIH but, because of the excellent results obtained with clodronate and even more with pamidronate, their clinical interest should be more evident for the long-term management of metastatic bone disease.

Metastatic bone pain

Palliation of bone pain can be quite difficult, especially in patients with widespread, often previously irradiated, sites of pain. Oral bisphosphonates are generally unable to reduce metastatic bone pain in a clinically significant manner. This was recently confirmed in a placebo-controlled study of oral clodronate in patients with progressing bone metastases, mainly from breast cancer.[36] Moreover, treatment compliance is generally poor because of difficulty with swallowing the capsules and occasional digestive side-effects.

Intravenous bisphosphonates can exert clinically relevant analgesic effects in patients with metastatic bone pain, although these compounds are still unfortunately viewed by some oncologists as expensive analgesics. Metastatic bone pain is traditionally attributed to various factors, notably the release of chemical mediators, increased pressure within the bone, microfractures, stretching of periosteum, reactive muscle spasm, nerve root infiltration, and/or compression.[37] However, as suggested by the clinical and biochemical effects of bisphosphonates, the dramatic increase in bone resorption probably plays an important contributory role. When pooling the available data of phase-II trials with repeated pamidronate infusions, a relief of bone pain was observed in at least one half of the patients.[3] Short-term placebo-controlled studies have confirmed that intravenous clodronate or pamidronate can exert significant and rapid analgesic effects.[38] Responding patients also show an improvement in their quality of life.

The optimal dose needs to be defined, especially that it is probably a function of the disease stage. Specific markers of bone matrix resorption, such as the telopeptide NTx, appear to follow a similar time course than the pain score after pamidronate administration.[39] Moreover, the drop in the levels of such markers could be a predictor of pain relief, as an analgesic response has been more frequent in the patients in whom these markers remained in the normal range or returned to normal (53–63%, dependent on the marker) than in the patients whose markers did not return to normal (0–20% of analgesic response).[39] However, it remains unknown if higher doses could indeed lead to a more marked inhibition of bone resorption and a greater analgesic effect. A dose of 60–90 mg pamidronate every 3–4 weeks is currently recommended for palliation of bone pain. A recent double-blind study in a relatively small series of 62 patients, mostly with breast cancer or myeloma, demonstrated no difference in the analgesic response between the doses of 60 and 90 mg of pamidronate for the treatment of bone pain.[40] Interestingly, the response was essentially observed in patients with moderate or severe bone pain (visual analog scale, VAS ≥ 50 mm), suggesting that patients with less severe pain should probably not be treated with bisphosphonates just for that purpose. Also, most of the effect was obtained after only two infusions, which could suggest that further administrations are not useful in initial nonresponders, leading to a decrease in the costs of therapy.[41] However, the analgesic activity of bisphosphonates must be viewed in the larger framework of the prevention of the complications of tumor-induced bone disease.

Prevention of the complications of metastatic bone disease

Two large-scale studies in patients with breast cancer metastatic to the skeleton, one with clodronate and one with pamidronate, indicate that the prolonged administration of oral bisphosphonates until death can significantly reduce the frequency of morbid skeletal events. The clodronate study was randomized, double-blind, placebo-controlled, and included 173 patients with breast cancer metastatic to bone.[42] In the clodronate-treated group (1600 mg/day), there was a significant reduction in the incidence of hypercalcemic episodes, in the number of vertebral fractures, and in the rate of vertebral deformities. The combined rate of all morbid skeletal events was reduced by 28%. In an open study, it was reported that the prolonged administration of oral pamidronate (300 mg/day) could reduce the frequency of bone complications by 38%. The incidence of hypercalcemia, bone pain, and symptomatic imminent fractures was reduced by 65%, 30%, and 50%, respectively.[43] The highest dose of 600 mg daily appears to be more efficient but could not be maintained because of gastrointestinal side-effects, which demonstrates the need for more potent compounds than pamidronate, at least for the oral route.

Regular pamidronate infusions can induce a recalcification or sclerosis of osteolytic lesions, achieving a partial objective response by conventional UICC criteria in approximately one fifth of the patients.[3] Although the clinical benefit of these observations remains unproven, this phenomenon of recalcification appears to be similar to what can be achieved by conventional hormono- or chemotherapy. Similarly, an increase in the objective bone response rate to chemotherapy has been shown in a large randomized clinical trial where patients were receiving chemotherapy plus pamidronate as compared to chemotherapy alone, 33% vs 18%, respectively.[44] Three randomized studies of regular pamidronate infusions have recently been completed.[45,46] Conte and collaborators evaluated the effects of infusions of 45 mg of pamidronate every 3 weeks in addition to standard first-line chemotherapy compared to chemotherapy alone in patients with breast cancer and bone metastases. The study was stopped when the disease progressed in the skeleton. In the 224 assessable patients, there was an increase of 48% in the median time to progression in bone. Improvement in bone pain was also seen more often in the pamidronate group but the decrease in other skeletal-related events was not significant.[45] These somewhat disappointing results can be explained by the high activity of first-line chemotherapy in breast cancer, by the premature cessation of bisphosphonate administration, and by the choice of too low a dose for pamidronate. The results of double-blind, randomized, placebo-controlled trials comparing 90 mg pamidronate infusions every 4 weeks to placebo infusions for 1 or 2 years in addition to chemo- or hormonotherapy in a large series of breast cancer patients with at least one lytic bone metastasis establish that bisphosphonates can reduce the skeletal morbidity rate in a clinically significant manner.[46]

The results were particularly impressive in the chemotherapy trial which included 382 patients.[44] Of the 380 patients, 60–62% had no metastatic site other than bone. Skeletal-related events (SREs) were defined as pathological fractures, spinal cord compression, vertebral collapse, radiation for pain relief or for treatment of pathological fractures or spinal cord compres-

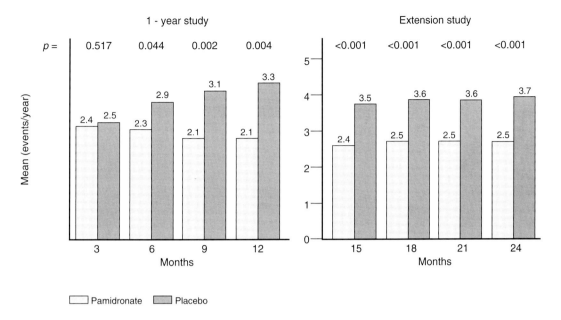

Fig. 16.1 Skeletal morbidity rate (mean number of skeletal-related events per year) in 382 women with metastatic breast cancer and lytic bone lesions treated by chemotherapy and randomly assigned to receive either 90 mg pamidronate or placebo infusions q 3–4 weeks for up to 2 years in a double-blind manner. (From refs 45 and 46.)

sion, or surgery to bone. The median time to the occurrence of the first SRE was increased by 47% in the pamidronate group (13 vs 7 months). There was a significant reduction in the proportion of patients having any SRE (43% vs 56%), in the number of nonvertebral pathological fractures (by 60%), and in the proportion of patients having radiation to bone (by 45%) or surgery on bone (by 52%). The follow-up of this trial indicates that the mean skeletal morbidity rate (number of SREs per year) has been 2.1 in the pamidronate group compared to 3.3 in the placebo group for up to 2 years ($p < 0.005$; Fig. 16.1). Pain, quality of life, and performance status worsened significantly less at the end of the 2-year evaluation in the pamidronate group.[44] The mean skeletal morbidity rates in the hormone therapy trial were 2.4 and 3.6 ($p < 0.01$) in the pamidronate and placebo groups, respectively.[46] There were also favorable effects on the quality of life and, at the end of the evaluation, there was a significant decrease in the pain score and in the analgesic requirement in both trials. Because the odds ratio of having an SRE while receiving pamidronate in the endocrine study was not significantly different from the odds ratio in the chemotherapy study, the data of the two studies have been pooled.[46] In this combined analysis of 751 patients, the proportion of patients having any SRE (not including TIH) was reduced from 64% to 51% by the end of the 24 monthly cycles ($p < 0.001$). The mean skeletal morbidity rate was reduced from 3.7 to 2.4 events/year ($p < 0.001$) and the time to the first SRE increased from 7 to 12.7 months ($p < 0.001$).

This patient cohort had advanced breast cancer at study entry. Even greater benefit might be possible if bisphosphonates are introduced earlier in the course of the disease, before bone metastases are widespread. Much of the financial burden for oncological care results from the time spent in hospital for the complications of the disease rather than for the anti-neoplastic treatment itself.[47] Moreover, metastatic skeletal disease accounts for the largest component of hospital costs and totals almost two thirds of the expenses in advanced breast cancer.[48] Limited cost-benefit analyses suggest that the prolonged administration of bisphosphonates, at least by the oral route, can lead to significant cost savings.[49] However, systematic cost-effectiveness studies are lacking, whether for oral or for intravenous bisphosphonates. The cost/benefit ratio of an early and prolonged intervention is unfortunately unknown and will certainly be greatly influenced by local factors. On the other hand, long-term treatment could induce some 'resistance' to bisphosphonates or to a state of 'frozen bone' because of excessive reduction of the bone turnover, but this could be more a theoretical than a practical concern.

The results obtained with the intravenous route are more impressive than the ones obtained with oral compounds. However, the choice can depend on individual circumstances. For an aggressive osteolytic disease, the choice has to be given to the intravenous route. However, the oral route is preferred for many patients on hormonal therapy, especially if the bone disease is not rapidly evolving. The optimal therapeutic schedule for pamidronate is not known with certainty, but monthly infusions are clearly effective and this schedule, while not ideal, is compatible with palliation of advanced malignancy. Criteria for when in the course of metastatic bone disease bisphosphonates should be started and stopped need now to be determined. Because bisphosphonates are providing supportive care, reducing the rate of skeletal morbidity (but evidently not abolishing it), the criteria for stopping their administration have to be different from those used for classical anti-neoplastic drugs and they should not necessarily be stopped when metastatic bone disease is progressing. However, criteria are lacking to determine if and how long an individual patient benefits from their administration, and the decision to continue or stop bisphosphonate therapy or increase their dosage remains essentially empirical. New biochemical markers of bone resorption might help identify those patients continuing to benefit from therapy and those who might benefit from higher doses or more potent compounds. The essential question remains, however, 'when to start?' One has to hope that prospective randomized studies will be performed to answer this important question, taking into account both clinical and economical aspects.

The increased potency of newer agents such as ibandronate and zoledronate will obviously allow the use of much lower doses and, of more clinical importance, their administration as rapid intravenous injections rather than slow infusions. Several studies with repeated injections or infusions with these compounds in patients with bone metastases have just been completed or are in progress. Monthly 6 mg ibandronate infusions appear to achieve results comparable to the ones achieved with 90 mg pamidronate infusions but a full analysis of the beneficial effects of this recently completed study is awaited. These potent bisphosphonates will certainly allow more convenient therapeutic schemes but it remains unknown if this increased potency will lead to better clinical results.

Prevention of bone metastases

Another potential role for bisphosphonate treatment is the prevention or at least a delay in the development of bone metastases. Trials in patients with established bone metastases suggest that long-term administration of bisphosphonates could indeed fulfill this major objective. Additionally, animal models of bone metastases have shown that bisphosphonates could effectively inhibit the development of bone metastases and decrease the tumor burden in bone when they are injected at the same time as breast cancer cells, suggesting that the production of bone-destroying substances by the cancer cells can set up a vicious cycle that can be interrrupted by anti-osteoclastic drugs.[50]

A secondary prevention double-blind trial, continued for 3 years after extraskeletal recurrence in 133 women with breast cancer, has shown a significant reduction in the number of bone metastases in the clodronate group.[51] An open trial in 124 patients with breast cancer, most of whom had visceral metastases, has failed to show that 300 mg of pamidronate/day had any influence on the first clinical or radiological evidence of skeletal metastases.[52] However, the median follow-up of living patients in the pamidronate wing was only 19 months and the influence on the development of subsequent bone metastases was not examined. Moreover, this study had a limited sample size and it was probably not a true preventative trial because of the advanced nature of the disease in most patients and the likelihood of infraclinical bone involvement in many of them.

A preliminary report of a double-blind trial involving 1079 breast cancer patients after surgery indicates that a 2-year treatment with 1600 mg clodronate daily can indeed reduce the incidence of bone metastases. The median follow-up was 4 years and a significant reduction was observed in postmenopausal patients, 7.3% in the placebo group as compared to 3.3% in the clodronate group ($p = 0.04$).[53] In a randomized open trial involving 302 patients with primary breast cancer and tumor cells in the bone marrow, which is an adverse risk factor for the development of metastases, it was shown that 1600 mg clodronate daily for 2 years reduced the number of bone as well as nonbone metastases by about 50% after a median follow-up of 36 months.[54] The survival rate was also significantly prolonged. Despite the enthusiasm these data generated, one must remain cautious and confirmation is eagerly awaited. Nevertheless, as pointed out in an accompanying editorial, these spectacular results could be due to a reduction in tumor burden in bone by an alteration of the microenvironment induced by bisphosphonates which could interrrupt the osteolytic cycle by reducing local production of growth factors. For example, TGF-β is a major component of bone matrix and a potent stimulator of PTHrP production by breast cancer cells, and PTHrP certainly plays an important role in the process of breast cancer-induced osteolysis.[55] As summarized above, in opposition with the classical opinion that bisphosphonates only act on bone cells, some recent work suggests that they could also act on the tumor cells themselves. Bisphosphonate pretreatment of cortical bone slices partially inhibits breast carcinoma cell adhesion.[21] Pretreatment of breast and prostate carcinoma cells with bisphosphonates inhibits tumor cell adhesion to unmineralized and mineralized osteoblastic extracellular matrices in a dose-dependent manner.[22] Moreover, yet unpublished work from several groups, including ours, indicates that bisphosphonates can induce apoptosis of breast cancer cells.

It will be important to determine the patients at high risk of developing bone metastases before recommending a general primary preventative use of bisphosphonates. Classical prognostic factors, such as tumor size, axillary node involvement, receptor status, but also PTHrP expression by the tumor cells and selected investigational prognostic markers, will probably be relevant.

Preventative therapy with bisphosphonates could also have the additional beneficial effect of preventing postmenopausal osteoporosis in a population of women for whom estrogen replacement therapy is generally avoided.

BISPHOSPHONATES IN OTHER SOLID TUMORS

Although skeletal metastases from prostate cancer are typically osteoblastic, histomorphometric and biochemical studies have shown unequivocal evidence for a marked increase in bone resorption.[56,57] Because bone formation is most often even more stimulated than bone resorption, bone metastases of prostate cancer are often accompanied by a slight decrease in serum Ca, inducing a state of secondary hyperparathyroidism, which will decrease serum Pi levels. This decrease in serum Ca and Pi concentrations could be the cause of the reported development of osteomalacia.[58] Adding bisphosphonates to this therapy could logically further aggravate this tendency, which could explain, at least partly, the transiency of pain relief achieved with clodronate in patients with metastases from prostate cancer,[59] as the development of osteomalacia can worsen bone repair. Recent data indicate that the renal tubular reabsorption of phosphate could be positively related to the extent of bone metastatic load in prostate cancer, suggesting an adaptation of the kidney level to meet demands for minerals in the face of enhanced bone formation. The bone formation markers, but not the bone resorption markers, are accordingly higher in patients with a relatively higher renal tubular reabsorption of phospate.[57] A recent trial testing the efficacy of 1 month of oral clodronate in a placebo-controlled trial in 42 patients was associated with an increase in bone alkaline phosphatase (BAP) levels, explained by the authors by an increased recruitment of osteoblasts at sites undergoing bone resorption.[60] However, the most likely explanation was disease progression reflecting the inability of oral bisphosphonates to treat metastatic bone disease effectively in advanced prostate cancer.

It has been shown in open trials that pamidronate infusions could inhibit bone resorption and decrease bone pain in patients with bone metastases from prostate cancer.[16,61] The newer bisphosphonate olpadronate has also been shown to reduce biochemical parameters of bone resorption and to decrease bone pain, although this was not assessed in a prospective manner.[14] Occasional dramatic symptomatic responses have been observed by several investigators using iterative bisphosphonate infusions in patients with painful bony metastases, but there are as yet too few systematic data to advise the regular use of bisphosphonates in metastatic prostate cancer and no precise recommendations can be made on the dose to be used. Adjuvant trials with clodronate have been started in the UK and the results are eagerly awaited.

Although lung and kidney cancers often metastasize to the skeleton, there are very few data on the use of bisphosphonates in patients with osteolytic bone metastases from other cancers and no guidelines can be provided at the present time.[16]

REFERENCES

1. Watson J, Chuah SY. Technique for the primary culture of human breast cancer cells and measurement of their prostaglandin secretion. *Clin Sci* (1992) **83:** 347–52.
2. Mundy GR. Mechanisms of bone metastasis. *Cancer* (1997) **80:** 1546–56.
3. Body JJ, Coleman RE, Piccart M. Use of bisphosphonates in cancer patients. *Cancer Treat Rev* (1996) **22:** 265–87.
4. Body JJ, Dumon JC, Gineyts E, Delmas PD. Comparative evaluation of markers of bone resorption in patients with breast cancer-induced osteolysis before and after bisphosphonate therapy. *Br J Cancer* (1997) **75:** 408–12.
5. Hiraga T, Tanaka S, Ikegame M *et al*. Morphology of bone metastasis. *Eur J Cancer* (1998) **34:** 230–9.
6. Taube T, Elomaa I, Blomqvist C, Beneton MNC, Kanis JA. Histomorphometric evidence for osteoclast-mediated bone resorption in metastatic breast cancer. *Bone* (1994) **15:** 161–6.
7. Siwek B, Lacroix M, de Pollak C, Marie P, Body JJ. Secretory products of breast cancer cells affect human osteoblastic cells: partial characterization of active factors. *J Bone Miner Res* (1997) **12:** 552–60.
8. Grill V, Ho P, Body JJ *et al*. Parathyroid hormone-related protein: elevated levels in both humoral hypercalcemia of malignancy and hypercalcemia complicating metastatic breast cancer. *J Clin Endocrinol Metab* (1991) **73:** 1309–15.
9. Vargas SJ, Gillespie MT, Powell GJ *et al*. Localization of parathyroid hormone-related protein mRNA expression in breast cancer and metastatic lesions by in situ hybridization. *J Bone Miner Res* (1992) **7:** 971–9.
10. Bouizar Z, Spyratos F, Deytieux S, de Vernejoul MC, Jullienne A. Polymerase chain reaction analysis of parathyroid hormone-related protein gene expression in breast cancer patients and occurrence of bone metastases. *Cancer Res* (1993) **53:** 5076–8.
11. Rabbani SA, Gladu J, Liu B, Goltzman D. Regulation in vivo of the growth of Leydig cell tumors by antisense ribonucleic acid for parathyroid hormone-related peptide. *Endocrinology* (1995) **136:** 5416–22.
12. Lacroix M, Siwek B, Marie PJ, Body JJ. Production

of interleukin-11 by breast cancer cells. *Cancer Lett* (1998) **127**: 29–35.
13. Sano M, Kushida K, Takahashi M *et al*. Urinary pyridinoline and deoxypyridinoline in prostate carcinoma patients with bone metastasis. *Br J Cancer* (1994) **70**: 701–3.
14. Pelger RCM, Hamdy NAT, Zwinderman AH, Lycklama AAB, Nijeholt A, Papapoulos SE. Effects of the bisphosphonate olpadronate in patients with carcinoma of the prostate metastatic to the skeleton. *Bone* (1998) **22**: 403–8.
15. Goltzman D, Rabbani SA. Pathogenesis of osteoblastic metastases. In Body JJ (ed) *Tumor Bone Diseases and Osteoporosis in Cancer Patients* (New York: Marcel Dekker, in press).
16. Body JJ, Bartl R, Burckhardt P *et al*. for the International Bone and Cancer Study Group. Current use of bisphosphonates in oncology. *J Clin Oncol* (1998) **16**: 3890–9.
17. Zimolo Z, Wesolowski G, Rodan GA. Acid extrusion is induced by osteoclast attachment to bone. Inhibition by alendronate and calcitonin. *J Clin Invest* (1995) **96**: 2277–83.
18. Vitté C, Fleisch H, Guenther HL. Bisphosphonates induce osteoblasts to secrete an inhibitor of osteoclast-mediated resorption. *Endocrinology* (1996) **137**: 2324–33.
19. Frith JC, Mönkkönen J, Blackburn GM, Russel RGG, Rogers MJ. Clodronate and liposome-encapsulated clodronate are metabolized to a toxic ATP analog, adenosine 5'-(β, γ-dichloromethylene) triphosphate, by mammalian cells in vitro. *J Bone Miner Res* (1997) **12**: 1358–67.
20. Luckman SP, Hughes DE, Coxon FP, Russell RGG, Rogers MJ. Nitrogen-containing bisphosphonates inhibit the mevalonate pathway and prevent post-translational prenylation of GTP-binding proteins, including ras. *J Bone Miner Res* (1998) **13**: 581–9.
21. van der Pluijm G, Vloedgraven H, van Beek E, van der Wee Pals L, Lowik C, Papapoulos S. Bisphosphonates inhibit the adhesion of breast cancer cells to bone matrices in vitro. *J Clin Invest* (1996) **98**: 698–705.
22. Boissier S, Magnetto S, Frappart L *et al*. Bisphosphonates inhibit prostate and breast carcinoma cell adhesion to unmineralized and mineralized bone extracellular matrices. *Cancer Res* (1997) **57**: 3890–4.
23. Body JJ, Delmas PD. Urinary pyridinium crosslinks as markers of bone resorption in tumor-associated hypercalcemia. *J Clin Endocrinol Metab* (1992) **74**: 471–5.
24. Dumon JC, Wantier H, Mathieu F, Mantia M, Body JJ. Technical and clinical validation of a new immunoradiometric assay for human osteocalcin. *Eur J Endocrinol* (1996) **135**: 231–7.
25. Nakayama K, Fukumoto S, Takeda S *et al*. Differences in bone and vitamin D metabolism between primary hyperparathyroidism and malignancy-associated hypercalcemia. *J Clin Endocrinol Metab* (1996) **81**: 607–11.
26. Nagai Y, Yamato H, Akaogi K *et al*. Role of interleukin-6 in uncoupling of bone in vivo in a human squamous carcinoma coproducing parathyroid hormone-related peptide and interleukin-6. *J Bone Miner Res* (1998) **13**: 664–72.
27. Singer FR, Ritch PS, Lad TE *et al*. Treatment of hypercalcemia of malignancy with intravenous etidronate. A controlled, multicenter study. *Arch Intern Med* (1991) **151**: 471–6.
28. O'Rourke NP, McCloskey EV, Vasikaran S, Eyres K, Fern D, Kanis JA. Effective treatment of malignant hypercalcaemia with a single intravenous infusion of clodronate. *Br J Cancer* (1993) **67**: 560–3.
29. Walker P, Watanabe S, Lawlor P, Hanson J, Pereira J, Bruera E. Subcutaneous clodronate: a study evaluating efficacy in hypercalcemia of malignancy and local toxicity. *Ann Oncol* (1997) **8**: 915–16.
30. Harinck HIJ, Bijvoet OLM, Plantingh AST *et al*. Role of bone and kidney in tumor-induced hypercalcemia and its treatment with bisphosphonate and sodium chloride. *Am J Med* (1993) **82**: 1133–42.
31. Body JJ, Dumon JC. Treatment of tumor-induced hypercalcaemia with the bisphosphonate pamidronate: dose–response relationship and influence of the tumour type. *Ann Oncol* (1994) **5**: 359–63.
32. Neskovic-Konstantinovic Z, Mitrovic L, Petrovic J, Stamatovic L, Ristovic Z. Treatment of tumour-induced hypercalcaemia in advanced breast cancer patients with three different doses of disodium pamidronate adapted to the initial level of calcaemia. *Supp Care Cancer* (1995) **3**: 422–4.
33. Purohit OP, Radstone CR, Anthony C, Kanis JA, Coleman RE. A randomised double-blind comparison of intravenous pamidronate and clodronate in the hypercalcaemia of malignancy. *Br J Cancer* (1995) **72**: 1289–93.
34. Ralston SH, Thiébaud D, Herrmann Z *et al*. Dose–response study of ibandronate in treatment

of cancer-associated hypercalcaemia. *Br J Cancer* (1997) **75:** 295–300.
35. Body JJ. Clinical research update: zoledronate. *Cancer* (1997) **80:** 1699–701.
36. Robertson AG, Reed NS, Ralston SH. Effect of oral clodronate on metastatic bone pain: a double-blind, placebo-controlled study. *J Clin Oncol* (1995) **13:** 2427–30.
37. Mercadante S. Malignant bone pain: pathophysiology and treatment. *Pain* (1997) **69:** 1–18.
38. Ernst DS, Brasher P, Hagen N, Paterson AH, MacDonald RN, Bruera E. A randomized, controlled trial of intravenous clodronate in patients with metastatic bone disease and pain. *J Pain Symptom Manage* (1997) **13:** 319–26.
39. Vinholes JJF, Purohit OP, Abbey ME, Eastell R, Coleman RE. Relationships between biochemical and symptomatic response in a double-blind randomised trial of pamidronate for metastatic bone disease. *Ann Oncol* (1997) **8:** 1243–50.
40. Koeberle D, Bacchus L, Thuerlimann B, Senn HJ. Pamidronate treatment in patients with malignant osteolytic bone disease and pain: a prospective randomized double-blind trial. *Supp Care Cancer* (1999) **7:** 21–7.
41. Body JJ. Bisphosphonates for metastatic bone pain. *Supp Care Cancer* (1999) **7:** 1–3.
42. Paterson AHG, Powles TJ, Kanis JA, McCloskey E, Hanson J, Ashley S. Double-blind controlled trial of oral clodronate in patients with bone metastases from breast cancer. *J Clin Oncol* (1993) **11:** 59–65.
43. Van Holten-Verzantvoort ATM, Kroon HM, Bijvoet OLM *et al.* Palliative pamidronate treatment in patients with bone metastases from breast cancer. *J Clin Oncol* (1993) **11:** 491–8.
44. Hortobagyi GN, Theriault RL, Lipton A *et al.* for the Protocol 19 Aredia Breast Cancer Study Group. Long-term prevention of skeletal complications of metastatic breast cancer with pamidronate. *J Clin Oncol* (1998) **16:** 2038–44.
45. Conte PF, Latreille J, Mauriac L *et al.* Delay in progression of bone metastases in breast cancer patients treated with intravenous pamidronate: results from a multinational randomised controlled trial. *J Clin Oncol* (1996) **14:** 2552–9.
46. Lipton A. Aredia: the once-monthly infusion for the treatment of bone metastases. *Curr Opin Oncol* (1998) **10 (Suppl 1):** S1–S5.
47. Richards MA, Braysher S, Gregory WM, Rubens RD. Advanced breast cancer: use of resources and cost implications. *Br J Cancer* (1993) **67:** 856–60.
48. Biermann WA, Cantor RI, Fellin FM, Jakobowski J, Hopkins L, Newbold RC. An evaluation of the potential cost reductions resulting from the use of clodronate in the treatment of metastatic carcinoma of the breast. *Bone* (1991) **12 (Suppl 1):** 37–42.
49. Elomaa I, Blomqvist C. Clodronate and other bisphosphonates as supportive therapy in osteolysis due to malignancy. *Acta Oncol* (1995) **34:** 629–36.
50. Yoneda T, Sasaki A, Dunstan C *et al.* Inhibition of osteolytic bone metastasis of breast cancer by combined treatment with the bisphosphonate ibandronate and tissue inhibitor of the matrix metalloproteinase-2. *J Clin Invest* (1997) **99:** 2509–17.
51. Kanis JA, Powles T, Paterson AHG, McCloskey EV, Ashley S. Clodronate decreases the frequency of skeletal metastases in women with breast cancer. *Bone* (1996) **19:** 663–7.
52. Van Holten-Verzantvoort ATM, Hermans J, Beex LVAM *et al.* Does supportive pamidronate treatment prevent or delay the first manifestation of bone metastases in breast cancer patients? *Eur J Cancer* (1996) **32A:** 450–4.
53. Powles TJ, Paterson AHG, Nevantaus A *et al.* Adjuvant clodronate reduces the incidence of bone metastases in patients with primary operable breast cancer. Proceedings ASCO (abstract 468). *J Clin Oncol* (1998) **17:** 123a.
54. Diel IJ, Solomayer EF, Costa SD *et al.* Reduction in new metastases in breast cancer with adjuvant clodronate treatment. *N Engl J Med* (1998) **339:** 357–63.
55. Mundy GR, Yoneda T. Bisphosphonates as anticancer drugs. *N Engl J Med* (1998) **6:** 398–400.
56. Miyamoto KK, McSherry SA, Robins SP, Besterman JM, Mohler JL. Collagen cross-link metabolites in urine as markers of bone metastases in prostatic carcinoma. *J Urol* (1994) **151:** 909–13.
57. Buchs N, Bonjour JP, Rizzoli R. Renal tubular reabsorption of phosphate is positively related to the extent of bone metastatic load in patients with prostate cancer. *J Clin Endocrinol Metab* (1998) **83:** 1535–41.
58. Taube T, Kylmälä T, Lamberg-Allardt C, Tammela TLJ, Elomaa I. The effect of clodronate on bone in metastatic prostate cancer. Histomorphometric report of a double-blind randomised placebo-controlled study. *Eur J Cancer* (1994) **30A:** 751–8.

59. Kylmälä T, Tammela T, Risteli L, Risteli J, Taube T, Elomaa I. Evaluation of the effect of oral clodronate on skeletal metastases with type 1 collagen metabolites. A controlled trial of the Finnish Prostate Cancer Group. *Eur J Cancer* (1993) **29A:** 821–5.
60. Magnusson P, Larsson L, Englund G, Larsson B, Strang P, Selin-Sjögren L. Differences of bone alkaline phosphatase isoforms in metastatic bone disease and discrepant effects of clodronate on different skeletal sites indicated by the location of pain. *Clin Chem* (1998) **44:** 1621–8.
61. Purohit OP, Anthony C, Radstone CR, Owen J, Coleman RE. High-dose intravenous pamidronate for metastatic bone pain. *Br J Cancer* (1994) **70:** 554–8.

17

Spinal stabilization

Kevin D Harrington

Pathophysiology • **Nonoperative treatment** • **Clinical course** • **Diagnosis** • **Operative treatment** • **Results** • **Conclusion**

The spine is the most common site for skeletal metastases irrespective of the primary tumor involved. The vertebral body typically is affected first,[1,2] although the initial radiographic finding often will be destruction of a pedicle. This discrepancy is explainable by the fact that, in the absence of a blastic or sclerotic reaction within the vertebral cancellous bone, between 30% and 50% of a vertebral body must be destroyed before any change can be recognized radiographically.[3] In contrast, minimal lysis of pedicular bone can be appreciated because the pedicle cortex tends to be involved early and because the pedicle can be seen well in cross-section on an anteroposterior roentgenogram.

It has been demonstrated that between 40% and 70% of patients dying from cancer have evidence of vertebral metastases by careful postmortem examination[3,4] but that the posterior elements are involved only one seventh as often as the vertebral body.[3] Seventy-five per cent of vertebral metastases originate in carcinomas of the breast, prostate, kidney, or lung, or from lymphomas or myelomas. Carcinomas of the breast and lung most commonly metastasize to the thoracic area, whereas prostatic carcinomas typically affect the lumbar spine, sacrum, and pelvis.[5] The breast drains principally by the azygous venous system, communicating with Batson's paravertebral venous plexus initially in the thoracic region.[6–8] In contrast, the prostate drains through the pelvis venous plexus communicating with the same valveless venous plexus about the lower spine.[9] The lung primarily drains via the pulmonary vein into the left heart and showers its tumor emboli in a generalized pattern throughout the skeleton. Tumors of the colon and rectum drain through the portal system, tending to seed the lung and liver with metastases much earlier and more frequently than they do bone.

PATHOPHYSIOLOGY

The vertebral bodies contain active bone marrow (red marrow) throughout life, unlike the peripheral skeleton which in adulthood contains a relatively avascular marrow (yellow marrow). The vascular sinusoidal system within red marrow of the dorsal vertebral body is particularly vulnerable to cancer cells, allowing them to escape within the circulation and become established within the cancellous network of bone. The ability of these cells to form a protective fibrin sheath and to secrete osteoclast-activating factors and perhaps lytic prostaglandins also appears to be enhanced within the red marrow of vertebrae.[10]

The posterior longitudinal ligament is the weakest soft tissue barrier histologically,[7] being

246 CANCER AND THE SKELETON

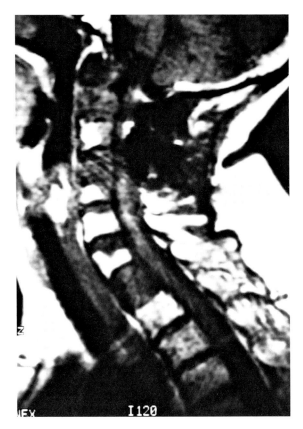

Fig. 17.1 Saggital T1-weighted MR image of the cervical spine of a 69-year-old woman with widely metastatic breast carcinoma. Multiple foci of abnormal replacement of the marrow signal are particularly apparent at the C1, C2, C4, and C8 vertebral bodies. Patient developed progressive long tract signs of secondary to the intrusion of tumor and bony detritus at the C2 level.

gradually destroyed by tumor cells at the point of perforating vessels. However, even after the destruction of such barrier soft tissues, most metastatic foci remain contained at least for some time by a thin fibrous reactive membrane.[1] It is for this reason that even when the spinal canal can be seen by imaging studies to be intruded upon by tumor tissue (Fig. 17.1), invasion of the dura or extension along the epidural space is relatively rare. Fujita *et al.* have demonstrated histologically that tumor meta-

stases spread to adjacent vertebrae beneath the longitudinal ligament or through the paravertebral muscles to the neighboring lamina.[1]

NONOPERATIVE TREATMENT

Vertebral metastases *per se* are often asymptomatic and may be discovered by routine bone scintigraphy or magnetic resonance (MR) imaging. MR imaging is particularly sensitive in demonstrating multifocal spinal metastases, even in asymptomatic patients,[11,12] and this fact has been used to support the concept of spinal decompression or stabilization[4,13,14] or of vertebral embolization[15,16] in an effort to prevent the development of intractable spine pain, instability, and progressive neurological compromise. In this author's opinion, however, patients with evidence scintigraphically or by bone imaging studies of vertebral metastases without either bony collapse or neurological impairment should not be considered candidates for operative intervention. There is no easy technique available for prophylactic operative control of spinal metastases, and most such patients can be effectively managed by noninvasive techniques. Even recently so-called minimally invasive operative techniques such as vertebroplasty by injection with polymethylmethacrylate (PMMA)[17] or endoscopic spinal decompression and stabilization[18] are fraught with significant risk and morbidity. Arterial embolization of spinal tumors has been effective in controlling the progression of some spinal metastases temporarily, but has also been complicated by major iatrogenic neurological deficits.[16]

In asymptomatic patients with spinal metastases, radiotherapy is not indicated unless the lesion can be demonstrated to progress in spite of chemotherapy or hormonal manipulation. Unfortunately, in the single largest group (patients with spinal metastases from breast cancer), the response rate reported even for similar chemotherapy protocols varies from 0 to 84%.[19,20] Very few patients with breast cancer metastatic to the spine have radiographically demonstrable regression of spinal metastases after chemotherapy, and it is unlikely that

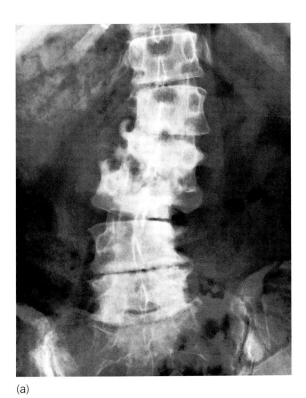 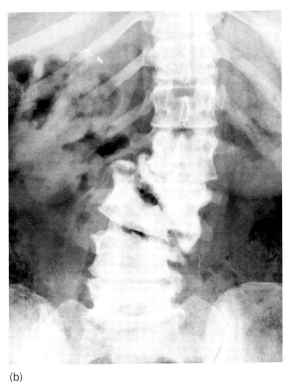

(a) (b)

Fig. 17.2 (a) Insufficiency fracture of the second and third lumbar vertebrae 6 years after extensive retroperitoneal irradiation for colon cancer. The patient had mild symptoms of lumbar spinal stenosis and foraminal stenosis at this point. (b) Seven months after an unfortunate three-level extensive posterior decompression which has resulted in worsening of the spinal instability and marked progression of the neurological deficit.

chemotherapy has any significant effect in enhancing restoration of cortical or cancellous bone destroyed by metastatic tumor. However, the overall survival time for these patients is significantly better than for those with untreated spinal metastases, even in the absence of pain or neurological compromise. Most such patients will also show symptomatic improvement of spinal pain, at least temporarily.

One caveat should be emphasized. There is a tendency among some oncologists to employ increasingly aggressive chemotherapeutic regimens for patients with spine pain unresponsive to more conventional therapy. Care should be taken to ensure that such uncontrolled pain is not indicative of microfractures, progressive vertebral collapse, or early neurological impairment. Not infrequently, patients who have already completed a full course of irradiation to affected vertebrae may actually develop these fractures and collapse as a complication of the radiation itself (the so-called insufficiency fracture), rather than as a result of recurrent tumor (Fig. 17.2). Conversely, when patients have not received irradiation, and the vertebral collapse has indeed occurred as a result of progressive tumor lysis, the oncologist must attempt to ensure that the options of irradiation or of surgical intervention have not been precluded by iatrogenic bone marrow depression caused by an overly aggressive regimen of chemotherapy.

Patients with spinal metastases can be divided into five categories, depending on the extent of neurological compromise or bone destruction:

Class I: No significant neurological involvement.
Class II: Bony involvement without collapse or instability.
Class III: Major neurological impairment (sensory or motor) without significant bony involvement.
Class IV: Vertebral collapse with mechanical pain or instability but without significant neurological compromise.
Class V: Vertebral collapse and instability combined with major neurological impairment.

Individuals in Classes I or II, with little or no neurological impairment and without evidence of vertebral collapse or instability, generally enjoy good relief from pain by chemotherapy or hormonal manipulation, or in the absence of success with these modalities, after local irradiation. Those in Class III, with neurological compromise in the absence of major bony destruction or spinal instability, usually will respond to radiotherapy alone. If the neurological compromise is of acute onset and relatively rapid, the radiotherapy should be augmented by systemic steroids.[21]

Spinal cord compression is reported to occur in approximately 5% of patients with widespread cancer.[21,22] The most common cause of cord or root compression is the extrusion of tumor tissue and bony detritus into the spinal canal following the partial collapse of a vertebral body infiltrated and weakened by a metastatic deposit (Fig. 17.3). On occasion, tumor tissue may break into the canal and compress the cord without causing significant destruction or collapse of the vertebral body (Fig. 17.4). Rarely a cord or root compression may result from a soft tissue mass growing into the spinal canal through a neural foramen, from intradural metastases, or from carcinomatous meningitis. However, as already noted, it is uncommon for the dura to be penetrated by metastatic tumor

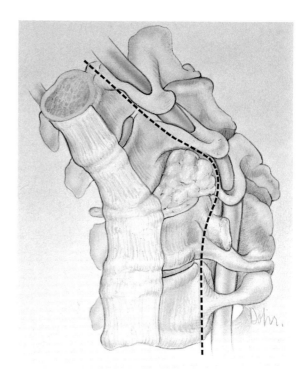

Fig. 17.3 Replacement of the vertebral body by tumor results in collapse of the body, increasing kyphosis, and extrusion of the tumor and bone fragments into the epidural space

tissue, although a reactive dural thickening is commonly encountered.

Because the metastatic tumor mass typically invades the canal from the vertebral body, the anterior cord motor functions are usually compromised first with sensory disturbances following as the cord is displaced posteriorly and impinges on the lamina. Although the lumbar vertebrae are most commonly affected by tumor metastases, it is in the thoracic spine that cord compression most commonly occurs. This is because the cord is largest here relative to canal diameter and thus suffers compression earliest from a given tumor mass. Extradural tumor may cause cord compression at more than one level in the same patients. Although clinically significant cord compromise is uncommon at multiple levels, this possibility must always

SPINAL STABILIZATION

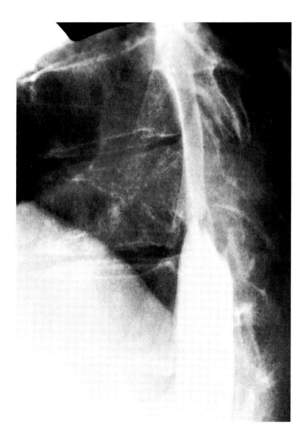

Fig. 17.4 Unusual 'napkin ring' constriction of the cord caused by a metastatic tumor within the spinal canal growing around the dura to compress the cord circumferentially

be considered before treatment is commenced and is one of the strongest arguments for preoperative cervical to lumbar MR imaging.[11,12]

Histological examination of spinal cords taken from patients dying with clinical evidence of metastatic cord compression reveals no consistent pattern. The pathological alterations are often minimal despite severe and long-standing clinical disease. Edema and cellular degeneration have been noted in the myelinated tissues at the level(s) compromised, but the gray matter generally is well preserved. The distribution of pathological changes usually does not conform to the arterial supply or venous drainage of the cord, although it has been suggested that venous occlusion is the most important factor leading to neuronal degeneration.[21]

CLINICAL COURSE

The most frequent manifestation of osseous metastasis is pain, usually localized, gradual in onset, relentlessly progressive, tender to percussion, and often worse at night. Radicular pain, when present, may assist the clinician in localizing the level of vertebral involvement. About half of all patients who ultimately develop cord impingement will complain of radicular pain for weeks or months before long-track signs become apparent. Loss of sphincter control is a late phenomenon, and usually occurs in patients with the most profound neurological deficits. In their series of 600 patients with spinal metastases and neurological compromise, Constans *et al.* found only 14 with isolated sphincter disturbances as a presenting symptom.[22] The sensory level is not a reliable indicator of the level of cord compromise, usually being recorded several segments below a myelographically demonstrable subarachnoid block.

The rapidity of onset of muscular weakness has considerable bearing on the ultimate prognosis. When there is a delay of less than 24 hours between the onset of symptoms and the appearance of the full-blown neurological syndrome, the prognosis is poor for recovery, no matter what treatment is offered.[2] Conversely, most patients whose neurological deficit has developed over a period of 7–10 days will respond favorably to cord decompression. Patients with rapid neurological deterioration most commonly have metastases involving the thoracic spine where the canal/cord ratio is smallest. Rapid neurological deterioration in this area may also be reflective of vascular compromise, and it has been demonstrated that cord blood supply is most tenuous between the T4 and T9 levels.[23]

DIAGNOSIS

Diagnostic studies must be considered before a focus of spinal metastases may be approached

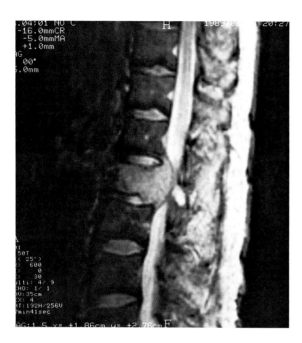

Fig. 17.5 Saggital T2-weighted MR image of the thoracolumbar junction revealing the L1 vertebral body to be completely replaced by tumor tissue which has extruded posteriorly markedly compressing the lower cord and completely obstructing the spinal canal

operatively. Bone scintigraphy is the most sensitive technique for demonstrating vertebral pathological fractures, but is rarely diagnostic of metastatic disease.[24] Patients with pathological vertebral fractures secondary to osteoporosis but not malignancy often show changes on scan which are indistinguishable from the effects of malignancy. False negative scans may occur when lytic lesions have prompted minimal reactive bone formation and where little if any vascular response has been elicited.[25] The most serious deficiency of bone scintigraphy is that it will often reflect multiple areas of vertebral involvement without clarifying which, if any, level is associated with progressive pain, neurological compromise, or vertebral collapse.[11]

MR imaging has become the preferred method for the evaluation of the extent of vertebral replacement by tumor and the extent of extraosseous extension, particularly within the spinal canal (Fig. 17.5). Computerized tomography (CT) remains the procedure of choice for examining fine cortical bone detail, including evaluation of spine fractures and assessing neural foraminal size, but it is much less sensitive than MR for detecting marrow-infiltrating disorders. There is still an occasional need for myelography, particularly in patients developing late recurrent neurological compromise long after initial decompression and stabilization with metal implants which degrade the CT or MR image.

OPERATIVE TREATMENT

When metastatic tumor has destroyed enough bone to result in vertebral collapse and progressive mechanical spine pain (Class IV) or neurological compromise (Class V), it is illogical to assume that any improvement can result from irradiation alone, no matter how radiosensitive the malignancy itself may be.

The indications for surgical intervention can be summarized as follows:

- Progressive spinal canal impingement and cord compression by radioresistant tumor, by recurrent tumor in an area already subjected to maximal irradiation, or by bone and soft tissue detritus extruded into the canal as a result of progressive spinal deformity. These patients require decompression anteriorly, anterolaterally, or posteriorly with or without spinal stabilization (Class V).
- Progressive kyphotic spinal deformity with intact posterior structures, but with intractable mechanical spine pain. These patients require anterior decompression and anterior stabilization (Class IV).
- Progressive kyphotic deformity associated with posterior element disruption and progressive shear deformity. These patients require anterior and posterior decompression and stabilization (Class IV or V).

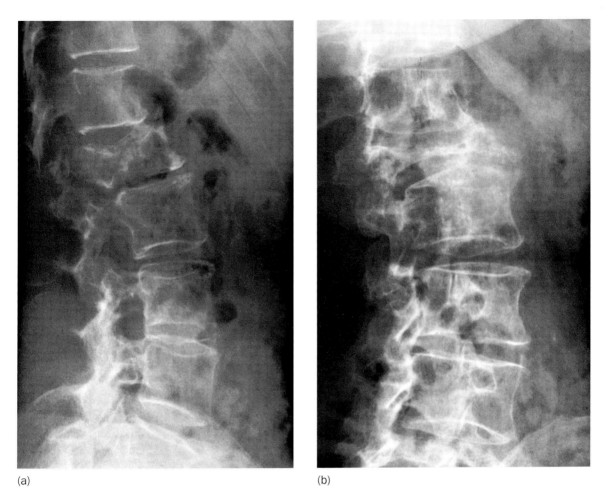

(a) (b)

Fig. 17.6 (a) Another postirradiation insufficiency fracture (of L1) in a 58-year-old woman with known breast cancer metastases in the lumbar spine. Two years earlier she had received local irradiation (3500 cGy) because of increasing back pain. The pain had resolved, but then returned in conjunction with the fracture apparent here. An additional 2000 cGy of radiation was given on the presumption that this was a pathological fracture from recurrent cancer. (b) Within 6 weeks, the vertebral body had collapsed completely and a severe cauda equina syndrome had developed with marked segmental instability. At operation, no evidence of tumor was noted, but there was histologic evidence of extensive radiation necrosis. A combination of anterior and posterior stabilization was required.

Denis and White have popularized the concept of the three-column spine, and have defined from both a biomechanical and a clinical viewpoint the extent of bony and soft tissue disruption necessary to result in true spinal instability.[26,27] Lytic destruction of an anterior vertebral body (anterior column only) is often the initial manifestation of metastatic involvement, but does not cause spinal instability and progressive deformity unless the posterior vertebral body (middle column) is destroyed as well. If the vertebral body begins to collapse, its ability to function as a weight-bearing fulcrum decreases, and the bending moment of the spine

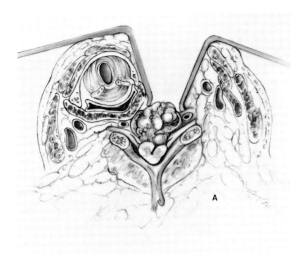
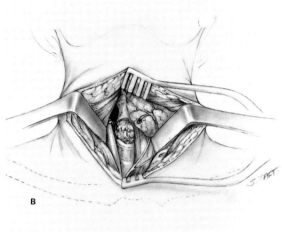

Fig. 17.7(a)–(e) Technique for anterior decompression and stabilization of the cervical spine. (a) Cross-sectional view of the neck demonstrating displacement and compression of the spinal cord by an expanding tumor mass. The anterior approach is shown with trachea, esophagus, and paratracheal muscles retracted medially and the sternocleidomastoid and the carotid sheath retracted laterally.

(b) Anterior view of the operative approach demonstrating the level of vertebral involvement (C5). The retracted thyroid gland and its ligated and transected middle thyroid vein are shown. The location of the recurrent laryngeal nerve is also indicated, although this is not invariably visualized.

shifts posteriorly with compression loads on the remaining vertebral body increasing geometrically. A progressive kyphotic deformity typically ensues, and the vector of this compression load encourages the extrusion of tumor tissue, disk, and bony debris posteriorly into the spinal canal (Fig. 17.3). If the posterior elements are minimally involved, and tensile stability of the third (posterior) column remains intact, spinal stability can be restored entirely through the anterior approach.[2,28,29]

The diseased anterior structures can be resected, the spinal canal decompressed, and the anterior and middle column stability restored by bone grafting or artificial constructs. However, if tumor destruction of the posterior elements is advanced as well, the greatly increased tensile loads posteriorly cannot be resisted, and a forward shearing deformity will develop, further compromising the spinal canal (Fig. 17.6(a) and (b)). This condition necessitates both an anterior and posterior decompression and stabilization.

The normal anatomy of the posterior longitudinal ligament is such that immediately behind the intervertebral disk the ligament is thick and broad, thereby minimizing the risk of central disk herniations under any circumstances. Behind the vertebral body, however, the posterior longitudinal ligament is thin and narrow, and it offers little resistance to posterior extrusion of tumor tissue or bone fragments against the cord. The technique of anterior decompression involves a complete vertebrectomy. The anterior two thirds of the vertebra can be removed with relative ease using a rongeur or large curette. As the surgeon approaches the posterior third of the vertebral body, and therefore the spinal canal, great care must be taken to remove tumor and bone debris without in any

SPINAL STABILIZATION 253

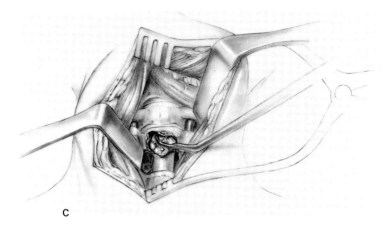

Fig. 17.7 continued
(c) The spinal cord has been decompressed anteriorly by resection of the tumor and C5 vertebral body remnants. In this instance the C4 vertebral body was found to be markedly weakened by tumor infiltration and was also removed piecemeal by an angled curette.

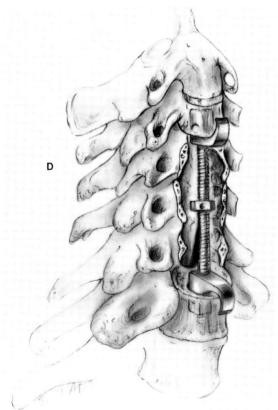

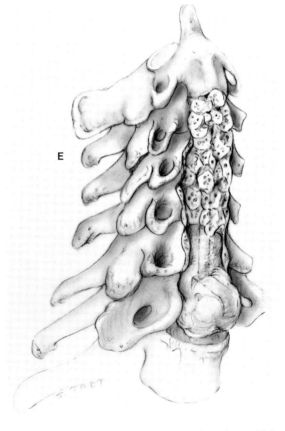

(d) Once the spinal canal has been decompressed completely and the endplates of the adjacent intact vertebral bodies have been perforated with a high-speed dental burr, the Knodt rod is positioned with its hooks embedded into the adjacent vertebral bodies and the previous vertebral height restored by twisting the rod

(e) The defect is filled with methylmethacrylate which polymerizes *in situ*, incorporating the rods and hooks. Care has been taken to prevent expansion of the acrylic into the spinal cavity by placing two malleable retractors behind the cement construct. In patients who have not been irradiated within 3 months preoperatively and who will not be irradiated within 3 months postoperatively, cancellous bone chips are packed anteriorly to the cement and metal construct in an effort to achieve a permanent bony arthrodesis.

way enhancing the already existing impingement on the spinal canal. An angled curette usually is the most effective instrument and allows material to be pulled forward out of the canal and away from the dura. For lesions of the cervical spine, an anterior approach is employed through the avascular interval between the sternocleidomastoid and carotid sheath laterally and the strap muscles, trachea, and esophagus medially (Fig. 17.7(a)). The middle thyroid vein is the only structure which usually requires ligation and transection, although care must be taken to avoid injury to the recurrent laryngeal nerve which runs obliquely through the lower field (Fig. 17.7(b)). If exposure of more than three cervical vertebrae is anticipated, a longitudinal incision can be used paralleling the anterior border of the sternocleidomastoid. In extreme circumstances, where an extensile exposure from C1 to T1 is required, the inverted L approach, popularized by Riley, can be employed.[30] Using longitudinal blunt dissection, one exposes the anterior longitudinal ligament and then gently reflects the longus coli to either side. This reveals the transverse processes and the canal for the vertebral artery. When the patient has received local irradiation preoperatively, particular care must be taken in retracting the esophagus which may be friable and prone to perforation.

The narrowed vertebral height and forward bulge of the tumor tissue (Fig. 17.7(b)) will usually be apparent and are helpful in identifying the level or levels of vertebral collapse. The major advantage of the anterior approach is in the surgeon's ability to resect the tumor focus directly, decompress the neurological structures from the side of their compromise, and jack open the collapsed vertebral space, thereby correcting the kyphotic deformity at its source.

Initial removal of tumor and destroyed bone can be expedited by using a rongeur; care should be taken to avoid damage to the intact vertebral bodies above and below the level(s) to be resected. When approximately two thirds of the body has been resected, it is safer to proceed thenceforth with an angled curette whose smooth rounded back surface is not likely to penetrate the spinal canal (Fig. 17.7(c)). The angled curette is also an effective instrument for undercutting the vertebral endplates proximal and distal to the vertebrae resected to ensure that the canal is fully decompressed and that no gross tumor tissue is left within the spinal canal anteriorly. Usually, the posterior longitudinal ligament has been destroyed by the tumor, and the dura will be readily visualized. Depending on the duration of tumor impingement on the dura, and particularly if the patient has been irradiated preoperatively, the dura will be gray-white and markedly thickened, with tumor tissue and bony or soft tissue debris firmly adherent to its anterior surface. By careful dissection using a small angled curette, it is possible to strip away this tissue without much risk of perforating the surprisingly tough dura.

Once the cord and roots have been decompressed completely, stabilization follows. Some surgeons advocate the use of an anterior interbody corticocancellous bone graft, keyed into the adjacent vertebral endplates and stabilized by external immobilization until incorporation is complete.[31,32] The rationale for using this technique is that once graft incorporation is complete, there need be no further concern for spinal instability. However, in patients who are chronically debilitated and facing a limited life expectancy, the requirement for prolonged external immobilization in excess of 10 weeks postoperatively is a serious disadvantage. Moreover, in patients who have received or will receive local irradiation within 3 or 4 months of operation, the likelihood of bone graft becoming incorporated at any point is markedly reduced.[2,28,33]

In an effort to achieve instant internal stability, not dependent on graft incorporation and not requiring external immobilization, many surgeons have begun using polymethylmethacrylate to create an artificial vertebral construct. Simple reconstruction of the vertebral body using this acrylic cement can be effective in preventing a recurrence of a kyphotic deformity, because, once polymerized, the cement has excellent resistance to compressive loads. However, it is difficult to correct the original deformity by using polymethylmethacrylate alone, and there is no means of affixing the cement mass effectively to the adjacent intact vertebral bodies. Attempts to secure the acrylic by a screw or wire are rarely effective, because the cement is a brittle material, and the screw will break out with repeated stresses. The use of anterior semi-tubular plates or intravertebral threaded pins to augment cement stabilization has been advocated by some,[18,34,35] but again these devices do not enhance restoration of normal vertebral body height before filling of the defect by cement. They have the additional disadvantage of protruding anterior to the vertebral column and potentially eroding the esophagus or, in the case of intravertebral pins, of migrating into the spinal canal.[36]

We have found the most adjustable and effective technique to be the use either of a Knodt distraction rod and hooks (Zimmer, Warsaw, Indiana, USA) (Fig. 17.7(d)) or the Rezaian spinal fixator (AMS, Hayward, California, USA) (see Fig. 17.10c), both of which effectively jack open the collapsed vertebral space(s) to an appropriate height, remain within the long axis of the vertebral column, and can be completely incorporated into the acrylic vertebral replacement[7,11,29] (Fig. 17.7(e)). The smaller Knodt distraction rods and hooks are best suited for the cervical and upper thoracic spine; the Rezaian fixator for the lower thoracic and lumbar spine.[37]

The endplates of the intact vertebral bodies above and below the area of decompression are penetrated using a high-speed power burr, and the cavity thus created enlarged to accept both the rod and the body of the hook (Fig. 17.7(d)). The tip of the hook protrudes slightly anterior to the vertebral body, but the remainder of the distraction device is incorporated by the acrylic cement (Fig. 17.8).

Although there are many patients who have survived for 3 or more years following stabilization without evidence of deterioration of their reconstruction, it is at least theoretically possible that many of these constructs, not reinforced by a bony arthrodesis, ultimately will fail. Consequently, for a patient with a projected survival in excess of 2 years, reinforcement of

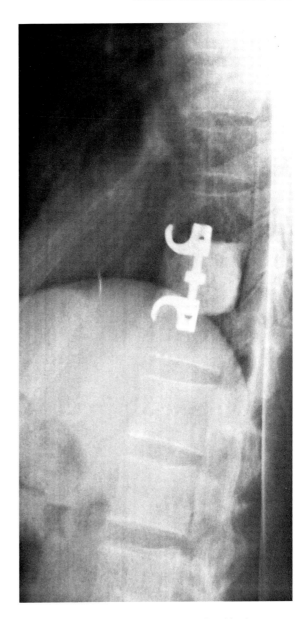

Fig. 17.8 Lateral X-ray demonstrating ideal positioning of the Knodt rod and methylmethacrylate after decompression and stabilization of the mid-thoracic spine

the vertebral replacement by anterior cancellous bone grafting is advocated. The graft can be packed over the remaining lateral elements of the resected vertebrae, as well as proximally and

256 CANCER AND THE SKELETON

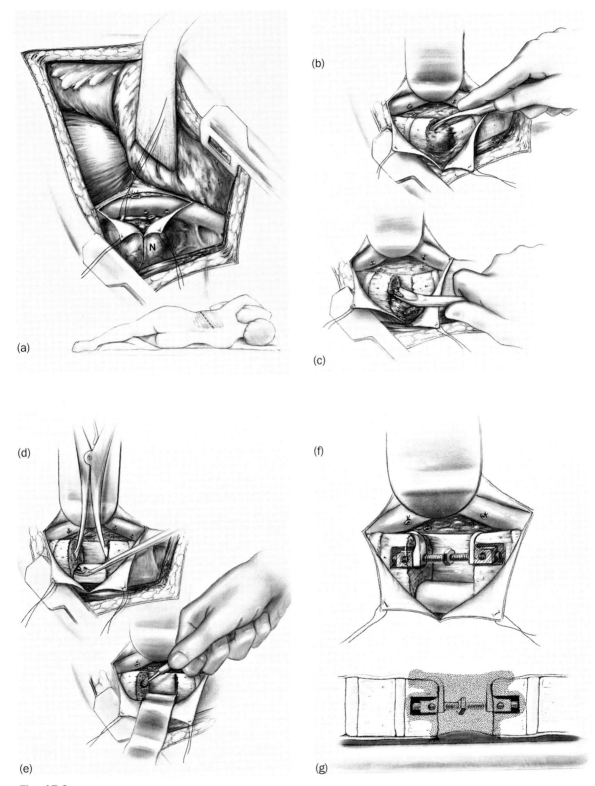

Fig. 17.9

Fig. 17.9 (a) Anterior decompression of the thoracic spine is accomplished by a thoracotomy with the patient in the lateral decubitus position. The aorta has been exposed and the segmental vessels ligated and transected. A prominent vertebral extrapleural tumor mass is apparent (N) and assists in localizing the focus of destruction.
(b) Most of the tumor and bone/disk debris has been removed using a small periosteal elevator.
(c) As the surgeon approaches the level of the posterior cortical margin, further decompression is accomplished using an angled gouge or curette. All disk material adherent to the adjacent vertebral body is removed.
(d) The vertebral space has been recreated using a lamina spreader. A small angled curette is used to complete decompression of the spinal canal and to round off the edges of the posterior cortex of the adjacent vertebrae.
(e) The endplates of adjacent vertebrae are undercut using a high-speed burr in order to allow the ends of the Knodt rod and the bodies of its hooks to be buried within the vertebral bone.
(f) The Knodt rod has been positioned with the resected space. As the rod was twisted, the hooks were distracted and their bodies now are firmly impacted within the adjacent vertebral bone. Only the tips of the hooks extend anterior to the vertebral cortex.
(g) The defect is filled with methylmethacrylate polymerizing *in situ*, incorporating the rods and hooks. As with the cervical spine, a malleable retractor, placed behind the expanding cement mass, prevents compression of the cord and intrusion on the epidural space.

distally over the exposed cortices of the intact vertebrae above and below the level of decompression (Fig. 17.7(e)). If a patient is irradiated within 2 months of his or her operation, it is unlikely that the cancellous graft will be incorporated. However, in patients who do not require further irradiation, the incidence of graft incorporation and the development of a mature bony arthrodesis has been high.[11]

Anterior decompression and stabilization of the thoracic spine require a thoracotomy, but once the heart, lung, and great vessels have been retracted, the vertebral bodies are readily approachable from T3 to L2 (Fig. 17.9). The upper thoracic spine (T1–T3) can be exposed using a thoracoplasty approach by mobilizing the scapula anteriorly and by resecting the second rib.

The lumbar spine is the most common location of spinal metastases, but the least likely area to require surgical decompression. This is fortunate because it is also the area where anterior exposure is the most difficult, at least for the L4, L5, and S1 vertebrae. Because of the prominent lordotic curve, particularly at the lumbosacral junction, and because of the increased torque mobility of the lumbar spine, both anterior and posterior stabilization ordinarily is required after anterior decompression. The combination usually chosen consists of anterior distraction fixation with the Rezaian device and PMMA, followed by posterior stabilization by pedicle screw/rod constructs or by the Luque rods with sublaminar wire fixation if pedicular bone is deficient (Fig. 17.10(a)–(c)). Alternative techniques for spinal decompression and stabilization include laminectomy with or without posterior fixation, arterial embolization, endoscopic decompression, and percutaneous vertebroplasty using injected PMMA. In a retrospective series based on 20 years' experience, Gilbert *et al.* reported that radiation alone was as effective as decompressive laminectomy, with or without irradiation, in the treatment of epidural cord compression. They measured the success of treatment in terms of overall function, noting that slightly less than 50% of patients regained the ability to walk, and also noting that more patients regained the ability to walk after irradiation alone than after irradiation with laminectomy decompression.[5] Since the publication of Gilbert's work, attempts to decompress the anteriorly compressed neural canal by posterior laminectomy thankfully are uncommon, although some authors continue to advocate the approach for selected patients who are debilitated or have multiple vertebrae involved.[38–41] The rate of local tumor recurrence and renewed neurological compromise is significantly higher using this approach.[38] In addition, a

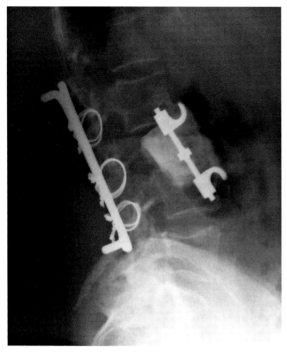

(a)

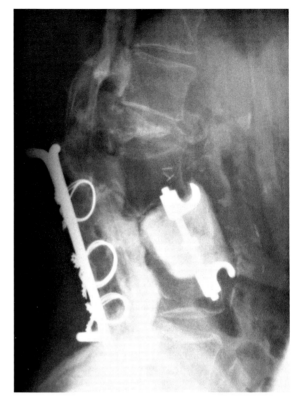

(b)

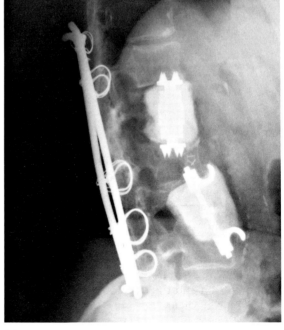

(c)

Fig. 17.10 (a) Radiograph of a 65-year-old woman with multiple myeloma, progressive tumor infiltration, and collapse of the L3 vertebral body. The patient presented with a rapidly progressive cauda equina syndrome (Frankel Grade C) despite 4500 cGy of local irradiation. After anterior L3 vertebrectomy and replacement by methylmethacrylate incorporating a Knodt rod, a posterior four-level stabilization was accomplished with Luque rods and sublaminar wire fixation. The patient enjoyed a complete neurologic recovery.
(b) Six years later, a new compression fracture appeared at L1, again associated with a progressive cauda equina syndrome.
(c) The L1 vertebral body was replaced using methylmethacrylate incorporating a Rezaian vertebral distractor. An attempt was made to replace the entire anterior vertebral construct with a longer Rezaian distractor and cement, but because of the extensive previous irradiation, the great vessels were so scarred down to the previous operative site that exposing it was impossible. The original Luque rods were replaced with longer rods and sublaminar wiring spanning seven levels.

major disadvantage of the posterior approach in previously irradiated patients is the fact that posterior soft tissue coverage of the spine often has become retracted and poorly vascularized as a result of the radiation, and the risk of major postoperative wound healing complications is high. For all these reasons, the author restricts use of the posterior approach to those patients with circumferential dural compression (Fig. 17.4) and to patients requiring combined anterior and posterior stabilization.

Arterial embolization techniques, usually employed serially for the control of the growth of expansile tumor metastases in vertebrae, have been successful in some hands.[15,42] However, the technique is fraught with complications, particularly in inexperienced hands.[16] To date, the author has had no experience with endoscopic anterior spinal decompression or with endoscopic-assisted anterior decompression with stabilization. Initial published studies have demonstrated the potential of this technique, although the complication rate remains high.[8,18] Percutaneous injection vertebroplasty can effectively stabilize collapsing vertebral bodies and, at least transiently, can relieve spinal pain in debilitated patients. However, no neurological decompression can be achieved by this technique, and again the complication rate is significant.[17]

RESULTS

It is essential to discuss, at least briefly, the overall results for the treatment of patients with spinal instability and neurological compromise from metastatic malignancy. Only by such an assessment can the reader determine for him or herself whether the aggressive techniques described here for selected instances of cord and root decompression and for spinal stabilization seem justified.

Frankel et al.[43] established a classification system for quantitating neurological compromise (Table 17.1). With the use of this system, the extent of sensory and motor dysfunction can be conveniently discussed, and the results of various treatment regimens can be compared. Although the Frankel classification relates

Table 17.1 Frankel classification system for neurological compromise

Grade A	Complete motor and sensory loss
Grade B	Complete motor loss; incomplete sensory loss
Grade C	Some motor function below the level of involvement; incomplete sensory loss
Grade D	Useful motor function below the level of involvement; incomplete sensory loss
Grade E	Normal motor and sensory function

primarily to acute trauma, rather than gradually progressive spinal cord compromise, it is nevertheless useful as a means of comparing the efficacy of different techniques for treating metastatic spine disease.

Using this system, Nather and Bose reported that fewer than 5% of patients with Frankel Grade A, B, or C lesions recovered normal (Grade E) or near-normal (Grade D) function after laminectomy decompression.[7] By comparison, in the author's series of 77 patients treated by techniques of anterior decompression described herein, 62% improved to the level of either Grade D or Grade E.[29] Of the 14 patients with complete paraplegia or quadriplegia (Grade A), eight improved at least two grades, and six regained the ability to walk and have normal bowel and bladder function.[7] The mean postoperative survival period for patients with breast metastases, myeloma, and lymphoma was approximately 28 months. At the other extreme, patients with lung cancer metastases had a mean postoperative survival period of only 8 months. Nineteen patients survived for more than 4 years postoperatively. Twelve had major neurological compromise preoperatively, and all 12 had improved at least two grades postoperatively. As expected, the long-term survivors had primarily malignant conditions with good prognoses for survival, including breast carcinoma in 10 patients and multiple myeloma in 6.

Ten of the 19 survivors required additional operations for the sequellae of other metastases, including four with distant spinal metastases and two with late local recurrence. Two patients suffered posterior wound sloughs through previous irradiated tissue. There were no wound-healing problems with anterior spine approaches. This fact reinforces the concern about wound-healing problems following posterior decompression or stabilization attempts. The author's experience seems comparable with that of other clinical investigators who used similar decompression and stabilization techniques.[35,44–47]

CONCLUSION

Based on these results, the author believes that patients with major neurological compromise or intractable mechanical spine pain from vertebral collapse or instability should be considered for decompression and stabilization, assuming their general medical condition does not preclude such aggressive treatment. The majority can be treated with the anterior approach alone. However, the author's enthusiasm for this procedure must not be construed as an advocacy for surgical management of all spinal metastases. Most patients do not continue to suffer severe pain after vertebral collapse once they have completed an initial period of rest and a course of local irradiation. Most do not experience significant neurological compromise, and many with spinal involvement, even when associated with severe local pain or neurological compromise, do not enjoy a sufficiently long-life expectancy to warrant operative intervention of this magnitude.

REFERENCES

1. Fujita T, Ueda Y, Kawahara N, Baba H, Tomita K. Local spread of metastatic vertebral tumors. A histologic study. *Spine* (1997) **22**: 1905–12.
2. Harrington KD. Metastatic disease of the spine. *J Bone Joint Surg* (1986) **68 (A)**: 1110–15.
3. Jaffe WL. *Tumors and Tumorous Conditions of the Bones and Joints* (Philadelphia, PA: Lea & Febiger, 1985).
4. Taneichi H, Kaneda K, Takeda N, Abumi K, Satoh S. Risk factors and probability of vertebral body collapse in metastases of the thoracic and lumbar spine. *Spine* (1997) **22**: 239–45.
5. Gilbert RW, Kim JH, Posner JB. Epidural spinal cord compression from metastatic tumor: diagnosis and treatment. *Ann Neurol* (1978) **3**: 40–51.
6. Geldof AA. Models for cancer skeletal metastasis: a reappraisal of Batson's plexus. *Anticancer Res* (1997) **17**: 1535–9.
7. Harrington KD. *Orthopaedic Management of Metastatic Bone Disease* (St Louis, MO: CV Mosby, 1988).
8. Huang TJ, Hsu RW, Liu HP, Liao YS, Shih HN. Technique of video-assisted thoracoscopic surgery for the spine: new approach. *World J Surg* (1997) **21**: 358–62.
9. Batson OV. The role of the vertebral veins in metastatic process. *Ann Intern Med* (1942) **16**: 38–45.
10. Galasko CSB, Bennett A. Relationship of bone destruction in skeletal metastases to osteoclast activation and prostaglandins. *Nature* (1976) **263**: 508–10.
11. Harrington KD. Metastatic tumors of the spine: diagnosis and treatment. *J Am Acad Orthop Surg* (1993) **1**: 76–86.
12. Heldmann U, Myschetzky PS, Thomsen HS. Frequency of unexpected multifocal metastasis in patients with acute spinal cord compression. Evaluation by low-field MR imaging in cancer patients. *Acta Radiologica* (1997) **38**: 372–5.
13. Onimus M, Schraub S, Bertin D, Bosset JF, Guidet M. Surgical treatment of vertebral metastases. *Spine* (1986) **11**: 883–94.
14. Windhagen HJ, Hipp JA, Silva MJ, Lipson SJ, Hayes WC. Predicting failure of thoracic vertebrae with simulated and actual metastatic defects. *Clin Orthop* (1997) **344**: 313–19.
15. Hess T, Kramann B, Schmidt E, Rupp S. Use of preoperative vascular embolization in spinal metastasis resection. *Arch Orthop Trauma Surg* (1997) **116**: 279–82.
16. Vetter SC, Strecker EP, Ackermann LW, Harms J. Preoperative embolization of cervical spine tumors. *Cardiovasc Intervent Radiol* (1997) **20**: 343–7.

17. Cortet B, Cotten A, Boutry N et al. Percutaneous vertebroplasty in patients with osteolytic metastases or multiple myeloma. *Rev Rhum Engl Ed* (1997) **64**: 177–83.
18. Huang TJ, Hsu RW, Liu HP, Liao YS, Hsu KY, Shih HN. Analysis of techniques for video-assisted thoracoscopic internal fixation of the spine. *Arch Orthop Trauma Surg* (1998) **117**: 92–5.
19. Carter SK. Methodology of data reporting in advanced breast cancer trials. *Cancer Chemother Pharmacol* (1979) **3**: 1–5.
20. Chlebowski RT, Irwin LE, Pugh RP, Sadoff L, Hestorff R. Survival of patients with metastatic breast cancer treated with either combination or sequential chemotherapy. *Cancer Res* (1979) **39**: 4503–6.
21. Boland PJ, Lane JM, Sundaresan N. Metastatic disease of the spine. *Clin Orthop* (1982) **169**: 95–102.
22. Constans JP, De Vitis E, Donzelli R, Spaciank R, Meder JP, Haye C. Spinal metastases with neurological manifestations. *J Neurosurg* (1983) **59**: 111–18.
23. Dommisse GF. The blood supply of the spinal cord: a critical vascular zone in spinal surgery. *J Bone Joint Surg* (1974) **56 (B)**: 225–35.
24. Tatsui H, Onomura T, Morishita S, Oketa M, Inoue T. Survival rates of patients with metastatic spinal cancer after scintigraphic detection of abnormal radioactive accumulation. *Spine* (1996) **21**: 2143–8.
25. Kinoshita T, Ishii K, Imai Y. Disappearance of 99mTc-MDP accumulation in metastatic bone disease during bone scintigraphy. *Radiat Med* (1997) **15**: 235–7.
26. Denis F. Spinal instability as defined by the three-column spine concept in acute spinal trauma. *Clin Orthop* (1984) **189**: 65–76.
27. White III AA, Panjabi MM. *Clinical Biomechanics of the Spine* (Philadelphia, PA: Lippincott, 1978): 394, 424–5.
28. Harrington KD. Anterior cord decompression and spine stabilization for patients with metastatic lesions of the spine. *J Neurosurg* (1984) **61**: 107–17.
29. Harrington KD. Anterior decompression and stabilization of the spine as treatment for vertebral collapse and spinal cord compression from metastatic malignancy. *Clin Orthop* (1988) **233**: 177–97.
30. Riley L. Surgical approaches to the anterior structures of the cervical spine. *Clin Orthop* (1973) **91**: 16–20.
31. Johnson JR, Leatherman KD, Holt RT. Anterior decompression of the spinal cord for neurological deficit. *Spine* (1983) **8**: 396–405.
32. Walsh GL, Gokaslan ZL, McCutcheon IE et al. Anterior approaches to the thoracic spine in patients with cancer: indications and results. *Ann Thorac Surg* (1997) **64**: 1611–18.
33. Fidler MW. Anterior decompression and stabilization of metastatic spinal fractures. *J Bone Joint Surg* (1986) **68 (B)**: 83–90.
34. Kostuik JP. Anterior spinal cord decompression for lesions of the thoracic and lumbar spine, techniques, new methods of internal fixation, results. *Spine* (1983) **8**: 512–31.
35. Sundaresan N, Galicich JH, Lane JM, Barnes MS, McCormack P. Treatment of neoplastic epidural cord compression by vertebral body resection and stabilization. *J Neurosurg* (1985) **63**: 676–84.
36. McAfee PC, Bohlman HH, Ducker T. Failure of stabilization of the spine with methylmethacrylate: a retrospective analysis of twenty-four cases. *J Bone Joint Surg Am* (1986) **68**: 1145–57.
37. Rezaian SM. Rezaian spinal fixator for management of fractures of the thoracolumbar spine. *J Neurol Orthop Med Surg* (1991) **12**: 307–14.
38. Bauer HC. Posterior decompression and stabilization for spinal metastases: analysis of sixty-seven consecutive patients. *J Bone Joint Surg* (1997) **79 (A)**: 514–22.
39. Lee CK, Rosa R, Fernand R. Surgical treatment of tumors of the spine. *Spine* (1986) **11**: 20–30.
40. Sapkas G, Kyratzoulis J, Papaioannou N, Babis G, Rologis D, Tzanis S. Spinal cord decompression and stabilization in malignant lesions of the spine. *Acta Orthop Scand Suppl* (1997) **275**: 97–100.
41. Siegal T, Siegal T. Surgical decompression of anterior and posterior malignant epidural tumors compressing the spinal cord: a prospective study. *Neurosurgery* (1985) **17**: 424–32.
42. Olerud C, Jonsson H, Lofberg AM. Embolization of spinal metastases reduces perioperative blood loss: twenty-one patients operated for renal cell carcinoma. *Acta Orthop Scand* (1993) **64**: 9–12.
43. Frankel HL, Hancock DO, Hyslop G. The value of postural reduction in the initial management of closed injuries of the spine with paraplegia and tetraplegia. *Paraplegia* (1969) **7**: 179–92.
44. Bohlman HH, Sachs BL, Carter JR. Primary neoplasms of the cervical spine: diagnosis and treatment of twenty-three patients. *J Bone Joint Surg* (1986) **68 (A)**: 483–94.

45. Siegal T, Tiqva P, Siegal T. Vertebral body resection for epidural compression by malignant tumors: results of forty-seven consecutive operative procedures. *J Bone Joint Surg Am* (1985) **67**: 375–82.
46. Sundaresan N, Galicich JH, Lane JM. Harrington rod stabilization for pathological fractures of the spine. *J Neurosurg* (1984) **60**: 282–6.
47. Weinstein JN, Kostuik JP. Differential diagnosis and surgical treatment of metastatic spine tumors. In Frymoyer JW (ed) *The Adult Spine: Principles and Practice* (New York: Raven Press, 1991): 861–88.

18

Osteoporosis in cancer patients

Aurélie Fontana and Pierre D Delmas

Direct effects of cancer treatment on bone loss • Indirect effects of cancer treatment on bone loss • Prevention of osteoporosis in patients with cancer • Breast cancer and bone loss: a major problem of management • Conclusion

Bone metabolism is characterized by two opposite activities: the formation of new bone by osteoblasts and the resorption of old bone by osteoclasts. Both are normally tightly coupled in time and space and bone mass depends on the balance between resorption and formation. Cancer itself may induce bone loss. Histomorphometric studies in hematological malignancies such as myeloma and chronic lymphoid leukemia have shown an increased bone resorption in the area invaded by malignant B-cells.[1,2] Moreover, studies of biological markers of bone turnover in solid tumors have shown increased bone resorption in patients presenting with cancer without bone metastases.[3] Breast carcinoma and other tumors increase osteoclastic activity probably by increasing the release of transforming growth factor (TGFα or β), parathyroid hormone related protein (PTHrP), and cytokines. Cancer treatment may also have direct or indirect effects on bone loss. With the improvement in cancer treatment, the number of long-term survivors increases, and the long-term consequences of adverse effects of treatment on bone become significant. In particular, osteoporosis is now a common finding in long-term survivors from breast cancer, the diagnosis and management of which are a source of problems for the clinician.

DIRECT EFFECTS OF CANCER TREATMENT ON BONE LOSS

A review of children treated with high doses of methotrexate has suggested that methotrexate could have a deleterious effect on bone with fractures and osteoporosis. Pathogenesis was not clear but an increase excretion of urinary calcium was noted in several cases.[4] The direct effects of the chemotherapeutic agents doxorubicin and methotrexate have been studied in the rat.[5] Histomorphometric analysis of bone revealed a reduction of osteoid parameters with a decrease of the absolute osteoid volume but with no change of osteoblastic surfaces, suggesting that the matrix produced per osteoblast was reduced. Resorption parameters were increased with methotrexate and unchanged with doxorubicin. The trabecular bone volume was markedly reduced by both treatments and the overall bone formation rate was decreased by about 60%. Thus, these chemotherapeutic agents appear to have adverse effects on bone remodeling, especially on bone formation. In contrast, some authors have recently reported a possible beneficial effect of chlorambucil on bone with an increased bone mineral density (BMD) in patients treated with chlorambucil and corticoids for chronic lymphoid leukemia compared with a control group treated with corticoids only.[6]

A direct effect of suppressive thyroxine therapy on bone loss in patients with thyroid cancer has also been reported.[7] Hyperthyroidism is a classical cause of osteoporosis and thyroxine therapy is often associated with subclinical hyperthyroidism. Several studies of the effects of suppressive doses of thyroxine on bone density have been conducted, with conflicting results. A meta-analysis including 33 studies of the effects of thyroid hormone therapy (suppressive or replacement therapy) on bone mass concluded that suppressive thyroid hormone therapy is associated with significant bone loss in postmenopausal women. BMD was reduced on average by 7% at the lumbar spine, 5% at the femoral neck, and 9% at the trochanter of the hip. The theoretical risk of hip and spine fracture was about 1.6 higher in postmenopausal women treated by suppressive thyroid therapy than in controls.[8] In premenopausal women, the only longitudinal study in patients with suppressive doses of thyroxine for thyroid cancer or goitre, has shown an accelerated spinal bone loss during the 3 years of the follow-up (about 2.6%/year vs 0.2%/year in controls).[9] More recently, a randomized trial using intravenous pamidronate (30 mg every 3 months during 2 years) in patients treated with suppressive doses of T4 for thyroid cancer showed no significant bone loss at any site of the skeleton (spine, hip, radius, and total body) in the placebo group compared with a control group not treated by thyroxine. The group treated with pamidronate had a significant increase of BMD.[10]

Glucocorticoids are widely used in cancer, especially to control emesis induced by chemotherapy. In hematologic malignant diseases, glucocorticoids are also often used in association with other chemotherapeutic agents, e.g. dexamethasone in multiple myeloma. Large doses of glucocorticoids over a prolonged period of time induce a rapid and severe bone loss, resulting in osteoporotic fractures through two mechanisms. A dose-dependent inhibition of bone formation has been widely documented.

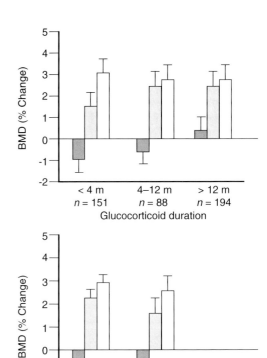

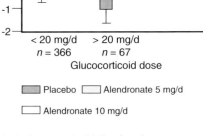

Fig. 18.1 Changes in BMD after 1 year according to the dose and the duration of glucocorticoid treatment. The change in BMD between the two doses of alendronate and the placebo is significant. (Adapted from ref. 13.)

An increase in osteoclastic bone resorption may occur with high doses – either directly or indirectly through secondary hyperparathyroidism related to the effects of glucocorticoids on calcium transport in the gut and kidney.[11] A prospective randomized study has shown that even low doses of glucocorticoid (mean of 7.5 mg per day) could induce a significant decrease in spine BMD in patients with rheumatoid arthritis after 20 weeks of treatment.[12] A double-blind, placebo-controlled study on the effect of alendronate in corticosteroid users showed that the decrease of spine BMD is more pronounced in newly treated patients with high-dose glucocorticoids, i.e. within 4 months and with a dose of prednisone ≥ 20 mg per day (Fig. 18.1).[13]

Some authors suggested that central nervous system irradiation could induce osteoporosis in children. Osteopenia is a common finding in children treated for brain tumors with a compromised health-related quality of life.[14] The study of 42 children treated for acute lymphoblastic leukemia has shown that irradiated patients had a significant decreased BMD measured by quantitative computed tomography compared with a nonirradiated group. The BMD of the nonirradiated group did not differ significantly from a group of healthy controls.[15] Growth hormone (GH) deficiency could be implicated as patients with GH deficiency induced by cranial or craniospinal irradiation for intracranial malignancy or acute leukemia have a significantly lower BMD if they are not treated by GH compared with patients treated by GH.[16]

INDIRECT EFFECTS OF CANCER TREATMENT ON BONE LOSS

Cancer treatment also has indirect effects on bone loss; chemotherapy may induce hypogonadism, and castration (surgical or by radiotherapy) is commonly used. Hypogonadism in men is known to induce bone loss with a large decrease of BMD during the first 2 years, about 7% per year.[17] This effect has been reported in men treated for Hodgkin's disease in whom BMD was measured on average 3–4 years after chemotherapy.[18] Men were in complete remission and all had azoospermia with raised luteinizing hormone (LH) and follicle stimulating hormone (FSH) levels, but no significant decrease in testosterone level. BMD was significantly reduced at the lumbar spine, femoral neck, and forearm with a positive correlation between serum testosterone level and lumbar spine and femoral neck BMD. Osteoporosis after orchidectomy for prostate cancer has also been

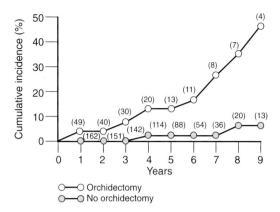

Fig. 18.2 Cumulative incidence of first osteoporotic fractures in men with prostate cancer with and without orchidectomy. Numbers in parentheses indicate patients remaining at each interval. (Adapted from ref. 19.)

reported.[19] About 14% of men treated by orchidectomy had osteoporotic fractures with a decrease of femoral neck BMD compared to 1% in men without orchidectomy. The cumulative incidence of first osteoporotic fractures was significantly increased in men with orchidectomy compared with men without orchidectomy (Fig. 18.2). Bone loss has also been observed in women treated for Hodgkin's disease; young women with premature ovarian failure induced by treatment had the same BMD compared with older postmenopausal women and they had a significantly lower BMD compared with those with a normal ovarian function after treatment.[20] Moreover, women treated by bone marrow transplantation for hematological malignancies generally undergo amenorrhea induced by total body irradiation[21] and cytotoxic drugs.[22] Estrogen deficiency induces accelerated bone loss within 5–8 years followed by a linear rate of bone loss. The age-related decrease in osteoblast activity within each remodeling unit combined with an increase in the number of remodeling units activated per unit time explains the magnitude of bone loss in postmenopausal women.[23]

PREVENTION OF OSTEOPOROSIS IN PATIENTS WITH CANCER

Oral contraceptives have been used to protect ovarian function in premenopausal women treated for Hodgkin's disease.[24] Chemotherapy often induces ovarian failure with destruction of ova and follicular elements of the ovary. When oral contraceptives were started at the time of chemotherapy, ovarian biopsies made after treatment did not show a decreased number of follicules contrasting with findings in women not so treated.

Amongst the various treatments of osteoporosis, bisphosphonates and estrogens (in postmenopausal women) appear to be the most effective. Hormone replacement therapy (HRT) is effective in slowing bone loss. During the first 2 years, HRT induces a significant increase in BMD which is more pronounced in cancellous bone than in cortical bone. Although the effects of HRT on incident fractures have been relatively little studied, cohort and case–control studies suggest strongly that HRT significantly decreases osteoporotic fractures. In most studies the relative risk of vertebral, hip, and wrist fractures ranges from 0.3 to 0.8 with an average of 0.6.[25]

Bisphosphonates are synthetic compounds which decrease bone resorption. They are known to prevent bone loss in a number of experimental osteoporosis models. They decrease bone turnover and increase bone balance at the basic multicellular unit (BMU) level. Several clinical studies have shown an increased BMD under bisphosphonate therapy; etidronate and alendronate are currently used in the treatment of osteoporosis in many countries. Their efficacy was also demonstrated in steroid osteoporosis. Some 117 patients with long-term corticosteroids were randomly assigned to receive a cyclical treatment of etidronate (400 mg/day). The lumbar spine BMD was maintained in the treated group compared with a significant decrease in the placebo group. The two groups had a decrease of the femoral neck BMD.[26] In a prospective, randomized, placebo-controlled study, glucocorticoid users treated with 5–10 mg alendronate showed a significant increase in spine BMD compared with placebo, with a significant decrease in the incidence of vertebral fracture (0.7% and 6.8% in the alendronate and placebo-treated groups, respectively)[27,28] (Fig. 18.1).

BREAST CANCER AND BONE LOSS: A MAJOR PROBLEM OF MANAGEMENT

Osteoporosis in breast cancer patients is a growing problem because it is the most frequent cancer in women and because a long survival is common. Seventy-one per cent of women after adjuvant chemotherapy for premenopausal breast cancer have premature ovarian failure and their BMD is significantly decreased compared with premenopausal women with breast cancer not treated by adjuvant chemotherapy.[29] A recent cross-sectional pilot study in 27 patients showed that more than 50% of premenopausal breast cancer patients had become amenorrheic after adjuvant chemotherapy and the lumbar spine BMD of these women was 14% lower compared with women who maintained normal ovarian function after chemotherapy.[30] Thus, the occurrence of vertebral and other fractures in breast cancer patients is not always due to bone metastases but can be related to osteoporosis. In such patients, osteoporotic fracture may be difficult to differentiate from metastatic fracture. Bone scintigraphy could be helpful in the presence of multiple areas of increased uptake. Magnetic resonance imaging, particularly in vertebral lesions, can differentiate benign fracture from malignant ones by detecting malignant infiltration of the bone marrow. Cancer markers such as breast carcinoma antigen (CA15-3) may also be helpful. An osteoporotic fracture will be associated with a decreased BMD at different sites of measurement by dual energy X-ray absorptiometry (DXA) although cancer with or without bone metastasis could also be associated with general bone loss.

In breast cancer, estrogen therapy is usually contraindicated because estrogens are closely related to the development of breast cancer.

Tamoxifen, a synthetic anti-estrogen, is widely used in breast cancer treatment and significantly reduces the risk of recurrence and death when used as adjuvant therapy. In premenopausal women, tamoxifen acts as an anti-estrogen on bone tissue and results in bone loss.[31] In contrast, several studies have shown a prevention of bone loss in postmenopausal breast cancer patients treated by tamoxifen compared with healthy postmenopausal controls, suggesting an estrogen-like effect on bone despite anti-estrogenic activity on the breast. The beneficial effects of tamoxifen on BMD in postmenopausal women are more pronounced in late than in early postmenopausal women and more in cancellous than in cortical bone. Love et al.[32] have shown in a large prospective, double-blind, randomized, controlled study an increased BMD at the spine in breast cancer patients treated with tamoxifen (20 mg/day) compared with a decreased BMD in the placebo group. This effect was related to a decrease of bone turnover as shown by the decrease of serum osteocalcin. Recently, a large placebo-controlled study[33] using tamoxifen (20 mg/day) in the prevention of breast cancer in more than 13 000 patients at high risk showed a non-significant reduction in hip, Colles', and spine fracture of about 20% in tamoxifen users. The reduction was greater in women more than 50 years of age. Tamoxifen has also been shown to reduce bone loss by about 50% in patients with an artificial menopause due to adjuvant chemotherapy of breast cancer, and the use of a cyclic treatment with risedronate, a new bisphosphonate, results in an increased BMD in these women.[34]

Bisphosphonates represent an effective alternative therapy for prevention of bone loss in patients with breast cancer. Some 148 premenopausal breast cancer patients treated with adjuvant cyclophosphamide, methotrexate, and fluorouracil have been randomized to receive oral clodronate (1600 mg/day) or to a control group. The decrease of lumbar spine and femoral neck BMD was about 6% and 2%, respectively, during 2 years in the control group and was prevented by clodronate with average changes of –2.2% and +0.9%, respectively, at the lumbar spine and femoral neck.[35] Bisphosphonates have also been shown to reduce the skeletal morbidity (hypercalcemia, pathologic fractures, surgery, and radiotherapy on bone) in patients with bone metastases from breast cancer[36,37] and in patients with multiple myeloma.[38]

Based on the clinical observation that tamoxifen can be an estrogen agonist on the skeleton, new compounds are currently being developed, named selective estrogen receptor modulators (SERMs). These interact with the estrogen receptor but act as either estrogen agonists or antagonists depending on the tissue and the hormonal status. Their mechanism of action is not yet fully understood. Like tamoxifen, SERMs have estrogen antagonist effects on the breast and estrogen agonist effects on bone and lipid metabolism. In contrast to tamoxifen, which can be regarded as the first-generation SERMs, new SERMs should have a neutral effect on the endometrium. Several compounds have been evaluated clinically.

Droloxifen and idoxifen have been used in metastatic breast cancer but there is still limited information about the effect of these compounds on the uterus and skeleton.[39,40] A double-blind, placebo-controlled, randomized phase-III study has evaluated the effect of a long-term treatment with raloxifene (30, 60, or 150 mg/day) for 2 years in 601 healthy menopausal women. Each dose of raloxifene was associated with a significant increase in BMD at the lumbar spine, hip, and total body whereas those receiving placebo had a decrease in BMD at all sites. Serum total and low-density lipoprotein cholesterol concentrations decreased significantly in all raloxifene groups whereas high-density lipoprotein cholesterol and triglyceride concentrations remained unchanged. Endometrial thickness was similar in raloxifene and placebo groups (Table 18.1).[41] After 3 years of treatment results remained the same.[42]

Regarding the risk of fracture, the MORE study performed in more than 7500 osteoporotic women (with or without fractures) treated by raloxifene, 60 or 120 mg/day or placebo, showed at 2 and 3 years a significant reduction of about 50% of the vertebral fracture incidence

Table 18.1 Effects of raloxifene on BMD, serum cholesterol, and uterine endometrium in postmenopausal women compared with placebo

	Placebo	30 mg/day	60 mg/day	150 mg/day
BMD (mean % change from baseline to end-point)				
Lumbar spine	−0.78	1.28[a]	1.64[a]	2.21[a]
Femoral neck	−1.34	0.55[a]	1.16[a]	1.48[a]
Total body	−0.55	1.26[a]	1.42[a]	1.86[a]
Serum lipids (median % change from baseline to end-point)				
Total cholesterol	−1.2	−5.2[a]	−6.4[a]	−9.7[a]
LDL-C	−1.0	−6.2[a]	−10.1[a]	−14.1[a]
Total C: HDL-C	2.4	−1.4	−4.9[a]	−6.1[a]
Triglycerides	0	0	3.2	0.5
Endometrial thickness (actual change from baseline to end-point)				
	0.3 mm	0.2 mm	0.2 mm	0.3 mm

[a] = $p < 0.01$ compared with placebo.
BMD = bone mineral density; LDL-C = low-density lipoprotein cholesterol; Total C = total cholesterol; HDL-C = high-density lipoprotein cholesterol.
Source: Adapted from Delmas et al.[34]

in the treated group compared with placebo. Results are comparable in patients with or without fractures at baseline.[43,44] No difference was seen on the nonvertebral fracture between the treatment group and the placebo. Raloxifene induces an increased risk of deep vein thrombosis similar to that of HRT and tamoxifen, with an incidence of 28/100 000 patients. Hot flashes and cramps were mildly increased in the raloxifene group. The incidence of breast cancer was significantly reduced by about 50% in patients treated by raloxifene.[45,46] Tamoxifen and raloxifene, in the situation of estrogen deficiency, appear to act as estrogen agonists in bone. SERMs are likely to play an important role in the near future for the prevention of osteoporosis in patients with breast cancer.

CONCLUSION

In conclusion, osteoporosis is a common and multifactorial finding in patients with a history of cancer. In cancer patients with good prognosis who are at high risk of developing osteoporosis, BMD should be assessed by DXA and treatment decisions should be made accordingly. Concerning the treatment of estrogen deficiency in women surviving breast cancer, a consensus statement has been recently published[47] that states that an alternative to estrogen treatment is necessary to reduce the risk of cardiovascular disease and osteoporosis. Bisphosphonates and new compounds such as SERMs are likely to improve the management of osteoporosis in those patients.

REFERENCES

1. Marcelli C, Chappard D, Rossi JF et al. Histologic evidence of an abnormal bone remodeling in B-cell malignancies other than multiple myeloma. *Cancer* (1988) **62**: 1163–70.
2. Mundy GR, Raisz LG, Cooper RA, Schechter GP, Salmon SE. Evidence for the secretion of an osteoclast stimulating factor in myeloma. *N Engl J Med* (1974) **291**: 1041–6.
3. Pecherstorfer M, Zimmer-Roth I, Schilling T et al. The diagnostic value of urinary pyridinium cross-links of collagen, serum total alkaline phosphatase, and urinary calcium excretion in neoplastic bone disease. *J Clin Endocrinol Metab* (1995) **80**: 97–103.
4. Nesbit M, Krivit W, Heyn R, Sharp H. Acute and chronic effects of methotrexate on hepatic, pulmonary, and skeletal systems. *Cancer* (1976) **37**: 1048–54.
5. Friedlaender GE, Tross RB, Doganis AC et al. Effects of chemotherapeutic agents on bone. *J Bone Joint Surg* (1984) **66A**: 602–7.
6. Leone J, Vilque J-P, Pignon B et al. Effect of chlorambucil on bone mineral density in the course of chronic lymphoid leukemia. *Eur J Haematol* (1998) **61**: 135–9.
7. Diamond T, Nery L, Hales I. A therapeutic dilemma: suppressive doses of thyroxine significantly reduce bone mineral measurements in both premenopausal and post menopausal women with thyroid carcinoma. *J Clin Endocrinol Metab* (1990) **72**: 1184–8.
8. Uzzan B, Campos J, Cucherat M et al. Effects on bone mass of long term treatment with thyroid hormones: a meta-analysis. *J Clin Endocrinol Metab* (1996) **81**: 4278–89.
9. Pioli G, Pedrazzoni M, Palummeri E et al. Longitudinal study of bone loss after thyroidectomy and suppressive thyroxine therapy in premenopausal women. *Acta Endocrinol* (1992) **126**: 238–42.
10. Rosen HN, Moses AC, Garber J et al. Randomized trial of pamidronate in patients with thyroid cancer: bone density is not reduced by suppressive doses of thyroxine, but is increased by cyclic intravenous pamidronate. *J Clin Endocrinol Metab* (1998) **83**: 2324–30.
11. Lukert BP. Glucocorticoid and drug-induced osteoporosis. In Favus MJ (ed) *Primer on the Metabolic Bone Diseases and Disorders of Mineral Metabolism* (3rd edn) (Philadelphia, PA, and New York: Lippincott-Raven, 1996): 278–82.
12. Laan R, van Riel P, van de Putte L, van Erning L, van't Hof M, Lemmens JA. Low-dose prednisone induces rapid reversible axial bone loss in patients with rheumatoid arthritis. *Ann Intern Med* (1993) **119**: 963–8.
13. Goemaere S, Correa-Rotter R, Saag K et al. Alendronate increases spine BMD irrespective of glucocorticoid dose or duration. *J Bone Miner Res* (1998) **23 (Suppl 182)**: 1140 (abst).
14. Barr RD, Simpson T, Webber CE et al. Osteopenia in children surviving brain tumours. *Eur J Cancer* (1998) **34**: 873–7.
15. Gilsanz V, Carlson ME, Roe TF, Ortega JA. Osteoporosis after cranial irradiation for acute lymphoblastic leukemia. *J Pediatr* (1990) **117**: 238–44.
16. Nussey SS, Hyer SL, Brada M, Leiper AD. Bone mineralization after treatment of growth hormone deficiency in survivors of childhood malignancy. *Acta Paediatr* (1994) **399 (Suppl)**: 9.
17. Stepan J, Lachman M, Zverina J et al. Castrated men exhibit bone loss: effect of calcitonin treatment on biochemical indices of bone remodeling. *J Clin Endocrinol Metab* (1989) **69**: 523–7.
18. Holmes SJ, Whitehouse RW, Clark ST et al. Reduced bone mineral density in men following chemotherapy for Hodgkin's disease. *Br J Cancer* (1994) **70**: 371–5.
19. Daniell HW. Osteoporosis after orchiectomy for prostate cancer. *J Urol* (1997) **157**: 439–44.
20. Redman JR, Bajorunas DR, Wong G et al. Bone mineralization in women following successful treatment of Hodgkin's disease. *Am J Med* (1988) **85**: 65–72.
21. Cust MP, Whitehead MI, Powles R, Hunter M, Milliken S. Consequences and treatment of ovarian failure after total body irradiation for leukaemia. *Br Med J* (1989) **299**: 1494–7.
22. Castaneda S, Carmona L, Carvajal I, Arranz R, Diaz A, Garcia-Vadillo A. Reduction of bone mass in women after bone marrow transplantation. *Calcif Tissue Int* (1997) **60**: 343–7.
23. Kanis JA. Pathogenesis of osteoporosis and fracture. In *Osteoporosis* (London: Blackwell Science Ltd, 1997): 22–55.
24. Chapman RM, Sutcliffe SB. Protection of ovarian function by oral contraceptives in women receiving chemotherapy for Hodgkin's disease. *Blood* (1981) **58**: 849–51.
25. Delmas PD. Hormone replacement therapy in the

26. Rout C, Oriente P, Laan R et al. Randomized trial of effect of cyclical etidronate in the prevention of corticosteroid-induced bone loss. *J Clin Endocrinol Metab* (1998) **83**: 1128–33.
27. Saag K, Emkey R, Cividino A et al. Effects of alendronate for two years on BMD and fractures in patients receiving glucocorticoids. *J Bone Miner Res* (1998) **23 (Suppl 182)**: 1141 (abst).
28. Saag KG, Emkey R, Schnitzer TJ et al. Alendronate for the prevention and treatment of glucocorticoid-induced osteoporosis. *N Engl J Med* (1998) **339**: 292–9.
29. Bruning PF, Pit MJ, de Jong-Bakker M et al. Bone mineral density after adjuvant chemotherapy for premenopausal breast cancer. *Br J Cancer* (1990) **61**: 308–10.
30. Headley JA, Theriault RL, Leblanc AD, Vassilopoulou-Sellin R, Hortobagyi GN. Pilot study of bone mineral density in breast cancer patients treated with adjuvant chemotherapy. *Cancer Invest* (1998) **16**: 6–11.
31. Powles TJ, Hickish T, Kanis JA et al. Effect of tamoxifen on bone mineral density measured by dual energy X-ray absorptiometry in healthy premenopausal and postmenopausal women. *J Clin Oncol* (1996) **14**: 78–84.
32. Love RR, Mazess RB, Barden HS et al. Effects of tamoxifen on bone mineral density in postmenopausal women with breast cancer. *N Engl J Med* (1992) **326**: 852–6.
33. Fisher B, Costantino JP, Wickerham DL et al. Tamoxifen for prevention of breast cancer: report of the National Surgical Adjuvant Breast and Bowel Project P-1 study. *J Natl Cancer Inst* (1998) **90**: 1371–88.
34. Delmas PD, Balena R, Confavreux E et al. Bisphosphonate risedronate prevents bone loss in women with artificial menopause due to chemotherapy of breast cancer: a double blind, placebo-controlled study. *J Clin Oncol* (1997) **15**: 955–62.
35. Saarto T, Blomqvist C, Valimaki M, Makela P, Sarna S, Elomaa I. Chemical castration induced by adjuvant cyclophosphamide, methotrexate, and fluorouracil chemotherapy causes rapid bone loss that is reduced by clodronate: a randomized study in premenopausal breast cancer patients. *J Clin Oncol* (1997) **15**: 1341–7.
36. Hortobagyi GN, Theriault RL, Porter L et al. Efficacy of pamidronate in reducing skeletal complications in patients with breast cancer and lytic bone metastase. *N Engl J Med* (1996) **335**: 1785–91.
37. Paterson AHG, Powles TJ, Kanis JA et al. Double-blind controlled trial of oral clodronate in patients with bone metastases from breast cancer. *J Clin Oncol* (1993) **11**: 59–65.
38. Berenson JR, Lichtenstein A, Porter L et al. Efficacy of pamidronate in reducing skeletal events in patients with advanced multiple myeloma. *N Engl J Med* (1996) **334**: 488–93.
39. Rauschining W, Pritchard KI. Droloxifen, a new antiestrogen, its role in metastatic breast cancer. *Breast Cancer Res Treat* (1994) **31**: 83–94.
40. Coombes RC, Haynes BP, Dowset M et al. Idoxifen: report of a phase I study in patients with metastatic breast cancer. *Cancer Res* (1995) **55**: 1070–4.
41. Delmas PD, Bjarnason NH, Mitlak BH et al. The effects of raloxifene on bone mineral density, serum cholesterol, and uterine endometrium in postmenopausal women. *N Engl J Med* (1997) **337**: 1641–7.
42. Bjarnason NH, Delmas PD, Mitlak BH et al. Raloxifene maintains favourable effects on bone mineral density, bone turnover and serum lipids without endometrial stimulation in postmenopausal women. 3-years study results. *Osteoporos Int* (1998) **8**: 11.
43. Ettinger B, Black D, Cummings H et al. for the MORE study group. Raloxifene reduces the risk of incident vertebral fractures: 24-month interim analyses. *Osteoporos Int* (1998) **8**: 11.
44. Ensrud K, Black D, Recker R et al. The effect of 2 and 3 years of raloxifene on vertebral and non-vertebral fractures in postmenopausal women with osteoporosis. *J Bone Miner Res* (1998) **23**: S174 (abst).
45. Jordan VC, Glusman JE, Eckert S et al. Incident primary breast cancers are reduced by raloxifene: integrated data from multicenter, double-blind, randomized trials in 12000 postmenopausal women. *Proceedings of ASCO* (1998) **17**: 122a (abst).
46. Cummings SR, Norton L, Eckert S et al. Raloxifene reduces the risk of breast cancer and may decrease the risk of endometrial cancer in post-menopausal women, two-year findings from the multiple outcomes of raloxifene evaluation (MORE) trial. *Proceedings of ASCO* (1998) **17**: 2a (abst).
47. Consensus statement. Treatment of estrogen deficiency symptoms in women surviving breast cancer. *J Clin Endocrinol Metab* (1998) **83**: 1993–2000.

Index

A375 human melanoma cells 72
  metastases 51
  osteoclastogenesis 67–8
  reactive bone formation 66–7
  vitronectin receptor 49
ablative therapy 56
acetaminophen therapy 185–6
active bone marrow 245
  see also red marrow
acute lymphoblastic leukaemia (ALL) 127
acute myelogenous leukaemia (AML) 127–8
adamantinoma 122
adenocarcinoma mouse prostate model, transgenic (TRAMP) 58
age-related bone loss, pathophysiology 2–3
alendronate 204
  intravenous 146
  structure 202
alendronate/placebo, treatment 264
alkaline phosphatase (ALP) 14, 68–9, 220
  activity stimulation 58
  bone (BAP) 240
  isoenzyme estimation (ALP-BI) 138–9
alkalosis, hypokalemic, hypochloremic 77–8
ALL, acute lymphoblastic leukaemia 127
aminoglutethimide, desmolase enzyme inhibitor 153
AML, acute myelogenous leukaemia 127–8
amorphous calcification, CT detection 122
anabolic steroids 139
analgesics 162, 223
  analgesic consumption (A) 146
  anti-androgen combination 154
  examples 187, 190
    nonopioid 187
  for severe pain, examples 190
  World Health Organisation ladder 186
  see also NSAIDs
anastrozole Type II aromatase inhibitor 153
androgens, antagonizing estrogens 152, 154
angiogenesis, cytokine requirement 69

angiography 113
angiosarcomas 122
animal models
  B16/F1 mouse melanoma cells 67, 69
  bisphosphonates 71–2, 208–9
  bone metastases 232, 238
  bone morphogenetic proteins (BMPs) 59
  bone-derived tumor growth factors 54–6
  hemopoietic tissue, transplantation to osteopetrotic recipients 4–6
  human myeloma 26–7
  hypercalcemia, myeloma 27
  Madin–Darby canine kidney (MDCK) cells, E-cadherin treatment 50
  Mat Ly/Lu variant of rat Dunning prostate cancer model 58
  metastases 49, 232
  morphology of bone metastases 66–7
  murine model of myeloma 26–7
  osteolytic bone disease 27
  osteopetrosis, and donor-derived osteoclasts 6
  osteoporosis, bone loss prevention 266
  osteosclerotic lesions 27, 29
  prostate adenocarcinoma (PA III), spontaneous 58
  transgenic adenocarcinoma mouse prostate (TRAMP) 58
anthracycline-resistant disease, taxoids 153
anthracyclines (doxirubicin and epirubicin) 153
anticoagulants, coumadin class 50
anticonvulsant therapy
  addiction/TCA alternative, neuropathic pain 193
  neuropathic pain 193
APD *see* pamidronate disodium
apoptotic osteoclast, ibandronate, metastatic lesion, MDA-231 human breast cancer 71
arginine-glycine-asparagine (RGD) 4, 10
aromatase inhibitors 152–3
Askin's tumor 121
avascular sinusoidal system 245
azoospermia 265

B16/F1 mouse melanoma cells
  intertrabecular type of metastatic bone disease 67
  tumor-mediated osteolysis 69
backache 130
BAP see bone alkaline phosphatase
Batson's plexus 45, 231
Bence Jones protein 21
  protein excretion 28
benign cortical defect, examples 114
benign prostatic hyperplasia (BPH) 58, 141, 156
benzodiazepine therapy 191
BGP see osteocalcin bone protein
biochemical markers 137–47
  bone formation 137–8, 140
  bone resorption 138–141
    N-terminal Ntx assay 139–41, 143
  breast cancer 145
  Crosslaps 139, 145
  diagnosis of metastatic bone disease 140–1
  differentiation markers, osteoblasts 14
  metastases 140–1, 156
  myeloma 28, 144–5
  osteolytic lesions 28
  patient evaluation 142–5
  prostate cancer 143–4
  technical aspects 139–40
  tumors 141
  urine vs serum markers (list) 137
  see also metastatic bone disease
biochemical response assessment 142–5
biopsy
  FN 134
  image-guided 133–5
  open surgical biopsy 134–5
bisphosphonate–calcium complex 84
bisphosphonates 52, 56, 84, 142
  action mechanisms 201–26, 232–4
    bone formation effect 208
    in myeloma 225
    pharmocokinetics 208
    side effects 209
  animal models 71–2
    toxicology 208–9
  bone formation 208
  bone resorption 203–5
    anti-resorbing properties 205, 266
    reduction methods 71
    seed and soil mechanisms 207
    tumoral 207–8
    in vitro 203
    in vivo 203–4
  breast cancer 231–40
  calcification, effects 203

  chemical structure
    effect 204–5
    P-C-P bond 201
  chemical structures 202, 221
  as combination therapy 163
  cortical bone slice, pretreatment 233–4
  DEXA assessment 219
  efficacy 27
  metastatic bone disease 70–3, 145–7, 195–6
    hypercalcaemia 145
    monitoring, markers 145–7
    prevention/delay 236–8
  myeloma bone disease 221–25
    randomized long-term studies 222
  pharmacokinetics 208
  pharmacology 221–2
  pretreatment, cortical bone 233–4
  pyrophosphate structure 201
  blood coagulation mechanism 50
BMD see bone mineral density
bone
  cancellous/cortical 25, 57
    and age 1–3
    remodeling 2–3
  cortex, 'saucerization' 121
  cortical bone 3
  Gla protein 13
  histomorphometry 219
  lining cells see trabecular bone
  volume regulation 3
bone cells see osteoblasts; osteoclasts
bone destruction see metastatic bone disease; osteolytic bone disease
bone formation
  biochemical markers 137–8, 140, 220
    post pamidronate infusion 147
  dose-dependent inhibition 264
bone formation/resorption coupling process
  humoral hypothesis 12
  osteoblastotropic factors 13–15
bone lesions
  diagnostic approach 113–15
  pathophysiology 22–4
bone loss see bone resorption; osteoporosis
bone marrow
  autologous cell support 153
  cavity, paracrine secretion 137
  density (BMD), raloxifene 268
  depression, iatrogenic 247
  inoculation 27
  metastases 33
  monocyte-macrophage lineage 4–5
  MRI 123–7
  primary tumors 121, 127–33

red
  distribution 123
  paucity 93
  scintigraphy 93
  stroma, composition 68
  stromal cells, MMP-1/2 production 218
  suppression 42
  transplantation 265
bone mass
  and age 1–2
  defined 1
bone metabolism, characteristics 263
bone metastases *see* metastatic bone disease
bone mineral density (BMD) 263, 265
  densitometry 219
  diminished 128
bone morphogenetic proteins (BMPs) 13–14, 59, 66, 232
  BMP-3 gene 58
bone remodeling process 1, 3
  bone structural unit (BSU) 4
  cellular events 3–4
  normal cancellous bone surface 5
  sequence, cellular events, formation phase 13
  TGFß superfamily, potential role 11
bone resorption
  biochemical evidence, in tumor type 141
  biochemical markers 138–141, 220
  bisphosphonates 203–5
  bone resorption factors in myeloma 216–18
  by osteoclasts, oxygen-derived free radicals involvement 10
  and calcium homeostasis, interleukin-6 effects 24
  deoxypyridinoline crosslinks of collagen 28
  formation/resorption coupling process, osteoblastotropic factors 12–15
  glucocorticoids 264–5
  hypercalcemia 23
  inhibition 205–7
  lymphotoxin increase 24
  methotrexate 263
  molecular mechanisms 7–10
  seed and soil mechanisms 207
  tumor mechanisms 69–72
  tumoral, action mechanisms 207–8
bone scintigraphy 91–107
  bone disease status 218
  breast cancer, metastases 101–3, 125
  complication factor 100–1
  detection and distribution of metastatic bone disease 44
  detection of osteoblastic activity 45
  diagnostic patterns 94–9
  flare phenomenon 100
  lung cancer 92
  myeloma 92
  role, for specific tumors 100–5
  scanning agents 91, 107, 174–7
  technique sensitivity 96
  see also named agents; specific organs;
bone scintigraphy, therapy *see* radioisotope therapy
bone sialoprotein II 10
bone structural unit (BSU) 4
bone tumors, primary, classification 118
bone-derived tumor growth factors 54–6
BPH *see* benign prostatic hypertrophy
breast cancer 12, 75, 128, 142
  see also breast cancer metastases *(below)*
  anthracycline-resistant disease, taxoids 153
  biochemical markers 145
  biochemical response assessment 142–3
  bisphosphonates 231–9
  bone loss
    management 266–8
    MDP scan pre/post chemotherapy 103
    see also osteoporosis
  bone relapse/patient survival, post herpetic relapse 35
  bone scintigraphy 101–3, 125, 101–3
  cell surface mucins, expression 141
  cells causing bone resorption 52
  gene expression 51
  growth factors expressed 69
  Her-2/Neu oncogene expression 50
  incidence 101
  MCF-7 cells 50
  MDA-MB-231 cells 50, 52–4, 56, 67, 69, 50, 56, 67, 69
    and hsp-27 51
    low E-cadherin expression 50
    osteolytic lesion radiograph 67
  molecular mechanisms 55
  normocalcemic patient 79
  receptor status, estrogen and progesterone 152
  staging 101–3
  systemic anti-tumor treatment 151–4
breast cancer antigen (CA15-3) 266
breast cancer metastases 125–6
  bone scintigraphy 101–3, 125
  breast/spine spread 37
  breastbone 39, 125, 128, 140
  E-cadherin 48
  epidemiology 33–4
  and hypercalcemia, MDP bone scan 93, 100
  lytic bone lesions
    long bone fracture 38
    lumbar spine 251

breast cancer metastases (contd)
  pathological fracture 39
  skeletal morbidity rate 237
  seed and soil concept 232
  site frequency, first relapse 35
  therapies
    osteoporotic predisposition 39
    response 142–3
  treatment
    bisphosphonates 231–40
      indications 233
    first-line chemotherapy, response rate 153–4
  visceral metastases 72
  see also metastatic bone disease
Burkitt's lymphoma 129

c-cbl cytoskeletal protein 9
c-fos 9
  over-expression/lack of expression, defects arising 10
c-src 9
  role integration model, osteoclast bone resorption 9
C-telopeptide crosslinks assay (ICTP) 139, 143, 220
calcitonin
  labeled 68
  treatment of hypercalcemia 84
calcitonin therapy 28, 84
  and bone pain 196
calcium
  measurement 138
    rapid rise 234
    small decrease 239
  renal handling 140
  tumor-induced hypercalcemia (TIH) 232, 234–5
  urinary calcium (uCa) excretion 41, 138, 142–3
    breast cancer 142
    elevation 41
calcium ion, properties 75
CAMs see cell adhesion molecules
cancer
  and bone formation/resorption coupling process 12–15
  clinical consequences, skeletal involvement 46–7
cancer pain 183–97
  anaesthetic and neurosurgical approaches 194
  assessment 185
  characteristics 37–8
  diagnosis 194–5
  incident pain, definition 196
  intensity (P) 146
    analgesic consumption (A) questionnaire 146
    assessment tools 185
  intractable spinal pain 246

  management 185–93, 195–6
    see also analgesics; clodronate; radiotherapy
  mechanisms, assessment and management 183–97
  metastatic bone disease 235–6
  NSAIDs 195–6
  opiates 195–6
  orthopaedic stabilization 38
  palliation
    chemotherapy 145
    radionuclides 172–80
    radiotherapy 155
    responses 174
  pamidronate, clinical trials 141
  pelvic and femoral lesions 37
  radiotherapy 161–4, 173
  referred pain 37
  score (PPA) 146
  spinal, aggressive chemotherapeutic regimens 247
  symptomatic assessment, scoring system 157
  syndromes 196–7
    see also spinal nerve compression
  WHO ladder 186
cancer-associated serum antigen (CASA) 143
candidiasis 193
carbamazepine therapy 193
carbonic anhydrase Type II 7
  and CSF-1, normal osteoclast function 9
  deficiency, osteopetrosis 8–9
carcinoembryonic antigen (CEA) 141
carcinoid tumor, metastatic bone disease, MIBG scan 94
carcinoma antigen (CA) 141
cardiac injection model 67
cardio-vascular toxicity 153
CASA, cancer-associated serum antigen 143
cathepsin K, osteoclasts 8
cathepsins, B, K, L, S, in osteoclasts 8
cauda equina/spinal cord compression 39–41, 46, 166
CEA see carcinoembryonic antigen
cell adhesion molecules (CAMs) 48–51
cell motility 51
cervical spine
  anterior decompression and stabilization 252–3
  craniocervical chordoma 122
  lesions 254
  MR scan, gross vertebral destruction 167
CFU-GM see granulocyte–macrophage-committed progenitor cells
chemoresistant carcinomas, examples 155
chemotaxis
  directed migrational 50
  unidirectional migration 4

chemotherapy *see* cytotoxic chemotherapy
cholesterol biosynthesis 71
chondroblastoma, radiographical characteristics 117
chondroid originating tumors 120
chondroma, radiographical characteristics 117
chondrosarcoma
　clear cell 120
　low-grade 116–17
chordoma 122
chromosome-17 and -18 50
chronic lymphatic leukemia (CLL) 128–9, 263
chronic myelocytic leukemia (CML) 128
circulating luteinizing hormone 154
cisplatinum 179
clear cell chondrosarcoma 120
CLL *see* chronic lymphatic leukemia
clodronate 28, 204, 220, 239
　as adjuvant therapy 72
　analgesic effects 235
　breast cancer metastases 234–5
　hypercalcemia of malignancy 145
　management of bone pain 223
　multiple myeloma, randomized long-term studies 223
　structure 202
　tumor-induced hypercalcemia (TIH) 234
CML *see* chronic myelocytic leukemia
coanalgesics 193
codeine opiate, WHO analgesic ladder Step (2) 190
Codman's triangle 116, 118
collagen
　amino-terminal propeptide of Type I procollagen (PINP) 220
　cross-links pyridinoline (Pyr) 231–2
　synthesis 138
　Type I collagen 10, 13–14, 51, 137, 139
　　C-terminal telopeptide (ICTP) 139, 143, 220
　　propeptides 139
　Type I procollagen (PICP) synthesis 138
　Type IV collagenase 50–1
colon carcinomas
　chromosome-17 and -18 deletions 50
　post-retroperitoneal irradiation 247
colony-stimulating factors (CSFs) 6
　CSF-1 coding abnormality, osteopetrosis 9
　exogenous CSF-1 therapy 9
coma and drowsiness, hypercalcemia 76
compact bone *see* cortical bone
complete vertebrectomy 252
computed tomography (CT)
　bone metabolism markers 143
　response assessment 142
cortactin protein 9

corticosteroid therapy
　neuropathic pain 193
　somatic pain 193
coumadins 50
cranial nerve metastases, radiotherapy 168
cranial nerve palsies, metastatic bone disease 37, 41
Crosslaps, biochemical marker assay 139, 145
crosslinks excretion 139, 141, 143, 145
CSFs *see* colony-stimulating factors
cyclic AMP, measurement of PTHrP 47
cyclo-oxygenase inhibitors, (COX-1 and -2) 186–7
cyclophosphamide 153
cyproterone acetate, as anti-androgen 154
cysteine proteinase 8
cytokines
　angiogenesis 69
　lymphotoxin (tumor necrosis factor ß) 24, 216
　production enhancement 25
　stimulation of osteoclastic bone resorption 69
　see also interleukins; specific named types
cytotoxic chemotherapy 72, 101–2, 105, 135, 142
　and bone pain 196
　breast cancer 152–4
　Class I spinal metastases 248
　cytotoxic agents
　　combination examples 153
　　principal examples 153
　induced ovarian failure 39
　side-effects 154
　visceral disease progression 152
　see also specific names

deoxypyridinoline
　crosslinks of collagen, measurement of bone resorption 28
　(Dpd) amino acid 138, 143, 145, 220
　　level elevation 141
　(DPyr) 231
　free (F-Dpd) 139, 145
depressed bone formation *see* myeloma bone disease, multiple myeloma
DEXA *see* dual energy X-ray absorptiometry
diagnostic efficiency (DE), prediction of PD 143–4
differentiation markers, osteoblasts 14
distraction rod and hooks, Knodt 255
diuretics *see* frusemide
divalent cation, effects 139
doxorubicin 153
Dpd biochemical marker 139, 145
droloxifen therapy 267
dual energy X-ray absorptiometry (DEXA) 219
Durie–Salmon Stage III multiple myeloma bone disease 132, 224
DXA *see* X-ray absorptiometry

E-cadherin 49–51
 involvement in metastasis 48–9
 MCF-7 breast cancer cells 50
 MDA-MB-231 breast cancer line 50
EB 1053, structure 202
echistatin, inhibition of arginine-glycine-asparagine (RGD) 10
ECM *see* extracellular matrix
EDTA *see* ethylenediamine tetra-acetic acid
EDTMP *see* ethylenediaminetetramethylenephosphonate
EGF *see* epidermal growth factor
electron microscopy scanning 10
ELISA *see* enzyme linked immunoassays
enchondroma 114, 120
 second metacarpal 114
endocrine therapy 102, 142–3, 151
 breast cancer 152–3
 prostate cancer 154
 second-line
  examples 153
  norethisterone acetate agent 153
 steroid receptor-positive tumors 152
endometrial cells 26
endometrial density 267
endoscopic spinal decompression and stabilization 246
endosteal bone resorption 3
endothelin-1 46, 59
enzyme linked immunoassays (ELISA) 139, 145
epidermal growth factor (EGF) 7
epidural opiates 193
epidural spinal cord compression 196–7
epirubicin 153
esophageal ulcers 222
esophagitis 222
estrogen 153
 deficiency 265
 synthesis, inhibitors 152
estrogen replacement therapy, post-menopause 3, 266
ethacrynic acid, hypercalcemia 84
ethylenediamine tetraacetic acid (EDTA) 139
ethylenediamine tetramethylenephosphonate (EDTMP) 177
etidronate 204, 222–3
 structure 202
Ewing's sarcoma 116–18, 121–2, 129
 'hair on end' characteristic 116
 MRI 134–5
 sunburst calcification 116
exemestane Type I inhibitor 153
external beam radiotherapy 161
 hemibody 164
 pain relief 162

extracellular matrix (ECM), between tumor cells and osteoclast precursor cells 68–9
extradural tumor 248
extraosseous disease 151

F-Pyr and F-Dpd markers, pyridinoline 139, 145, 220
femoral shaft metastatic bone disease, radiographical images 124
fenantyl opiate, WHO analgesic ladder step (3) 190–1
fever 130
fibroblast growth factor (FGFs) 14, 58–9
fibronectin 49
fibrosarcoma 120
fibrous cortical defects 114
fibrous dysplasia 114
fibrous histiocytoma 120–1
fine needle biopsy 134
fluid retention 193
fluoride therapy 12
fluorodeoxyglucose-18 (FDG) 91–2, 99, 105, 107
 PET 105, 107
fluorouracil 5, 153
focal tumor-induced osteolysis, secondary 145
follicle-stimulating hormone (FSH) 154, 265
follicular thyroid carcinoma, management 172
formestane (4-hydroxyandrostenedione) Type I inhibitor 153
Frankel classification, neurological compromise 259
frusemide, hypercalcemia 84

gabapentin therapy, neuropathic pain 193
gallium nitrate 52
 bone resorption inhibitor, side effects 84
gallium-67 91
gamma camera imaging 94, 97
gastritis 193
gastrointestinal metastases 35
gastrointestinal primary tumor 99
gastrointestinal toxicity 153, 222
geographic lesions 115
germ cell tumors 155
 tumor markers 141
glioma 123
glomerular filtration rate 47
 compromised, hypercalcemia association 23
 filtration status 28
glucocorticoid anti-inflammatory agent 193, 264
 administration 84, 219
 alendronate 146, 204
 alendronate/placebo 264
glucocorticoids
 bone loss 264–5
 and radiotherapy 221

gonadotrophins 152
goserelin 152
granulocyte–macrophage-committed progenitor cells (CFU-GM) 6
growth factors, reactive bone formation 66

'hair on end' appearance, Ewing's sarcoma 116
Hand–Schüller–Christian disease 132
HARA see human lung squamous cell carcinoma cell line
heat shock protein (hsp-27) 51
HEDP see hydroxyethylidene diphosphonate
hemangiocortical defects 114
hemangioendothelioma see angiosarcomas
hematological malignancies
   hypercalcemia 75, 82–3
   see also myeloma
hematopoietic stem cells 12
hemibody radiotherapy 163
hemopoietic cell transplantation, and osteopetrosis 4, 6
hemopoietic growth factors 153
heparan sulfate proteoglycan (HSPG), TRAPase-positive cells 69
heparin-binding growth factors
   examples 69
   FGFs 13
hepatic metastases 152
hepatocyte growth factor (HGF) 216
hepatotoxicity 84, 186
Her-2/Neu oncogene expression, breast cancer 50
HHM see humoral hypercalcemia of malignancy
high-dose steroidal therapy 37
histiocytoma, malignant fibrous (MFH) 120–1
histiocytosis 121
   Langerhans' cell 132–3
   skull, plain radiograph 132
histiocytosis X 132
Hodgkin's disease 83, 129, 265–6
   and BMD 265–6
   lesion types 45
hormonal therapy manipulation, Class I spinal metastases 248
hormone replacement therapy (HRT) 266
Howship's lacunae 52
HPLC (reverse-phase) 139
HPOA see hypertrophic pulmonary osteoarthropathy
HSPG see heparan sulfate proteoglycan
human lung squamous cell carcinoma cell line (HARA) 69
   reactive bone formation 66
human melanoma bone disease, osteolytic lesion formation 48–9

human T-cell lymphotrophic virus Type I (HTLV-1) 79, 83
hydrocodone 190
hydromorphone opiate 190–1
hydroxy-lysylpyridinoline amino acid 138
hydroxyethylidene diphosphonate (HEDP) 178
hydroxyproline (Hyp) excretion 140–1, 143
hypercalcemia 22, 41–2, 46–7, 71, 75–85, 145
   and bone metastases 81–2
   and breast cancer, MDP bone scan 100
   causes 75, 77
      primary hyperparathyroidism 75
   clinical features 75–6
   differential diagnosis 76–7
   hematological malignancies 75, 82–3
   humoral hypercalcemia of malignancy (HHM) 46, 77–83, 234
      biochemical features 77
      hypokalemic alkalosis 80
      plasma phosphate, below range 76–7
      PTH level suppression 77
      PTH-rP 52, 79–82
      squamous cell carcinoma, lung 78
   interleukin-6 24
   lymphoplasmacytic neoplasia 82
   in myeloma 27–8
   nonparathyroid, PTH level suppression 77
   soft tissue uptake 99
hypercalcemia (contd)
   symptoms
      early recognition 81
      gastrointestinal symptoms 76
      neurological manifestations 76
      psychiatric symptoms 76
      renal manifestations 76, 204
      and signs 76
   syndrome categories 77–8
   treatment 83–5
      bisphosphonates 84–5, 145
         PTHrP, response predictor 84–5–5
      calcitonin 84–5
      gallium nitrate 84
      mithramycin 84–5
      pamidronate 84–5
   tumor-induced (TIH) 232, 234–5
   see also bone resorption; humoral hypercalcemia of malignancy (HHM)
hypercalciuria 204
hyperchloremic acidosis 77
hyperglycemia 193
hyperparathyroidism see primary hyperparathyroidism
hyperresorptive bone disease, examples 70–1
hyperthyroidism 11

hypertrophic breast tissue 79
hypertrophic pulmonary osteoarthropathy (HPOA) 97
hypocalcemia, osteoblastic metastases, predomination 138
hypogonadism 265
hypokalemic, hypochloremic alkalosis 77–8
hypokalemic alkalosis 80
hypophysectomy 152

I-metaiodobenzylguanidine (MIBG) 91
iatrogenic bone marrow depression 247
ibandronate 238
   breast cancer 71
   crosslinks excretion 145
   myeloma 226
   structure 202
icandronate, structure 202
ICTP (serum C-telopeptide of Type I collagen) 139, 220
idoxifen therapy 267
IGFs see insulin-like growth factor
ilium, lytic lesions 165
image-guided biopsy 133–5
immunohistochemistry, PTH-rP identification 25
insufficiency fracture 247
insulin-like growth factor (IGFs) 232
   reactive bone formation 66
integral membrane proteins (integrins) 4, 10
   vitronectin receptor 48–9
interleukins
   IL-1 10, 24
   IL-1β 23, 24, 25, 216
   IL-1α 24
   IL-3 6
   IL-6 6, 23–5, 216–17
International Myeloma Foundation 29
intertrabecular type of metastatic bone disease 66–7
iodine scintigraphy
   I-metaiodobenzylguanidine (MIBG) 91, 93–4
   thyroid cancers 93
iodine-131, properties 172

juxtacortical chondrosarcoma 120

Kahler's disease 21
Kaposi's sarcoma-related herpes virus 22, 25
Knodt distraction rod and hooks 255

laminar new bone, cortical thickening 116
laminin 48–9
   antagonists 56
   bone resorption effects 49
   YIGSR synthetic agonist 51

Langerhans' cell, histiocytosis 132–3
letrozole Type II inhibitor 153
leucoerythroblastic anemia 42
leukemias
   acute 127–8
   chronic 128–9, 263
leukopenia 42
LH see luteinizing hormone
lining cells, defined 10
liposarcoma 122
long bones
   adamantinoma 122
   metastatic disease, radiological follow-up 102
   pathological fractures 38, 46
      prophylactic surgery, indications 156
      radiotherapy 164–6
lumbar spine
   cancellous bone percentage 2
   cancellous bone remodeling 2
   insufficiency fracture 247
   sclerotic vertebral metastases 106, 257
lung cancer
   and fracture rate 39
   metastatic bone disease
      histological types 36
      statistical rates 104–5
   primary tumors 113
   scintigraphy 92, 104–5
luteinizing hormone (LH) 265
luteinizing hormone-releasing hormone (LH-RH) agonists 152
lymph node disease see Hodgkin's disease
lymphangitis carcinomatosa 152
lymphomas 122, 127, 129–30
   bone involved, MRI examinations 133
lymphoplasmacytic neoplasia, hypercalcemia associated 82
lymphotoxin cytokine (tumor necrosis factor ß) 23–4, 216
lysosomal enzymes, maximal proteolytic activity 8
lysyl-pyridinoline amino acid 138
lytic lesions see osteolytic lesions

macrophage colony stimulating factor (M-CSF) 216
magnetic resonance imaging (MRI) 113–35
   bone marrow 123–7
   bone metastases, neurological complications 166–7
   indications 126
   myeloma 219
   spinal stabilization 246
malignant bone disease see specific types
malignant fibrous histiocytoma (MFH) 120–1

marble bone disease *see* osteopetrosis
marrow dendritic cells, myeloma viral link 25
Mat Ly/Lu variant of rat Dunning prostate cancer model 58
matrix metalloproteinases (MMPs) 216
  bone resorption stimulation 218
  mediation of bone resorption 70
  MMP-2, TIMP-2 55, 57
MCF-7 breast cancer cells, E-cadherin effect 50
MDA-MB-231 cells *see* breast cancer
MDP *see* methylene diphosphonate
Medical Research Council (MRC) 223
  European myeloma trial 29
medrogesterone acetate agent, second-line endocrine therapy 153
medullary thyroid cancers, I-metaiodobenzylguanidine (MIBG) 93
megestrol acetate, second-line endocrine therapy 153
melanoma bone disease, osteolytic lesion formation 48–9
melanoma cells, A375 49
menopause 152
  bone loss 1–2
  estrogen withdrawal 2
menstrual cycle 139
meperidine semisynthetic opiate 191
mesenchymal chondrosarcoma 120
metastatic bone disease 33–42, 43–59
  animal models 49, 66–73, 232
  biochemical markers
    bone formation 140
    bone resorption 140–1
    tumors 141
  bone marrow suppression 42
    leucoerythroblastic anemia 42
  cancer types, at post mortem 33
  carcinoid tumor, MIBG scan 94
  causes 123
  classification 43
  clinical features 34–7
  clinical pain syndromes 37
  clinical stage/frequency 104
  complications 37–42
    prevention 236–8
  cranial nerve palsies 41
  diagnostic features 37, 123–7
  direct osteolytic effects 231
  distribution, and scintographic detection 44
  frequency
    common malignancy association 45
    and statistics 43–4
  hypercalcemia 41–2, 46–7
  incidence 33–4

lung cancer, fracture rate 39
lytic forms 141
morphology 65–73
  histopathological classification 65–7
  intertrabecular type 66–7
neurological complications 166–8
pathological fractures 38, 46
prevention/delay 238–9
radiology
  contrasted, post diagnosis survival 35
  and MRI 122–7
  photopenic lesions 92
scintigraphy
  diagnostic patterns 94–9
  MDP bone scan 106
spinal cord/cauda equina compression 39–41, 46, 166
  back pain 40
  with breast cancer, survival from diagnosis 41
  breast cancer complication 40
metastatic bone disease (*contd*)
  causes 39–40
  lung cancer 40
  lymphoma 40
  pain types 40
  prostatic cancer 40
  radiotherapy 40
  renal carcinoma 40
  thoracic spine, MRI scan 40
thrombocytopenia 42
treatment
  bisphosphonate 70–3, 145–7
  pain management, diagnostic issues 194–5
  prophylactic fixation therapy 39
  radiotherapy 40, 142, 159–68
  systemic 56–7, 151–6
urinary calcium excretion, elevation 41
vertebral body fractures 39
see also bone pain
methadone opiate 191
methotrexate 153, 263
  bone resorption 263
methylene diphosphonate (MDP) 91
MFH *see* malignant fibrous histiocytoma
MGUS *see* monoclonal gammopathy of undetermined significance
MIBG *see* I-metaiodobenzylguanidine
minimally invasive techniques *see* image-guided biopsy
minodronate, structure 202
mithramycin, treatment of hypercalcemia 84
mitogenesis stimulation 58
mitomycin C 153–4
mitozantrone 153, 154

MMPs *see* metalloproteinases
monoclonal gammopathy of undetermined significance (MGUS) 216
morphine opiate, WHO analgesic ladder Step (3) 190
moth-eaten lesions 116
multifocal osteosarcoma 119–20
multiple blastic metastases, ALP-BI 140
myelography 196
myeloma
  animal models 26–7
  assessment 218–20
    bone markers 28
    bone scintigraphy 92
    M-CSF presence in serum 218
    MRI 131, 219
    osteoclast activity 22
  biochemical markers 28, 144–5
  biology 216–18
  bone resorption factors 216–18
  differential diagnosis 127
  epidemiology 21–2
    transmission 27
  historical background 21
  imaging 218–20
  MRC European myeloma trial 29
  multiple myeloma 21, 82, 144–5
    bisphosphonates, randomized long-term studies 222
    common symptoms 130
    complication reduction 145
    definition 215
    Durie–Salmon Stage III 224, 132
    osteoclast activity increase 215
    PICP level 140
    residronate, (oral) 145
  osteoclastic bone resorption 12
    inhibition 70
  pathology
    asynchronous bone turnover 215
    biology 130, 216–18
    bone cortex, 'saucerization' 121
    bone destruction, potential factors 24–6
    bone formation rate reduction 23
    osteolysis, cellular mechanism 22–3
    osteolytic lesions 22, 45
    osteosclerosis, stimulation by osteoblasts 45
    renal impairment, causal examples 28
    symptoms/progressive deterioration 29
  pathophysiology 21–9
    ARH-77 human myeloma cells 27
    fracture susceptibility 22
    and hypercalcemia 23, 27–8
    in vitro cells, osteoclast activating factors, expression and secretion 23
    marrow dendritic cells, Kaposi sarcoma, related virus 25
    osteolytic lesions, histologic section 23
    punched-out lytic bone lesion, characteristic example 11–12, 130
  treatment 28–9, 220–25
    bisphosphonate 221–25
    radiotherapy 220–1
    response 143–4
    surgical intervention 221
    zoledronate induced apoptosis 72
myelotoxicity 176
myoclonic jerks 191

N-terminal Ntx assay 139–41, 145–7, 235
  parathyroid hormone-related protein (PTH-rP) 79
naloxone, respiratory depression, reversal 191
nausea 84
needle biopsies 133–4
neoplastin prostate tissue 59
nephrogenous cyclic AMP 52
  excretion 78
nephrotoxicosis 84, 222
neridronate, structure 202
nerve compression syndromes
  metastatic bone disease 46
  spinal cord compression 39–40, 166, 219, 248
neural pathways, nociceptive information transmission 184
neuroblastomas
  childhood, scintigraphy 105
  I-metaiodobenzylguanidine (MIBG) 93, 105
  Tc MDP 105
neurological complications
  bone metastases, MRI 166–7
  radiotherapy 166–8
neurological compromise
  (Class V), spinal stabilization 250
  Frankel classification 259
neurological deficit prevention, glucocorticosteroids and radiotherapy 221
neuropathic pain 183–4, 193
  anticonvulsant therapy, addiction/TCA alternative 193
  gabapentin therapy 193
  tricyclic antidepressant (TCAs) therapy 193
neurotoxicity 84
  plasma calcium normalization 84
neutropenia 164
nitric oxide synthase inhibitors 10
NM-23 oncogene, tumor metastatic inhibition 50
nociceptive information transmission, neural pathways 184
nociceptive pain 183–4

non-Hodgkin's lymphoma (NHL) 83, 129
nonoperative treatment, spinal stabilization 246–50
nonossifying fibroma
    example 114
    see also benign cortical defect, examples
nonparathyroid hypercalcemia, PTH level suppression 77
nonsteroidal anti-inflammatory drugs (NSAIDs)
    and acetaminophen therapy 185–6
    metastatic bone disease 195–6
    and opiates 195–6
    side effects 186
norethisterone acetate agent, second-line endocrine therapy 153
Ntx (N-terminal Ntx assay) 79, 139–41, 145–7, 235
nuclear medicine 91–107
    scanning methods 93–4
number needed to treat (NNT) 162

OCIF see osteoclastogenesis inhibitory factor
olpadronate, structure 202
oncology
    liver secondaries 113
    lung secondaries 113
    osteoblastic metastases, values 138
OPG see osteoprotegerin
opiates 187–93
    addiction, definition 190
    administration 188–90
        around the clock (ATC) schedule 188
        routes 192–3
    controlled release 188
    epidural 193
    examples 190
    physical dependence, definition 189–90
    side effects 188, 190–1
    tolerance, definition 189
opioid histamine release 192
oral candidiasis 193
oral contraceptive 266
orbital/parasellar lesion (skull) 41
osteoblast stimulating factor, examples 12
osteoblastic metastases 1, 45, 57–9
    solid tumor, marrow cavity deposits 57
    vertebral body sclerosis, X-ray 57
osteoblastic metastatic bone disease, development 57
osteoblasts
    bone resorption 10–11
    cell origin 12
    chemotaxis 13
    depositional activity 123
    differentiation markers, examples 14

function 3
    mitogenic factor 59
    proliferation 13
    stimulation of function, paracrine influences 137
    treatment response, criteria for evaluation 142
osteocalcin bone protein (BGP) 138–9, 220
    levels 140
    measurement 28, 51
    synthesis 13–14
osteocarcinoma, teenage 116
osteoclast precursor cells, extracellular matrix (ECM) 68
osteoclastogenesis
    c-fos 9
    differentiation-inducing factor (ODIF) 11, 86
    ECM role 69
    inhibitory factor (OCIF) 11
    tumor induced, ultrastructural cell changes 67–9
osteoclasts
    activity regulation 10–12, 123
    apoptosis 7, 13, 71
    bone resorption 12, 41, 52
        cytokine stimulators 69
        inhibition by bisphosphonates 70
        interleukin-1X and ß 24
    in breast cancer, ibandronate 71
    capacity, collagen degrading enzyme production 8
    cathepsin K 8
    cell lineage and origin 4–7, 12
    function 3
        carbonic anhydrase Type II isoenzyme and CSF-1 9
    function inhibition by anti cancer drugs 52
    matrix degradation 8
    osteoclastotropic cytokines 24
    stimulation by tumor cells at metastatic site 52–4
osteoid originating tumors 118–20
osteolytic lesions
    animal models 27
    B16/F1 melanoma cells 69
    CT value 115
    cytokines 67
    development and local bone turnover 55
    discrete, focal 128
    histological section 23
    human melanoma cells 48
    ilium lesion, pre-radiotherapy 165
    malignant 3
    markers 28
    metastases 92
        anterior vertebral body (anterior column) 251
        breast cancer 237
        tumor cell mediation 51–2
    myeloma 21–9

osteolytic lesions (contd)
  plasmacytoma, pelvic radiograph 129
  recalcification 215
  tumor-induced (TIO) 231
  see also metastatic bone disease
osteomyelitis, recurrent 116
osteopenia 22, 129, 265
osteopetrosis
  bone resorption, critical molecular mechanisms 8
  carbonic anhydrase Type II isoenzyme deficiency 8–9
  cell transplantation, hemopoietic tissue derived 4–5
  childhood, inherited 8
  colony-stimulating factors (CSFs), -1 coding abnormality 9
  and donor-derived osteoclasts 6
  and hemopoietic cell transplantation 6
  osteoclast formation defect 9
  renal tubular acidosis, childhood 8
osteopontin, extracellular bone constituent 4, 11
osteoporosis 71, 128, 219, 263–8
  cancer treatments
    direct effects 263–5
    indirect effects 265
  cortical bone loss
  differentiation from metastases 37
  in elderly, mean wall decrease 12
  models of bone loss prevention 266
  pathophysiology 12
  treatment examples 266
osteoprotegerin (OPG) 11, 86
osteosarcoma 118–20
  classical 117
  'cloud like calcification' 117–18
  conventional (high grade) 118–19
  'hair on end' appearance 116
  osteoblast phenotype 58
  pathological hallmark 118
  sunburst calcification 116
  synovial sarcoma 122
  telangiectatic 117, 119
  see also specific named types
osteosclerosis 23, 34
  myeloma bone disease 22, 27
  stimulation by osteoblasts 45
ovarian ablation 39, 152–3
ovarian cancer, E-cadherin 48
oxycodone opiate, WHO analgesic ladder Step (2) 190

P13 kinase enzyme 9
P-glycoprotein, overexpression 107
Paget's disease 7, 11, 70, 96
  differentiation from metastases 37
  management 139
  radiology 115
Paget's sarcoma 119
pain see cancer pain; neuropathic pain
palliative therapy
  chemotherapy 145
  radionuclides 172–80
  radiotherapy 155
pamidronate 28, 56, 72, 204–5, 223–5
  analgesic effects 235
  clinical trials 141
  hypercalcemia of malignancy 85, 145, 234
  (intravenous), biochemical response, clinical response probability 146
  metastatic bone disease monitoring 145–7
  multiple myeloma, randomized long-term studies 223–5
  myeloma 45, 223–5
  post-infusion changes 147
  recalcification/sclerosis induction 236
  structure 202
  treatment, hypercalcemia 84
papain cysteine protease superfamily 8
paraplegia 166
parathyroid adenomata 79
parathyroid hormone (PTH) 2–3, 7, 10, 14, 25, 138
  hypercalcemia of malignancy 78–80
  pre-treatment, uptake increase 173–4
parathyroid hormone-related protein (PTH-rP) 41, 47, 56, 59, 138
  amino acid sequence 79
  hypercalcemia of malignancy 52, 79–82
  identification, immunohistochemical 25
  metastatic bone disease site 69
  myeloma bone disease, implication 24–5
  N-terminal antibodies 80
  N-terminal RIA 79
  osteoclast activity 52–3
  prostate cancer 232
  PTH-rP plasma levels 52, 79–82
  tumor induced bone resorption 69
parathyroid hormone-releasing peptide (PTHRP) 217–18
pathological analysis, trephine methodology 134
pathological fractures 38, 46
  metastatic bone disease 38
  prophylactic surgery, indications 156
  radiotherapy 164–6
PDGF see platelet-derived growth factor
pelvic metastatic bone disease 124
  medulloblastoma deposits 124
peptic ulcer disease 186
periosteal bone formation 3

peripheral nerve metastases, radiotherapy 168
permeative lesions 116
PGE2/PG2a *see* prostaglandins
phosphoinositol metabolism 9
phosphorus, serum, increase 28
phosphorus-32, properties 172, 173–4
PICP *see* collagen
placenta growth factor 69
plasma cell disorders 130–2
plasma cell dyscrasias 219
plasmacytoma 127, 129–30
   definition 130
   lytic lesions 129
   solitary 22, 216, 220
plasminogen activator
   sequence 59
   urokinase-type (uPA) 58
platelet dysfunction 186
platelet-derived growth factor (PDGF) 13
   reactive bone formation 66
pleiotrophin 69
plicamycin therapy 52
pneumoencephalography 113
POEMs syndrome (polyneuropathy, organomegaly, endocrinopathy, M protein, and skin changes) 23
polymethylmethacrylate (PMMA) 246, 257
positron emission tomography (PET) 94, 99, 105, 107
post-menopause, estrogen replacement therapy 3
post-traumatic hematoma 115
postoperative radiotherapy 166
prednisolone therapy 153
primary bone marrow tumors 127–33
primary bone tumors 117–22
   see also specific types
primary chondrosarcoma 120
primary hyperparathyroidism 7, 234, 11
   biochemical features 77
   hypercalcemia 75
plasma phosphate, low 76–7
primary lymphoma 129
primary malignant bone tumors, classification 118
progestational agents, examples 153
progestogens 152
prophylactic wide-field radiotherapy 164, 166
proptosis 41
prostaglandins (PGE2, PGF2a), osteolytic bone disease 231
prostate, benign prostatic hyperplasia 58, 141, 156
prostate cancer 12, 46, 143–4
   biochemical markers 143–4
   bone scintigraphy 103–4
      axial distribution metastases 96

      MDP bone scan 95
   cell line PC3 59
   metastatic bone disease 33, 127, 140
      development 57
      epidemiology 34
      prostate–spine spread 37
      refractory metastatic 176
      skeletal metastases, characteristics 239
      staging, bone scintigraphy 103–4
   nerve compression 46
   osteoblastic responses 46, 57
   osteoporotic fracture 265
   osteosclerotic disease 34
   principal site 154–5
   SPECT imaging 95
   treatment
      endocrine treatment 154
      response 143–4
      systemic 154–5
prostate-specific antigen (PSA) 59, 103, 141, 156, 179
prostatitis 141, 156
protein–tyrosine phosphatase (PTP) 71
proteolytic enzyme
   digestion 57
   production by tumors 48, 51
PSA *see* prostate-specific antigen
pseudo-tumor, MRI and ultrasound value 115
PTH *see* parathyroid hormone
PTH-rP *see* parathyroid hormone-related protein
PTP *see* protein–tyrosine phosphatase
punched-out lesions 11, 130
Pyr biochemical marker 139, 145
pyrexia 121
pyridinoline (F-Pyr) 139, 220
pyridinoline markers 138–9, 141, 143, 145

Radiation Therapy Oncology Group (RTOG) 164
radiation therapy *see* radiotherapy
radioimmunoassay, cell surface mucins, expression 141
radioisotope therapy 171–80, 195
   cost benefits 179
   efficacy enhancement 179–80
   injected 159
   palliation, radionuclides 172
   patient treatment, response assessment 142
   side-effects 179
   site directed radiotherapy 172–3
   survival expectancy 179
radiology 92
   change, growth, examples 115
   and MRI 113–35
      diagnosis 113–15, 123–5
      metastatic bone disease 122–7

radiology (contd)
  plain radiographs 143, 223
    bone disease status 218
    patient treatment, response assessment 142
    sclerotic vertebral metastases 106
  principles 115–17
radionuclide scans see bone scintigraphy
radiopharmaceutical agents
  mechanisms of uptake 91–3
  PET 107
  radionuclides for palliation 172
radiosensitizers, example 179
radiotherapy 28–9, 50, 142, 159–68, 195
  beam arrangement 160
  bone pain
    localized 161–3, 173
    scattered 163–4
  Class III spinal metastases 248
  delivery process 159–61
  external beam 161–4
  history 161
  metastatic bone disease
    neurological complications 166–8
    pathological fracture 164–6
  myeloma bone disease 215, 220–1
  prophylactic wide-field 164, 166
  radiation beams, classification 159
  site-directed 172–3
  see also specific named types
raloxifene therapy 267–8
RANK ligand 11
receptor positive tumor, therapies associated 152
renal bisphosphonate–calcium complex 84
renal cell carcinoma, scintigraphy 104
renal cortical carcinoma 78
  hypercalcemia 75
renal function impairment 28
renal intercalated cellular, complex vacuolar ATPase 8
renal toxicity 84
renal tubular acidosis, carbonic anhydrase Type II isoenzyme deficiency 8
renal tubular calcium reabsorption 28, 46–7
residronate, (oral), multiple myeloma 145
respiratory depression 191
reticulo-endothelial disorders 127, 132–3
  histiocytic elements 132
reticulum cell sarcoma see malignant lymphoma
reverse-phase high-performance liquid chromatography (HPLC) 139
Rezaian spinal fixator 255, 257
RGD see arginine-glycine-asparagine
rhenium-186
  controlled studies 178

  properties 172
rheumatoid arthritis 186–7
rib fracture 39
risedronate 220
  structure 202
round cell neoplasms 121–2
RTOG see Radiation Therapy Oncology Group

S375 human melanoma cells 69
sacrum, large tumor, bone destruction, CT scan 129
samarium-153
  controlled studies 177–8
  properties 172
sarcoma see osteosarcoma
'saucerization', bone cortex 121
SCID see severe combined immunodeficiency
scintigraphic patterns, diagnostic, metastatic bone disease 94–9
second-line endocrine therapy, norethisterone acetate agent 153
secondary hyperparathyroidism 239
seizures 191
selective estrogen receptor modulators (SERMs) 267
serine protease, expression 59
serine protease urokinase (uPA) 59
serum biochemical markers (list) 137
serum resorption marker ICTP 144
severe combined immunodeficiency (SCID) 27
short tau inversion recovery (STIR) 125
single photon emission computed tomography (SPECT) 94–5, 99
site-directed radiotherapy 172–3
skeletal malignancy see metastatic bone disease
skeletal metastases, radioisotope therapy 173
skeletal related-events (SREs) 236
skeleton 1–15
  natural history 1–2
  remodeling 3–4
skip lesions 122
skull, orbital/parasellar lesion 41
skull metastases, diplopia 41
soft bone disease 21
soft tissue calcification, CT value 115
solid tumors
  bone destruction, osteoclast demonstration 52
  malignancy associated 12
solitary plasmacytoma 22, 216, 220
somatic pain 193
SORMs see selective estrogen receptor modulators
SPECT see single photon emission computed tomography
spinal canal, intrusion by tumor tissue 246
spinal classical lesion, vertebra plana 132–3

spinal cord compression 39–41, 46, 166, 248
   decompression and stabilization 246
   elevation 219
spinal metastases 106, 257
   categorised 248
   CT scan 160
   MRI study 125
   scintigraphy 99
   X-ray 160
   see also cervical; lumbar
spinal stabilization 245–59
   bony detritus 248
   and MRI 246
   neurological compromise (Class V) 250
   nonoperative treatment 246–9, 246–50
   operative treatment 250–9
   pathophysiology 245–6
spinal tumors
   arterial embolization 246
   metastases 37, 166–7
   see also spinal metastases; vertebral
spleen cell, transplantation 4
squamous cell carcinoma
   human lung cell line (HARA) 69
   hypercalcemia (HHM) 75, 78
   pamidronate 72
   reactive bone formation 66
src 9
SREs see skeletal related-events
steroid receptor-positive tumors, endocrine therapy
   option 152
steroids
   common side-effects 193
   high-dose therapy 37
STIR see short tau inversion recovery
stromal mesenchymal cells 12
strontium-85, bone scintigraphy 91
strontium-89
   characteristics 172
   properties 174–7
   randomized controlled trials 175
subperiosteal new bone formation 128
sunburst calcification
   Ewing's tumor 116
   osteosarcoma associated 116
super scan
   MDP bone scans, stages of disease 98
   nuclear medicine 97
surgical intervention, indications, summary 250
syndecan-1, heparin sulfate proteoglycan 218
systemic anti-tumor treatment
   specific 151–4
   steroidal therapies 248
   treatment response, assessment 155–6

T-cell leukemia/lymphoma 82
tamoxifen therapy 138, 152–3, 267
tartrate-resistant acid phosphatase (TRAPase) 67–8, 69
taxoids, anthracycline-resistant disease 153
TCA see tricyclic antidepressants
technetium-99m
   2-methoxyisobutylisonirile (MIBI) 220
   dimercaptosuccinic acid (V DMSA) 91, 93
   methylene disphosphonate scan (MDP) 91, 93, 96–8, 100, 105–7, 177
   sestamibi, myeloma 93, 105
telangiectatic osteosarcomas 117, 119
telopeptide Type I collagen (ICTP assay) 139, 143, 220
TENS see transcutaneous electrical nerve stimulation
testosterone 154
TGF see transforming growth factors
thallium-201 91
thrombocytopenia 84, 164
   metastatic bone disease 42
thyroid cancers
   I iodine 93
   I-metaiodobenzylguanidine (MIBG) 93
thyrotoxicosis 1
thyroxine therapy 264
tibia, pathological fractures, metastatic bone disease 38
TIH see tumor-induced hypercalcemia
tiludronate, structure 202
TIMPS, bone resorption inhibitors 218
tin-117m, properties 172
TIO see tumor-induced osteolysis
tongue weakness 41
trabecular bone (bone lining cells) 25, 57
   see also cancellous bone
TRANCE ligand see RANK ligand
TRANCE (RANK ligand) 11
transcutaneous electrical nerve stimulation (TENS) 168
transforming growth factors
   superfamily 13
   TGF-β2, prostate cancer cells 58
   TGF-β 14, 53–4, 59, 69, 216–18
      reactive bone formation 66
      role 11
   TGF-α 7, 13
transgenic adenocarcinoma mouse prostate model (TRAMP) 58
TRAPase see tartrate-resistant acid phosphatase
trephine methodology 134
tricyclic antidepressants (TCAs) 193
trigeminal neuropathy 41

tuberculosis 122
tumor(s)
  with CHO cells 25
  direct bone resorption, principal mechanisms 69–72
  extent/spread
    dissemination by vertebral venous plexus 45, 231
    MRI value 115
  hypoxia 92
  lysis, progressive 247
  mediation of bone destruction, at metastatic site 51–2
  metastatic capacity variation 50
  metastatic inhibition, NM-23 oncogene 50
  see also bisphosphonates
tumor cell motility, chemotactic factors 51
tumor growth factors, in bone 54–6
tumor markers see biochemical markers; bone formation markers
tumor necrosis factor
  TNF-β 25, 216
    see also lymphotoxin
  TNF-α 24, 217
tumor peptide see parathyroid hormone-related protein (PTH-rP)
tumor-induced hypercalcemia (TIH) see hypercalcemia
tumor-like disorders see specific names and types

UICC see Union Internationale Contre le Cancer
ultrasound imaging 113, 133
Union Internationale Contre le Cancer (UICC) 102
uPA see serine protease urokinase; urokinase-type plasminogen activator
urinary calcium (uCa) excretion 41, 138, 142–3
urinary hydroxyproline excretion 138
urinary pyridinolines, stability 139
urine biochemical markers (list) 137
urokinase 232
urokinase-type plasminogen activator (uPA) 58
uvomorulin see E-cadherin

V DMSA see technetium 99m, pentavalent dimercaptosuccinic acid
vascular endothelial growth factor (VEGF) 69
VCAM-1 mediation 26
venous embolism, retrograde 123
venous tumor emboli 122
vertebral, see also spinal
vertebral body
  fractures, scintigraphy 99
  lytic lesions 251
  sclerosis, radiology 57
  vertebra plana, spinal classical lesion 132–3
vertebral collapse
  differentiation from metastases 37
  mechanical spine pain (Class IV) 250
vertebral metastases 166–7
vertebral venous plexus 45, 231
vertebrectomy 252
vertebroplasty by injection 246
visceral lesions 152
visceral metastases 72
vitronectin receptor, A375 human melanoma cells 49
vomiting 84

Walker 256 carcinosarcoma cells 204
white cell disorders 127–30
wide field irradiation 163
wide-channeled marrow sinusoids 51
World Health Organisation 185–6
  analgesic ladder 186

X-ray absorptiometry (DXA) 266

yellow marrow see avascular marrow
YIGSR synthetic agonist 51
YM175 72
yttrium-90, properties 172

zoledronate
  apoptosis of osteoclasts 72
  structure 202
  therapy 226, 238